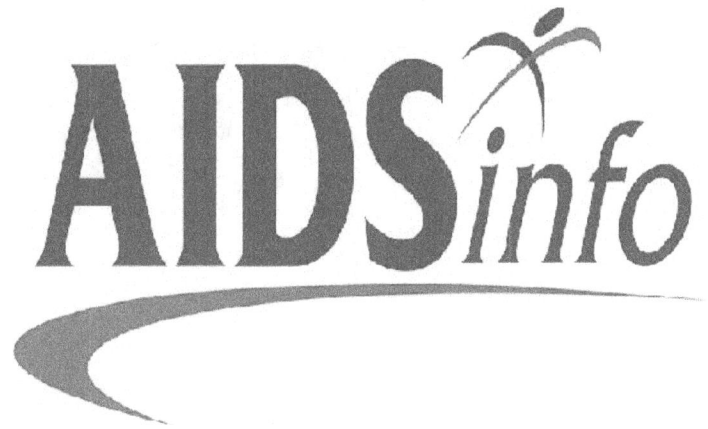

Guidelines for the Use of Antiretroviral Agents in HIV-1-Infected Adults and Adolescents

Guidelines for the Use of Antiretroviral Agents in HIV-1-Infected Adults and Adolescents

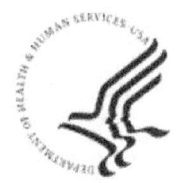

Developed by the HHS Panel on Antiretroviral Guidelines for Adults and Adolescents – A Working Group of the Office of AIDS Research Advisory Council (OARAC)

What's New in the Guidelines? (Last updated February 12, 2013; last reviewed February 12, 2013)

The following key changes were made to update the March 28, 2012, version of the guidelines. Significant updates are highlighted throughout the revised guidelines.

Drug-Resistance Testing

In persons failing INSTI-based regimens, the panel now recommends that a genotypic assay for INSTI resistance should be performed to determine whether to include a drug from this class in subsequent regimens **(AII)**. Previously, the Panel recommended that INSTI resistance testing should be considered **(BIII)** in this setting.

Co-Receptor Tropism Assay

A genotypic tropism assay is now commercially available. The assay predicts HIV-1 co-receptor usage based on sequencing of the V3-coding region of HIV-1 *env*, the principal determinant of co-receptor usage. The Panel recommends that a genotypic tropism assay be used as an alternative to a phenotypic tropism assay before initiation of a CCR5 antagonist-containing regimen **(BII)**.

Initiating ART in Treatment-Naive Patients

The Panel has updated its recommendations on initiation of ART in treatment-naive patients. The Panel's recommendations are listed below.

- Antiretroviral therapy (ART) is recommended for all HIV-infected individuals to reduce the risk of disease progression.

  The strength and evidence for this recommendation vary by pretreatment CD4 cell count: CD4 count <350 cells/mm^3 **(AI)**; CD4 count 350 cells/mm^3 to 500 cells/mm^3 **(AII)**; CD4 count >500 cells/mm^3 **(BIII)**.

- ART also is recommended for HIV-infected individuals for the prevention of transmission of HIV.

  The strength and evidence for this recommendation vary by transmission risks: perinatal transmission **(AI)**; heterosexual transmission **(AI)**; other transmission risk groups **(AIII)**.

- Patients starting ART should be willing and able to commit to treatment and understand the benefits and risks of therapy and the importance of adherence **(AIII)**. Patients may choose to postpone therapy, and providers, on a case-by-case basis, may elect to defer therapy on the basis of clinical and/or psychosocial factors.

What to Start: Initial Combination Regimen for Antiretroviral-Naive Patients

The following changes and updates were made to this section:

- A rilpivirine (RPV)-based regimen is now recommended as an alternative NNRTI-based regimen **only** in patients with pre-treatment HIV RNA ≤100,000 copies/mL **(BI)**. This is based on results from clinical trials that show that the proportion of patients who experienced virologic failure at 96 weeks was greater in patients with pre-treatment HIV RNA >100,000 copies/mL than in patients with pre-therapy HIV RNA ≤100,000 copies/mL.

- Elvitegravir/cobicistat/tenofovir/emtricitabine (EVG/COBI/TDF/FTC) as a fixed-dose combination product is recommended as an alternative regimen for ART-naive patients with pre-treatment creatinine clearance >70 mL/min **(BI)**.

- The discussion on 3-NRTI regimens was removed from this section because 3-NRTI regimens are no longer recommended regimens for ART-naive patients.
- Tables 5a, 5b, 6, and 7 were updated to reflect the above changes.

Acute and Recent (Early) HIV Infection

- The term "early" HIV infection is now used when describing both the acute phase of HIV infection (i.e., immediately after HIV infection and before seroconversion) and recent (i.e., within first 6 months) HIV infection.
- The recommendation for initiation of ART in patients with early infection was changed from "should be considered optional **(CIII)**" to "should be offered **(BII)**."
- The section was updated to include a summary of recent randomized controlled trials that examined the role of time-limited ART in patients with early HIV infection.

HIV-Infected Women

- The recommendation on use of efavirenz (EFV) during pregnancy was updated to be in accord with the recommendation in the *Perinatal Antiretroviral Guidelines*. The key update includes the following statement: "Because the risk of neural tube defects is restricted to the first 5 to 6 weeks of pregnancy and pregnancy is rarely recognized before 4 to 6 weeks of pregnancy, EFV can be continued in pregnant women receiving an EFV-based regimen who present for antenatal care in the first trimester, provided the regimen produces virologic suppression **(CIII)**."
- The Panel also recommends that intravenous zidovudine use during labor may be omitted in women who have HIV RNA < 400 copies/mL near delivery **(BII)**. Oral combination ART should be continued during labor.

Drug-Drug Interaction

- This section includes new information under the heading "Pharmacokinetic (PK) Enhancing." The additional text describes the roles and mechanisms of ritonavir (RTV) and cobicistat (COBI) as pharmacokinetic enhancers to increase the exposure of antiretroviral drugs.
- Tables 14_16c have been updated with new pharmacokinetic interaction data, including known and predicted interactions involving EVG/COBI/TDF/FTC and other drugs.

Additional Updates

Minor revisions have also been made to the following sections:

- Introduction
- Adverse Effects of Antiretroviral Agents (and Table 13)
- ARV Drug Characteristics and ARV Drug Cost Tables (Appendix B)

Table of Contents

HHS Panel on Antiretroviral Guidelines for Adults and Adolescents
Panel Roster (Last updated February 12, 2013; last reviewed February 12, 2013)

These Guidelines were developed by the Department of Health and Human Services (HHS) Panel on Antiretroviral Guidelines for Adults and Adolescents (a Working Group of the Office of AIDS Research Advisory Council).

Panel Co-Chairs

John G. Bartlett	Johns Hopkins University, Baltimore, MD
H. Clifford Lane	National Institutes of Health, Bethesda, MD

Executive Secretary

Alice K. Pau	National Institutes of Health, Bethesda, MD

Scientific Members

Judith Aberg	New York University, New York, NY
Adaora Adimora	University of North Carolina, Chapel Hill, NC
John T. Brooks	Centers for Disease Control and Prevention, Atlanta, GA
Deborah L. Cohan	University of California San Francisco, San Francisco, CA
Eric Daar	University of California Los Angeles, Harbor-UCLA Medical Center, Los Angeles, CA
Steven G. Deeks	University of California San Francisco, San Francisco, CA
Carlos del Rio	Emory University, Atlanta, GA
Robert T. Dodge	University of North Carolina, Chapel Hill, NC
Courtney V. Fletcher	University of Nebraska Medical Center, Omaha, NE
Gerald Friedland	Yale University School of Medicine, New Haven, CT
Joel E. Gallant	Johns Hopkins University, Baltimore, MD
Stephen J. Gange	Johns Hopkins University, Baltimore, MD
Christopher M. Gordon	National Institutes of Health, Bethesda, MD
Roy M. Gulick	Weill Medical College of Cornell University, New York, NY
W. Keith Henry	Hennepin County Medical Center & University of Minnesota, Minneapolis, MN
Michael D. Hughes	Harvard School of Public Health, Boston, MA
Bill G. Kapogiannis	National Institutes of Health, Bethesda, MD
Daniel R. Kuritzkes	Brigham and Women's Hospital & Harvard Medical School, Boston, MA
Richard W. Price	University of California San Francisco, San Francisco, CA
Michael Saag	University of Alabama at Birmingham, Birmingham, AL
Paul Sax	Brigham and Women's Hospital & Harvard Medical School, Boston, MA
Mark Sulkowski	Johns Hopkins University, Baltimore, MD
Zelalem Temesgen	Mayo Clinic, Rochester, MN
Phyllis Tien	University of California San Francisco, San Francisco, CA
Rochelle Walensky	Massachusetts General Hospital & Harvard Medical School, Boston, MA
David A. Wohl	University of North Carolina, Chapel Hill, NC

Community Members

Lei Chou	Treatment Action Group, New York, NY
Paul Dalton	San Francisco, CA
Heidi Nass	University of Wisconsin, Madison, WI
Jeff Taylor	AIDS Treatment Activists Coalition, Palm Springs, CA
Nelson Vergel	Program for Wellness Restoration, Houston, TX

Members Representing Department of Health and Human Services Agencies

Victoria Cargill	National Institutes of Health, Rockville, MD
Laura Cheever	Health Resources and Services Administration, Rockville, MD
Jonathan Kaplan	Centers for Disease Control and Prevention, Atlanta, GA
Kendall Marcus	Food and Drug Administration, Silver Spring, MD
Henry Masur	National Institutes of Health, Bethesda, MD
Lynne Mofenson	National Institutes of Health, Bethesda, MD
Kimberly Struble	Food and Drug Administration, Silver Spring, MD

Non-Voting Observer

Monica Calderon	National Institutes of Health, SAIC-Frederick, Inc., NCI-Frederick, Frederick, MD

Acknowledgement

The Panel would like to acknowledge the assistance of Sarita D. Boyd, Pharm.D. (Food and Drug Administration) for her assistance in updating the drug interaction tables, and Thomas Uldrick, M.D. (National Cancer Institute) for his assistance with the Malignancies discussion located in the Initiating Antiretroviral Therapy in Treatment-Naive Patients section.

Name	Panel Status*	Company	Relationship
Judith Aberg	M	• Janssen Therapeutics (formerly Tibotec Therapeutics) • Merck • ViiV	• Advisory Board • Advisory Board • Advisory Board
Adaora Adimora	M	None	N/A
John G. Bartlett	C	None	N/A
John T. Brooks	M	None	N/A
Victoria Ann Cargill	M	None	N/A
Laura W. Cheever	M	None	N/A
Lei Chou	M	None	N/A
Deborah Cohan	M	None	N/A
Eric Daar	M	• Abbvie (formerly Abbott) • Bristol-Myers Squibb • Gilead • Janssen Therapeutics (formerly Tibotec Therapeutics) • Merck • ViiV	• Research support • Consultant • Advisory Board; Research support • Advisory Board • Consultant; Research support • Consultant; Research support
Paul Dalton	M	None	N/A
Steven G. Deeks	M	• Boehringer Ingelheim • Bristol-Myers Squibb • Gilead • GlaxoSmithKline • Merck • Tobira • ViiV	• Advisory Board • Advisory Board • Honoraria; Research support • Advisory Board • Advisory Board • Advisory Board • Advisory Board
Carlos del Rio	M	• Gilead • Pfizer	• Advisory Board • Consultant
Robert Dodge	M	• Abbvie (formerly Abbott) • Boehringer Ingelheim • Gilead • Janssen Therapeutics (formerly Tibotec Therapeutics) • ViiV	• Speakers' Bureau • Speakers' Bureau • Advisory Board; Speakers' Bureau; Consultant • Advisory Board • Speakers' Bureau; Consultant
Courtney V. Fletcher	M	None	N/A

Guidelines for the Use of Antiretroviral Agents in HIV-1-Infected Adults and Adolescents

Name	Panel Status*	Company	Relationship
Gerald H. Friedland	M	None	N/A
Joel E. Gallant	M	• Bristol-Myers Squibb • GlaxoSmithKline • Gilead • Janssen Therapeutics (formerly Tibotec Therapeutics) • Merck • RAPID Pharmaceuticals • Sangamo Biosciences • Takara Bio Inc	• Advisory Board • Consultant • Advisory Board; Research support • Advisory Board • Advisory Board • Advisory Board • DSMB member • DSMB member
Stephen Gange	M	• Merck	• DSMB member
Christopher M. Gordon	M	None	N/A
Roy M. Gulick	M	• Bristol-Myers Squibb • Gilead • GlaxoSmithKline • Janssen Therapeutics (formerly Tibotec Therapeutics) • Koronis • Merck • Pfizer • ViiV • ViroStatics	• Consultant • Consultant • Consultant • Consultant; Research support • Consultant • Consultant • Research support • Consultant; Research support • Consultant
W. Keith Henry	M	• Gilead • GlaxoSmithKline/ViiV	• Advisory Board; Research support; Speakers' Bureau; Honoraria; Consultant • Research support
Michael D. Hughes	M	• Boehringer Ingelheim • Janssen Therapeutics (formerly Tibotec Therapeutics) • Medicines Development, LTD. • Pfizer	• DSMB member • DSMB member • DSMB member • DSMB member
Jonathan E. Kaplan	M	None	N/A

Name	Panel Status*	Company	Relationship
Bill Kapogiannis	M	None	N/A
Daniel R. Kuritzkes	M	• Abbvie (formerly Abbott) • Aileron • Avexa • Boehringer Ingelheim • Bristol-Myers Squibb • GlaxoSmithKline • Gilead • InnoVirvax • Koronis • Merck • Pathogenica • Roche • Roxane • Tobira • Vertex • ViiV • ViroStatics • VIRxSYS	• Consultant • Consultant • Consultant • Consultant • Advisory Board • Consultant • Advisory Board; Research support; Honoraria • Consultant • Consultant • Advisory Board; Research support • Consultant • Consultant; Honoraria • Consultant • Consultant • Consultant • Advisory Board • Advisory Board • Consultant
H. Clifford Lane	C	None	N/A
Kendall Marcus	M	None	N/A
Henry Masur	M	None	N/A
Lynne Mofenson	M	None	N/A
Heidi M. Nass	M	None	N/A
Alice Pau	ES	None	N/A
Richard W. Price	M	• Abbvie (formerly Abbott) • Merck	• Honoraria; Travel support • Research support
Michael Saag	M	• Ardea Biosciences • Boehringer Ingelheim • Bristol-Myers Squibb • Gilead • GlaxoSmithKline/ViiV • Janssen Therapeutics (formerly Tibotec Therapeutics) • Merck • Vertex	• Research support • Research support • Advisory Board; Consultant; Research support • Advisory Board; Consultant; Research support • Consultant; Research support • Consultant; Research support • Advisory Board; Consultant; Research support • Advisory Board; Research support

Name	Panel Status*	Company	Relationship
Paul E. Sax	M	• Bristol-Myers Squibb • Gilead • GlaxoSmithKline/ViiV • Janssen Therapeutics (formerly Tibotec Therapeutics) • Merck	• Advisory Board; Research support • Advisory Board; Research support • Advisory Board; Research support • Consultant • Advisory Board
Kimberly Struble	M	None	N/A
Mark Sulkowski	M	• Abbvie (formerly Abbott) • Boehringer Ingelheim • Bristol-Myers Squibb • Gilead • Janssen Therapeutics (formerly Tibotec Therapeutics) • Merck • Pfizer • Roche • Vertex	• Advisory Board; Research support • Advisory Board; Research support • Advisory Board; Research support • Advisory Board; Research support • Advisory Board; Research support • Advisory Board; Research support • Steering committee • Advisory Board; Research support • Advisory Board; Research support
Jeff Taylor	M	None	N/A
Zelalem Temesgen	M	• Gilead • Janssen Therapeutics (formerly Tibotec Therapeutics) • Merck • Pfizer • ViiV	• Educational grant; Research support • Education grant • Educational grant • Research support • Education grant
Phyllis Tien	M	• Gilead	• Advisory Board
Nelson R. Vergel	M	None	N/A
Rochelle Walensky	M	None	N/A
David Alain Wohl	M	• BMS • Gilead • GlaxoSmithKline • Janssen Therapeutics (formerly Tibotec Therapeutics) • Merck	• Advisory Board • Advisory Board • Research support • Advisory Board • Research support

* C = co-chair; ES = executive secretary; M=member; DSMB = Data Safety Monitoring Board; N/A = not applicable

Introduction

Antiretroviral therapy (ART) for the treatment of HIV infection has improved steadily since the advent of potent combination therapy in 1996. New drugs that offer new mechanisms of action, improvements in potency and activity even against multidrug-resistant viruses, dosing convenience, and tolerability have been approved. ART has dramatically reduced HIV-associated morbidity and mortality and has transformed HIV disease into a chronic, manageable condition. In addition, effective treatment of HIV-infected individuals with ART is highly effective at preventing transmission to sexual partners.[1] However, less than one-third of HIV-infected individuals in the United States have suppressed viral loads,[2] which is mostly a result of undiagnosed HIV infection and failure to link or retain diagnosed patients in care. Despite remarkable improvements in HIV treatment and prevention, economic and social barriers that result in continued morbidity, mortality, and new HIV infections persist.

The Department of Health and Human Services (HHS) Panel on Antiretroviral Guidelines for Adults and Adolescents (the Panel) is a working group of the Office of AIDS Research Advisory Council (OARAC). The primary goal of the Panel is to provide HIV care practitioners with recommendations based on current knowledge of antiretroviral (ARV) drugs used to treat adults and adolescents with HIV infection in the United States. The Panel reviews new evidence and updates recommendations in these guidelines when needed. The Panel's primary areas of attention have included baseline assessment, treatment goals, indications for initiation of ART, choice of the initial regimen for ART-naive patients, drugs or combinations to avoid, management of adverse effects and drug interactions, management of treatment failure, and special ART-related considerations in specific patient populations. For recommendations related to pre-exposure HIV prophylaxis (PrEP) for HIV-uninfected persons, please refer to recommendations from the Centers for Disease Control and Prevention (CDC).[3,4]

These guidelines generally represent the state of knowledge regarding the use of ARV agents. However, because the science of HIV evolves rapidly, the availability of new agents and new clinical data may change therapeutic options and preferences. Information included in these guidelines may not be consistent with approved labeling for the particular products or indications in question, and the use of the terms "safe" and "effective" may not be synonymous with the Food and Drug Administration (FDA)-defined legal standards for product approval. The Panel frequently updates the guidelines (current and archived versions of the guidelines are available on the AIDS*info* website at http://www.aidsinfo.nih.gov). However, the guidelines cannot always be updated apace with the rapid evolution of new data in the field of HIV and cannot offer guidance on care for all patients. Clinicians should exercise clinical judgment in management decisions tailored to unique patient circumstances.

The Panel recognizes the importance of clinical research in generating evidence to address unanswered questions related to the optimal safety and efficacy of ART. The Panel encourages both the development of protocols and patient participation in well-designed, Institutional Review Board (IRB)-approved clinical trials.

Guidelines Development Process

Table 1. Outline of the Guidelines Development Process

Topic	Comment
Goal of the guidelines	Provide guidance to HIV care practitioners on the optimal use of antiretroviral (ARV) agents for the treatment of HIV infection in adults and adolescents in the United States.
Panel members	The Panel is composed of approximately 40 voting members who have expertise in HIV care and research. The Panel includes at least one representative from each of the following U.S. Department of Health and Human Services (HHS) agencies: Centers for Disease Control and Prevention (CDC), Food and Drug Administration (FDA), Health Resource Services Administration (HRSA), and National Institutes of Health (NIH). Approximately two-thirds of the Panel members are non-governmental scientific members. The Panel also includes four to five community members with knowledge in HIV treatment and care. The U.S. government representatives are appointed by their respective agencies; other Panel members are selected after an open announcement to call for nominations. Each member serves on the Panel for a 4-year term with an option for reappointment for an additional term. A list of current members can be found in the Panel Roster.
Financial disclosure	All members of the Panel submit financial disclosure in writing annually, reporting any association with manufacturers of ARV drugs or diagnostics used for management of HIV infections. A list of the latest disclosures is available on the AIDS*info* website (http://aidsinfo.nih.gov/contentfiles/AA_financialDisclosures.pdf).
Users of the guidelines	HIV treatment providers
Developer	Panel on Antiretroviral Guidelines for Adults and Adolescents—a working group of the Office of AIDS Research Advisory Council (OARAC)
Funding source	Office of AIDS Research, NIH
Evidence collection	The recommendations in the guidelines are generally based on studies published in peer-reviewed journals. On some occasions, particularly when new information may affect patient safety, unpublished data presented at major conferences or prepared by the FDA and/or manufacturers as warnings to the public may be used as evidence to revise the guidelines.
Recommendation grading	As described in Table 2
Method of synthesizing data	Each section of the guidelines is assigned to a working group of Panel members with expertise in the area of interest. The working groups synthesize the available data and propose recommendations to the Panel. The Panel discusses all proposals during monthly teleconferences. Recommendations endorsed by the Panel are included in the guidelines as official recommendations.
Other guidelines	These guidelines focus on treatment for HIV-infected adults and adolescents. Included is a brief discussion on the management of women of reproductive age and pregnant women. For more detailed and up-to-date discussion on the use of antiretroviral therapy (ART) for these women, as well as for children, and other special populations, please refer to guidelines specific to these groups. The guidelines are also available on the AIDS*info* website (http://www.aidsinfo.nih.gov).
Update plan	The Panel meets monthly by teleconference to review data that may warrant modification of the guidelines. Updates may be prompted by new drug approvals (or new indications, dosing formulations, or frequency of dosing), new significant safety or efficacy data, or other information that may have a significant impact on the clinical care of patients. In the event of significant new data that may affect patient safety, the Panel may post a warning announcement with recommendations on the AIDS*info* website in the interim until the guidelines can be updated with the appropriate changes. Updated guidelines are available on the AIDS*info* website (http://www.aidsinfo.nih.gov).
Public comments	A 2-week public comment period follows release of the updated guidelines on the AIDS*info* website. The Panel reviews comments received to determine whether additional revisions to the guidelines are indicated. The public may also submit comments to the Panel at any time at contactus@aidsinfo.nih.gov.

Basis for Recommendations

Recommendations in these guidelines are based upon scientific evidence and expert opinion. Each recommended statement includes a letter (**A**, **B**, or **C**) that represents the strength of the recommendation and with a Roman numeral (**I**, **II**, or **III**) that represents the quality of the evidence that supports the recommendation (see Table 2).

Table 2. Rating Scheme for Recommendations

Strength of Recommendation		Quality of Evidence for Recommendation	
A:	Strong recommendation for the statement	**I:**	One or more randomized trials with clinical outcomes and/or validated laboratory endpoints
B:	Moderate recommendation for the statement	**II:**	One or more well-designed, non-randomized trials or observational cohort studies with long-term clinical outcomes
C:	Optional recommendation for the statement		
		III:	Expert opinion

HIV Expertise in Clinical Care

Many studies have demonstrated that outcomes achieved in HIV-infected outpatients are better when care is delivered by a clinician with HIV expertise,[5-10] which reflects the complexity of HIV infection and its treatment. Thus, appropriate training and experience, as well as ongoing continuing education, are important components of optimal care. Primary care providers without HIV experience, such as those who provide service in rural or underserved areas, should identify experts in their regions who will be available for consultation when needed.

References

1. Cohen MS, Chen YQ, McCauley M, et al. Prevention of HIV-1 infection with early antiretroviral therapy. *N Engl J Med*. 2011;365(6):493-505. Available at http://www.ncbi.nlm.nih.gov/pubmed/21767103.

2. Centers for Disease Control and Prevention. *HIV in the United States: The Stages of Care—CDC Fact Sheet*. 2012. Available at http://www.cdc.gov/nchhstp/newsroom/docs/2012/Stages-of-CareFactSheet-508.pdf. Accessed December 21, 2012.

3. Centers for Disease Control and Prevention. Interim guidance: Preexposure prophylaxis for the prevention of HIV infection in men who have sex with men. *MMWR Morb Mortal Wkly Rep*. 2011;60(3):65-68. Available at http://www.ncbi.nlm.nih.gov/pubmed/21270743.

4. Centers for Disease Control and Prevention. Interim guidance for clinicians considering the use of preexposure prophylaxis for the prevention of HIV infection in heterosexually active adults. *MMWR Morb Mortal Wkly Rep*. 2012;61(31):586-589. Available at http://www.ncbi.nlm.nih.gov/pubmed/22874836.

5. Kitahata MM, Koepsell TD, Deyo RA, Maxwell CL, Dodge WT, Wagner EH. Physicians' experience with the acquired immunodeficiency syndrome as a factor in patients' survival. *N Engl J Med*. 1996;334(11):701-706. Available at http://www.ncbi.nlm.nih.gov/entrez/query.fcgi?cmd=Retrieve&db=PubMed&dopt=Citation&list_uids=8594430.

6. Kitahata MM, Van Rompaey SE, Shields AW. Physician experience in the care of HIV-infected persons is associated with earlier adoption of new antiretroviral therapy. *J Acquir Immune Defic Syndr*. 2000;24(2):106-114. Available at http://www.ncbi.nlm.nih.gov/entrez/query.fcgi?cmd=Retrieve&db=PubMed&dopt=Citation&list_uids=10935685.

7. Landon BE, Wilson IB, McInnes K, et al. Physician specialization and the quality of care for human immunodeficiency virus infection. *Arch Intern Med*. 2005;165(10):1133-1139. Available at http://www.ncbi.nlm.nih.gov/entrez/query.fcgi?cmd=Retrieve&db=PubMed&dopt=Citation&list_uids=15911726.

8. Laine C, Markson LE, McKee LJ, Hauck WW, Fanning TR, Turner BJ. The relationship of clinic experience with advanced HIV and survival of women with AIDS. *AIDS*. 1998;12(4):417-424. Available at http://www.ncbi.nlm.nih.gov/entrez/query.fcgi?cmd=Retrieve&db=PubMed&dopt=Citation&list_uids=9520172.

9. Kitahata MM, Van Rompaey SE, Dillingham PW, et al. Primary care delivery is associated with greater physician experience and improved survival among persons with AIDS. *J Gen Intern Med*. 2003;18(2):95-103. Available at http://www.ncbi.nlm.nih.gov/entrez/query.fcgi?cmd=Retrieve&db=PubMed&dopt=Citation&list_uids=12542583.

10. Delgado J, Heath KV, Yip B, et al. Highly active antiretroviral therapy: Physician experience and enhanced adherence to prescription refill. *Antivir Ther*. 2003;8(5):471-478. Available at http://www.ncbi.nlm.nih.gov/entrez/query.fcgi?cmd=Retrieve&db=PubMed&dopt=Citation&list_uids=14640395.

Baseline Evaluation (Last updated February 12, 2013; last reviewed February 12, 2013)

Every HIV-infected patient entering into care should have a complete medical history, physical examination, and laboratory evaluation and should be counseled regarding the implications of HIV infection. The goals of the initial evaluation are to confirm the diagnosis of HIV infection, obtain appropriate baseline historical and laboratory data, ensure patient understanding about HIV infection and its transmission, and to initiate care as recommended in HIV primary care guidelines[1] and guidelines for prevention and treatment of HIV-associated opportunistic infections.[2] The initial evaluation also should include introductory discussion on the benefits of antiretroviral therapy (ART) for the patient's health and to prevent HIV transmission. Baseline information then can be used to define management goals and plans. In the case of previously treated patients who present for an initial evaluation with a new health care provider, it is critical to obtain a complete antiretroviral (ARV) history (including drug-resistance testing results, if available), preferably through the review of past medical records. Newly diagnosed patients should also be asked about any prior use of ARV agents for prevention of HIV infection.

The following laboratory tests performed during initial patient visits can be used to stage HIV disease and to assist in the selection of ARV drug regimens:

- HIV antibody testing (if prior documentation is not available or if HIV RNA is below the assay's limit of detection) **(AI)**;
- CD4 T-cell count (CD4 count) **(AI)**;
- Plasma HIV RNA (viral load) **(AI)**;
- Complete blood count, chemistry profile, transaminase levels, blood urea nitrogen (BUN), and creatinine, urinalysis, and serologies for hepatitis A, B, and C viruses **(AIII)**;
- Fasting blood glucose and serum lipids **(AIII)**; and
- Genotypic resistance testing at entry into care, regardless of whether ART will be initiated immediately **(AII)**. For patients who have HIV RNA levels <500 to 1,000 copies/mL, viral amplification for resistance testing may not always be successful **(BII)**.

In addition, other tests (including screening tests for sexually transmitted infections and tests for determining the risk of opportunistic infections and need for prophylaxis) should be performed as recommended in HIV primary care and opportunistic infections guidelines.[1, 2]

Patients living with HIV infection often must cope with many social, psychiatric, and medical issues that are best addressed through a patient-centered, multi-disciplinary approach to the disease. The baseline evaluation should include an evaluation of the patient's readiness for ART, including an assessment of high-risk behaviors, substance abuse, social support, mental illness, comorbidities, economic factors (e.g., unstable housing), medical insurance status and adequacy of coverage, and other factors that are known to impair adherence to ART and increase the risk of HIV transmission. Once evaluated, these factors should be managed accordingly. The baseline evaluation should also include a discussion of risk reduction and disclosure to sexual and/or needle sharing partners, especially with untreated patients who are still at high risk of HIV transmission.

Education about HIV risk behaviors and effective strategies to prevent HIV transmission should be provided at each patient visit (see Preventing Secondary Transmission of HIV).

References

1. Aberg JA, Kaplan JE, Libman H, et al. Primary care guidelines for the management of persons infected with human immunodeficiency virus: 2009 update by the HIV Medicine Association of the Infectious Diseases Society of America.

Clin Infect Dis. Sep 1 2009;49(5):651-681. Available at http://www.ncbi.nlm.nih.gov/entrez/query.fcgi?cmd=Retrieve&db=PubMed&dopt=Citation&list_uids=19640227.

2. Centers for Disease Control and Prevention (CDC). Guidelines for prevention and treatment of opportunistic infections in HIV-infected adults and adolescents: recommendations from CDC, the National Institutes of Health, and the HIV Medicine Association of the Infectious Diseases Society of America. *MMWR Recomm Rep.* Apr 10 2009;58(RR-4):1-207. Available at http://www.ncbi.nlm.nih.gov/entrez/query.fcgi?cmd=Retrieve&db=PubMed&dopt=Citation&list_uids=19357635.

Laboratory Testing

Laboratory Testing for Initial Assessment and Monitoring While on Antiretroviral Therapy (Last updated February 12, 2013; last reviewed February 12, 2013)

A number of laboratory tests are important for initial evaluation of HIV-infected patients upon entry into care, during follow-up (if antiretroviral therapy (ART) has not been initiated), and before and after the initiation or modification of therapy to assess virologic and immunologic efficacy of ART and to monitor for laboratory abnormalities that may be associated with antiretroviral (ARV) drugs. Table 3 outlines the Panel's recommendations for the frequency of testing. As noted in the table, some tests may be repeated more frequently if clinically indicated.

Two surrogate markers are routinely used to assess the immune function and level of HIV viremia: CD4 T-cell count (CD4 count) and plasma HIV RNA (viral load). Resistance testing should be used to guide selection of an ARV regimen; a viral tropism assay should be performed before initiation of a CCR5 antagonist; and HLA-B*5701 testing should be performed before initiation of abacavir (ABC). The rationale for and utility of these laboratory tests are discussed below.

Table 3. Laboratory Monitoring Schedule for Patients Before and After Initiation of Antiretroviral Therapy[a] (page 1 of 2)

	Entry into care	Follow-up before ART	ART initiation or modification[b]	Follow-up 2–8 weeks post-ART initiation or modification	Every 3–6 months	Every 6 months	Every 12 months	Treatment failure	Clinically indicated
HIV serology	√ If diagnosis has not been confirmed								
CD4 count	√	√ Every 3–6 months	√		√	In clinically stable patients with suppressed viral load, CD4 count can be monitored every 6–12 months (see text).		√	√
HIV viral load	√	√ Every 3–6 months	√	√c	√d			√	√
Resistance testing	√		√e					√	√
HLA-B*5701 testing			√ If considering ABC						
Tropism testing			√ If considering a CCR5 antagonist					√ If considering a CCR5 antagonist, or for failure of CCR5 antagonist-based regimen	√
Hepatitis B serology[f]	√		√ May repeat if HBsAg (-) and HBsAb (-) at baseline						√
Hepatitis C serology, with confirmation of positive results	√								√
Basic chemistry[g,h]	√	√ Every 6–12 months	√	√	√				√

	Entry into care	Follow-up before ART	ART initiation or modification[b]	Follow-up 2–8 weeks post-ART initiation or modification	Every 3–6 months	Every 6 months	Every 12 months	Treatment failure	Clinically indicated
ALT, AST, T. bilirubin	√	√ Every 6–12 months	√	√	√				√
CBC with differential	√	√ Every 3–6 months	√	√ If on ZDV	√				√
Fasting lipid profile	√	√ If normal, annually	√	√ Consider 4–8 weeks after starting new ART regimen that affects lipids		√ If abnormal at last measurement	√ If normal at last measurement		√
Fasting glucose or hemoglobin A1C	√	√ If normal, annually	√		√ If abnormal at last measurement	√ If normal at last measurement			√
Urinalysis[g]	√		√			√ If on TDF	√		√
Pregnancy test			√ If starting EFV						√

[a] This table pertains to laboratory tests done to select an ARV regimen and monitor for treatment responses or ART toxicities. Please refer to the HIV Primary Care guidelines for guidance on other laboratory tests generally recommended for primary health care maintenance of HIV patients.[1]

[b] ART may be modified for treatment failure, adverse effects, or regimen simplification.

[c] If HIV RNA is detectable at 2 to 8 weeks, repeat every 4 to 8 weeks until suppression to <200 copies/mL, then every 3 to 6 months.

[d] Viral load typically is measured every 3 to 4 months in patients on ART. However, for adherent patients with suppressed viral load and stable immunologic status for more than 2 to 3 years, monitoring at 6 month intervals may be considered.

[e] In ART-naive patients, if resistance testing was performed at entry into care, repeat testing before initiation of ART is optional. The exception is pregnant women; repeat testing is recommended in this case. For virologically suppressed patients who are switching therapy for toxicity or convenience, viral amplification will not be possible and therefore resistance testing should not be performed. Results from prior resistance testing can be used to help in the construction of a new regimen.

[f] If HBsAg is positive at baseline or before initiation of ART, TDF plus either FTC or 3TC should be used as part of the ARV regimen to treat both HBV and HIV infections. If HBsAg, and HBsAb, and anti-HBc are negative at baseline, hepatitis B vaccine series should be administered.

[g] Serum Na, K, HCO3, Cl, BUN, creatinine, glucose (preferably fasting). Some experts suggest monitoring the phosphorus levels of patients on TDF. Determination of renal function should include estimation of CrCl using Cockcroft-Gault equation or estimation of glomerular filtration rate based on MDRD equation.

[h] For patients with renal disease, consult the Guidelines for the Management of Chronic Kidney Disease in HIV-Infected Patients: Recommendations of the HIV Medicine Association of the Infectious Diseases Society of America.[2]

More frequent monitoring may be indicated for patients with evidence of kidney disease (e.g. proteinuria, decreased glomerular dysfunction) or increased risk of renal insufficiency (e.g., patients with diabetes, hypertension).

Acronyms: 3TC = lamivudine, ABC = abacavir, ALT = alanine aminotransferase, ART = antiretroviral therapy, AST = aspartate aminotranserase, CBC = complete blood count, CrCl = creatinine clearance, EFV = efavirenz, FTC = emtricitabine, HBsAb = hepatitis B surface antibody, HBsAg = hepatitis B surface antigen, HBV = hepatitis B virus, MDRD = modification of diet in renal disease (equation), TDF = tenofovir, ZDV = zidovudine

References

1. Aberg JA, Kaplan JE, Libman H, et al. Primary care guidelines for the management of persons infected with human immunodeficiency virus: 2009 update by the HIV medicine Association of the Infectious Diseases Society of America. *Clin Infect Dis*. Sep 1 2009;49(5):651-681. Available at http://www.ncbi.nlm.nih.gov/entrez/query.fcgi?cmd=Retrieve&db=PubMed&dopt=Citation&list_uids=19640227.

2. Gupta SK, Eustace JA, Winston JA, et al. Guidelines for the management of chronic kidney disease in HIV-infected patients: Recommendations of the HIV Medicine Association of the Infectious Diseases Society of America. *Clin Infect Dis*. Jun 1 2005;40(11):1559-1585. Available at http://www.ncbi.nlm.nih.gov/entrez/query.fcgi?cmd=Retrieve&db=PubMed&dopt=Citation&list_uids=15889353.

CD4 T-Cell Count (Last updated February 12, 2013; last reviewed February 12, 2013)

The CD4 T-cell count (CD4 count) serves as the major laboratory indicator of immune function in patients who have HIV infection. It is one of the key factors in determining both the urgency of antiretroviral therapy (ART) initiation and the need for prophylaxis for opportunistic infections. It is also the strongest predictor of subsequent disease progression and survival according to findings from clinical trials and cohort studies.[1, 2] CD4 counts are highly variable; a significant change (2 standard deviations) between 2 tests is approximately a 30% change in the absolute count, or an increase or decrease in CD4 percentage by 3 percentage points.

- **Use of CD4 Count for Initial Assessment.** The CD4 count is one of the most important factors in determining the urgency of ART initiation and the need for prophylaxis for opportunistic infections. All patients at entry into care should have a baseline CD4 count **(AI)**. Recommendations for initiation of ART can be found in the Initiating Antiretroviral Therapy in Antiretroviral-Naive Patients section of these guidelines.

- **Use of CD4 Count for Monitoring Therapeutic Response.** An adequate CD4 response for most patients on therapy is defined as an increase in CD4 count in the range of 50 to 150 cells/mm^3 per year, generally with an accelerated response in the first 3 months of treatment. Subsequent increases in patients with good virologic control average approximately 50 to 100 cells/mm^3 per year until a steady state level is reached.[3] Patients who initiate therapy with a low CD4 count[4] or at an older age[5] may have a blunted increase in their counts despite virologic suppression.

Frequency of CD4 Count Monitoring. ART now is recommended for all HIV-infected patients. In untreated patients, CD4 counts should be monitored every 3 to 6 months to determine the urgency of ART initiation. In patients on ART, the CD4 count is used to assess the immunologic response to ART and the need for initiation or discontinuation of prophylaxis for opportunistic infections **(AI)**.

The CD4 count response to ART varies widely, but a poor CD4 response is rarely an indication for modifying a virologically suppressive antiretroviral (ARV) regimen. In patients with consistently suppressed viral loads who have already experienced ART-related immune reconstitution, the CD4 cell count provides limited information, and frequent testing may cause unnecessary anxiety in patients with clinically inconsequential fluctuations. Thus, for the patient on a suppressive regimen whose CD4 cell count has increased well above the threshold for opportunistic infection risk, the CD4 count can be measured less frequently than the viral load. In such patients, CD4 count may be monitored every 6 to 12 months, unless there are changes in the patient's clinical status, such as new HIV-associated clinical symptoms or initiation of treatment with interferon, corticosteroids, or anti-neoplastic agents **(CIII)**.

Factors that affect absolute CD4 count. The absolute CD4 count is a calculated value based on the total white blood cell (WBC) count and the percentages of total and CD4+ T lymphocytes. This absolute number may fluctuate in individuals or may be influenced by factors that may affect the total WBC count and lymphocyte percentages, such as use of bone marrow-suppressive medications or the presence of acute infections. Splenectomy[6, 7] or co-infection with human T-lymphotropic virus type I (HTLV-1)[8] may cause misleadingly elevated absolute CD4 counts. Alpha-interferon, on the other hand, may reduce the absolute CD4 count without changing the CD4 percentage.[9] In all these cases, CD4 percentage remains stable and may be a more appropriate parameter to assess the patient's immune function.

References

1. Mellors JW, Munoz A, Giorgi JV, et al. Plasma viral load and CD4+ lymphocytes as prognostic markers of HIV-1 infection. *Ann Intern Med.* Jun 15 1997;126(12):946-954. Available at http://www.ncbi.nlm.nih.gov/entrez/query.fcgi?cmd=Retrieve&db=PubMed&dopt=Citation&list_uids=9182471.

2. Egger M, May M, Chene G, et al. Prognosis of HIV-1-infected patients starting highly active antiretroviral therapy: A collaborative analysis of prospective studies. *Lancet.* Jul 13 2002;360(9327):119-129. Available at http://www.ncbi.nlm.nih.gov/pubmed/12126821.

3. Kaufmann GR, Perrin L, Pantaleo G, et al. CD4 T-lymphocyte recovery in individuals with advanced HIV-1 infection receiving potent antiretroviral therapy for 4 years: The Swiss HIV Cohort Study. *Arch Intern Med.* Oct 13 2003;163(18):2187-2195. Available at http://www.ncbi.nlm.nih.gov/entrez/query.fcgi?cmd=Retrieve&db=PubMed&dopt=Citation&list_uids=14557216.

4. Moore RD, Keruly JC. CD4+ cell count 6 years after commencement of highly active antiretroviral therapy in persons with sustained virologic suppression. *Clin Infect Dis.* Feb 1 2007;44(3):441-446. Available at http://www.ncbi.nlm.nih.gov/entrez/query.fcgi?cmd=Retrieve&db=PubMed&dopt=Citation&list_uids=17205456.

5. Althoff KN, Justice AC, Gange SJ, et al. Virologic and immunologic response to HAART, by age and regimen class. *AIDS.* Oct 23 2010;24(16):2469-2479. Available at http://www.ncbi.nlm.nih.gov/pubmed/20829678.

6. Zurlo JJ, Wood L, Gaglione MM, Polis MA. Effect of splenectomy on T lymphocyte subsets in patients infected with the human immunodeficiency virus. *Clin Infect Dis.* Apr 1995;20(4):768-771. Available at http://www.ncbi.nlm.nih.gov/entrez/query.fcgi?cmd=Retrieve&db=PubMed&dopt=Citation&list_uids=7795071.

7. Bernard NF, Chernoff DN, Tsoukas CM. Effect of splenectomy on T-cell subsets and plasma HIV viral titers in HIV-infected patients. *J Hum Virol.* Jul-Aug 1998;1(5):338-345. Available at http://www.ncbi.nlm.nih.gov/entrez/query.fcgi?cmd=Retrieve&db=PubMed&dopt=Citation&list_uids=10195261.

8. Casseb J, Posada-Vergara MP, Montanheiro P, et al. T CD4+ cells count among patients co-infected with human immunodeficiency virus type 1 (HIV-1) and human T-cell leukemia virus type 1 (HTLV-1): High prevalence of tropical spastic paraparesis/HTLV-1-associated myelopathy (TSP/HAM). *Rev Inst Med Trop Sao Paulo.* Jul-Aug 2007;49(4):231-233. Available at http://www.ncbi.nlm.nih.gov/entrez/query.fcgi?cmd=Retrieve&db=PubMed&dopt=Citation&list_uids=17823752.

9. Berglund O, Engman K, Ehrnst A, et al. Combined treatment of symptomatic human immunodeficiency virus type 1 infection with native interferon-alpha and zidovudine. *J Infect Dis.* Apr 1991;163(4):710-715. Available at http://www.ncbi.nlm.nih.gov/entrez/query.fcgi?cmd=Retrieve&db=PubMed&dopt=Citation&list_uids=1672701.

Plasma HIV-1 RNA Testing (Last updated February 12, 2013; last reviewed February 12, 2013)

Plasma HIV-1 RNA (viral load) should be measured in all HIV-1-infected patients at baseline and on a regular basis thereafter, especially in patients who are on treatment, because viral load is the most important indicator of response to antiretroviral therapy (ART) (AI). Commercially available HIV-1 RNA assays do not detect HIV-2 viral load. For further discussion on HIV-2 RNA monitoring in patients with HIV-1/HIV-2 co-infection or HIV-2 mono-infection, see HIV-2 Infection. Analysis of 18 trials that included more than 5,000 participants with viral load monitoring showed a significant association between a decrease in plasma viremia and improved clinical outcome.[1] Thus, viral load testing serves as a surrogate marker for treatment response[2] and can be useful in predicting clinical progression.[3, 4] The minimal change in viral load considered to be statistically significant (2 standard deviations) is a threefold, or a $0.5 \log_{10}$ copies/mL change.

Optimal viral suppression is generally defined as a viral load persistently below the level of detection (<20 to 75 copies/mL, depending on the assay used). However, isolated blips (viral loads transiently detectable at low levels, typically <400 copies/mL) are not uncommon in successfully treated patients and are not thought to represent viral replication or to predict virologic failure.[5] In addition, low-level positive viral load results (typically <200 copies/mL) appear to be more common with some viral load assays than with others. Furthermore, there is no definitive evidence that patients with viral loads quantified as <200 copies/mL using these assays are at increased risk for virologic failure.[6-8] For the purposes of clinical trials, the AIDS Clinical Trials Group (ACTG) currently defines virologic failure as a confirmed viral load >200 copies/mL, which eliminates most cases of apparent viremia caused by blips or assay variability.[9] This definition also may be useful in clinical practice (see Virologic and Immunologic Failure).

For most individuals who are adherent to their antiretroviral (ARV) regimens and who do not harbor resistance mutations to the prescribed drugs, viral suppression is generally achieved in 12 to 24 weeks, although it may take longer in some patients. Recommendations for the frequency of viral load monitoring are summarized below.

- **At initiation or change in therapy.** Plasma viral load should be measured before initiation of therapy and preferably within 2 to 4 weeks, and not more than 8 weeks, after treatment initiation or after treatment modification (BI). Repeat viral load measurement should be performed at 4- to 8-week intervals until the level falls below the assay's limit of detection (BIII).

- **In virologically suppressed patients in whom therapy was modified because of drug toxicity or for regimen simplification.** Viral load measurement should be performed within 2 to 8 weeks after changing therapy. The purpose of viral load monitoring at this point is to confirm potency of the new regimen (BIII).

- **In patients on a stable ARV regimen.** Viral load should be repeated every 3 to 4 months or as clinically indicated (BII). Clinicians may extend the interval to every 6 months for adherent patients who have suppressed viral loads for more than 2 to 3 years and whose clinical and immunologic status is stable (BIII).

Monitoring in patients with suboptimal response. In addition to viral load monitoring, a number of additional factors should be assessed, such as adherence to prescribed medications, altered pharmacology, or drug interactions. Patients who fail to achieve viral suppression should undergo resistance testing to aid in the selection of an alternative regimen, as discussed in Drug-Resistance Testing and Virologic and Immunologic Failure (AI).

References

1. Murray JS, Elashoff MR, Iacono-Connors LC, Cvetkovich TA, Struble KA. The use of plasma HIV RNA as a study endpoint in efficacy trials of antiretroviral drugs. *AIDS*. May 7 1999;13(7):797-804. Available at http://www.ncbi.nlm.nih.gov/entrez/query.fcgi?cmd=Retrieve&db=PubMed&dopt=Citation&list_uids=10357378.

2. Hughes MD, Johnson VA, Hirsch MS, et al. Monitoring plasma HIV-1 RNA levels in addition to CD4+ lymphocyte count improves assessment of antiretroviral therapeutic response. ACTG 241 Protocol Virology Substudy Team. *Ann Intern Med*. Jun 15 1997;126(12):929-938. Available at http://www.ncbi.nlm.nih.gov/entrez/query.fcgi?cmd=Retrieve&db=PubMed&dopt=Citation&list_uids=9182469.

3. Marschner IC, Collier AC, Coombs RW, et al. Use of changes in plasma levels of human immunodeficiency virus type 1 RNA to assess the clinical benefit of antiretroviral therapy. *J Infect Dis*. Jan 1998;177(1):40-47. Available at http://www.ncbi.nlm.nih.gov/entrez/query.fcgi?cmd=Retrieve&db=PubMed&dopt=Citation&list_uids=9419168.

4. Thiebaut R, Morlat P, Jacqmin-Gadda H, et al. Clinical progression of HIV-1 infection according to the viral response during the first year of antiretroviral treatment. Groupe d'Epidemiologie du SIDA en Aquitaine (GECSA). *AIDS*. May 26 2000;14(8):971-978. Available at http://www.ncbi.nlm.nih.gov/entrez/query.fcgi?cmd=Retrieve&db=PubMed&dopt=Citation&list_uids=10853978.

5. Havlir DV, Bassett R, Levitan D, et al. Prevalence and predictive value of intermittent viremia with combination hiv therapy. *JAMA*. Jul 11 2001;286(2):171-179. Available at http://www.ncbi.nlm.nih.gov/entrez/query.fcgi?cmd=Retrieve&db=PubMed&dopt=Citation&list_uids=11448280.

6. Damond F, Roquebert B, Benard A, et al. Human immunodeficiency virus type 1 (HIV 1) plasma load discrepancies between the Roche COBAS AMPLICOR HIV-1 MONITOR Version 1.5 and the Roche COBAS AmpliPrep/COBAS TaqMan HIV-1 assays. *J Clin Microbiol*. Oct 2007;45(10):3436-3438. Available at http://www.ncbi.nlm.nih.gov/entrez/query.fcgi?cmd=Retrieve&db=PubMed&dopt=Citation&list_uids=17715371.

7. Gatanaga H, Tsukada K, Honda H, et al. Detection of HIV type 1 load by the Roche Cobas TaqMan assay in patients with viral loads previously undetectable by the Roche Cobas Amplicor Monitor. *Clin Infect Dis*. Jan 15 2009;48(2):260-262. Available at http://www.ncbi.nlm.nih.gov/entrez/query.fcgi?cmd=Retrieve&db=PubMed&dopt=Citation&list_uids=19113986.

8. Willig JH, Nevin CR, Raper JL, et al. Cost ramifications of increased reporting of detectable plasma HIV-1 RNA levels by the Roche COBAS AmpliPrep/COBAS TaqMan HIV-1 version 1.0 viral load test. *J Acquir Immune Defic Syndr*. Aug 1 2010;54(4):442-444. Available at http://www.ncbi.nlm.nih.gov/entrez/query.fcgi?cmd=Retrieve&db=PubMed&dopt=Citation&list_uids=20611035.

9. Ribaudo H, Lennox J, Currier J, al e. Virologic failure endpoint definition in clinical trials: Is using HIV-1 RNA threshold <200 copies/mL better than <50 copies/mL? An analysis of ACTG studies. Paper presented at: *16th Conference on Retroviruses and Opportunistic Infections*. Montreal, Canada, 2009.

Panel's Recommendations

- HIV drug-resistance testing is recommended in persons with HIV infection at entry into care regardless of whether antiretroviral therapy (ART) will be initiated immediately or deferred **(AII)**. If therapy is deferred, repeat testing should be considered at the time of ART initiation **(CIII)**.

- Genotypic testing is recommended as the preferred resistance testing to guide therapy in antiretroviral (ARV)-naive patients **(AIII)**.

- Standard genotypic drug-resistance testing in ARV-naive persons involves testing for mutations in the reverse transcriptase (RT) and protease (PR) genes. If transmitted integrase strand transfer inhibitor (INSTI) resistance is a concern, providers may wish to supplement standard genotypic resistance testing with an INSTI genotype test **(CIII)**.

- HIV drug-resistance testing should be performed to assist in the selection of active drugs when changing ARV regimens in persons with virologic failure and HIV RNA levels >1,000 copies/mL **(AI)**. In persons with HIV RNA levels >500 but <1,000 copies/mL, testing may be unsuccessful but should still be considered **(BII)**.

- Drug-resistance testing should also be performed when managing suboptimal viral load reduction **(AII)**.

- In persons failing INSTI-based regimens, genotypic testing for INSTI resistance should be performed to determine whether to include a drug from this class in subsequent regimens **(AII)**.

- Drug-resistance testing in the setting of virologic failure should be performed while the person is taking prescribed ARV drugs or, if not possible, within 4 weeks after discontinuing therapy **(AII)**.

- Genotypic testing is recommended as the preferred resistance testing to guide therapy in patients with suboptimal virologic responses or virologic failure while on first or second regimens **(AII)**.

- The addition of phenotypic to genotypic testing is generally preferred for persons with known or suspected complex drug-resistance mutation patterns, particularly to protease inhibitors (PIs) **(BIII)**.

- Genotypic resistance testing is recommended for all pregnant women before initiation of ART **(AIII)** and for those entering pregnancy with detectable HIV RNA levels while on therapy **(AI)** (see the *Perinatal Treatment Guidelines* for more detailed discussion).

Rating of Recommendations: A = Strong; B = Moderate; C = Optional

Rating of Evidence: I = Data from randomized controlled trials; II = Data from well-designed nonrandomized trials or observational cohort studies with long-term clinical outcomes; III = Expert opinion

Genotypic and Phenotypic Resistance Assays

Genotypic and phenotypic resistance assays are used to assess viral strains and inform selection of treatment strategies. Standard assays provide information on resistance to nucleoside reverse transcriptase inhibitors (NRTIs), non-nucleoside reverse transcriptase inhibitors (NNRTIs), and protease inhibitors (PIs). Testing for integrase and fusion inhibitor resistance can also be ordered separately from several commercial laboratories. Co-receptor tropism assays should be performed whenever the use of a CCR5 antagonist is being considered. Phenotypic co-receptor tropism assays have been used in clinical practice. A genotypic assay to predict co-receptor use is now commercially available (see Co-receptor Tropism Assays).

Genotypic Assays

Genotypic assays detect drug-resistance mutations present in relevant viral genes. Most genotypic assays involve sequencing of the RT and PR genes to detect mutations that are known to confer drug resistance. Genotypic assays that assess mutations in the integrase and gp41 (envelope) genes are also commercially available. Genotypic assays can be performed rapidly and results are available within 1 to 2 weeks of sample collection. Interpretation of test results requires knowledge of the mutations selected by different antiretroviral (ARV) drugs and of the potential for cross resistance to other drugs conferred by certain mutations. The International AIDS Society-USA (IAS-USA) maintains an updated list of significant resistance-associated mutations in the RT, PR, integrase, and envelope genes (see

The Stanford University HIV Drug Resistance Database (http://hivdb.stanford.edu) also provides helpful guidance for interpreting genotypic resistance test results. Various tools to assist the provider in interpreting genotypic test results are now available.[2-5] Clinical trials have demonstrated that consultation with specialists in HIV drug resistance improves virologic outcomes.[6] Clinicians are thus encouraged to consult a specialist to facilitate interpretation of genotypic test results and design of an optimal new regimen.

Phenotypic Assays

Phenotypic assays measure the ability of a virus to grow in different concentrations of ARV drugs. RT and PR gene sequences and, more recently, integrase and envelope sequences derived from patient plasma HIV RNA are inserted into the backbone of a laboratory clone of HIV or used to generate pseudotyped viruses that express the patient-derived HIV genes of interest. Replication of these viruses at different drug concentrations is monitored by expression of a reporter gene and is compared with replication of a reference HIV strain. The drug concentration that inhibits viral replication by 50% (i.e., the median inhibitory concentration [IC_{50}]) is calculated, and the ratio of the IC_{50} of test and reference viruses is reported as the fold increase in IC_{50} (i.e., fold resistance).

Automated phenotypic assays that can produce results in 2 to 3 weeks are commercially available, but they cost more to perform than genotypic assays. In addition, interpretation of phenotypic assay results is complicated by incomplete information regarding the specific resistance level (i.e., fold increase in IC_{50}) that is associated with drug failure, although clinically significant fold increase cutoffs are now available for some drugs.[7-11] Again, consultation with a specialist to interpret test results can be helpful.

Further limitations of both genotypic and phenotypic assays include lack of uniform quality assurance testing for all available assays, relatively high cost, and insensitivity to minor viral species. Despite being present, drug-resistant viruses that constitute less than 10% to 20% of the circulating virus population will probably not be detected by commercially available assays. This limitation is important because after drugs exerting selective pressure on drug-resistant populations are discontinued, a wild-type virus often re-emerges as the predominant population in the plasma. As a consequence, the proportion of virus with resistance mutations decreases to below the 10% to 20% threshold.[12-14] In the case of some drugs, this reversion to predominantly wild-type virus can occur in the first 4 to 6 weeks after the drugs are discontinued. Prospective clinical studies have shown that despite this plasma reversion, re-initiation of the same ARV agents (or those sharing similar resistance pathways) is usually associated with early drug failure, and that the virus present at failure is derived from previously archived resistant virus.[15] Therefore, resistance testing is of greatest value when performed before or within 4 weeks after drugs are discontinued **(AII)**. Because resistant virus may persist in the plasma of some patients for longer periods of time, resistance testing done 4 to 6 weeks after discontinuation of drugs may still detect mutations. However, the absence of detectable resistance in such patients must be interpreted with caution when designing subsequent ARV regimens.

Use of Resistance Assays in Clinical Practice (See Table 4)

Use of Resistance Assays in Determining Initial Treatment

Transmission of drug-resistant HIV strains is well documented and associated with suboptimal virologic response to initial antiretroviral therapy (ART).[16-19] The likelihood that a patient will acquire drug-resistant virus is related to the prevalence of drug resistance in HIV-infected persons engaging in high-risk behaviors in the community. In the United States and Europe, recent studies suggest that the risk that transmitted virus will be resistant to at least one ARV drug is in the range of 6% to 16%.[20-25] Up to 8%, but generally less than 5% of transmitted viruses will exhibit resistance to drugs from more than one class.[24, 26-28]

If the decision is made to initiate therapy in a person with early HIV infection, resistance testing at baseline can guide regimen selection to optimize virologic response. Therefore, resistance testing in this situation is recommended **(AII)**. A genotypic assay is preferred for this purpose **(AIII)**. In this setting, treatment initiation should not be delayed pending resistance testing results. Once results are obtained, the treatment regimen can be modified if warranted (see Acute and Recent HIV Infection). In the absence of therapy, resistant viruses may decline over time to less than the detection limit of standard resistance tests, but when therapy is eventually initiated, resistant viruses even at a low level may still increase the risk of treatment failure.[29-31] Therefore, if therapy is deferred, resistance testing should still be done during acute HIV infection **(AIII)**. In this situation, the genotypic resistance test result may be kept on record until the patient is to be started on ART. Repeat resistance testing at the time treatment is started should be considered because it is possible for a patient to acquire drug-resistant virus (i.e., superinfection) between entry into care and initiation of ART **(CIII)**.

Performing drug-resistance testing before ART initiation in patients with chronic HIV infection is less straightforward. The rate at which transmitted resistance-associated mutations revert to wild-type virus has not been completely delineated, but mutations present at the time of HIV transmission are more stable than those selected under drug pressure. It is often possible to detect resistance-associated mutations in viruses that were transmitted several years earlier.[32-34] No prospective trial has addressed whether drug-resistance testing before initiation of therapy confers benefit in this population. However, data from several, but not all, studies suggest that virologic responses in persons with baseline resistance mutations are suboptimal.[16-19, 35-37] In addition, a cost-effectiveness analysis of early genotypic resistance testing suggests that baseline testing in this population should be performed.[38] Therefore, resistance testing in chronically infected persons is recommended at the time of entry into HIV care **(AII)**. Although no definitive prospective data exist to support the choice of one type of resistance testing over another, genotypic testing is generally preferred in this situation because of lower cost, more rapid turnaround time, the assay's ability to detect mixtures of wild-type and resistant virus, and the relative ease of interpreting test results **(AIII)**. If therapy is deferred, repeat testing soon before initiation of ART should be considered because the patient may have acquired drug-resistant virus (i.e., superinfection) **(CIII)**.

Standard genotypic drug-resistance testing in ARV-naive persons involves testing for mutations in the RT and PR genes. Although transmission of integrase strand transfer inhibitor (INSTI)-resistant virus has rarely been reported, as use of INSTIs increases, the potential for transmission of INSTI-resistant virus may also increase. Therefore, when INSTI resistance is suspected, providers may wish to supplement standard baseline genotypic resistance testing with genotypic testing for resistance to this class of drugs **(CIII)**.

Use of Resistance Assays in the Event of Virologic Failure

Resistance assays are useful in guiding treatment decisions for patients who experience virologic failure while on ART. Several prospective studies assessed the utility of resistance testing to guide ARV drug selection in patients with virologic failure. These studies involved genotypic assays, phenotypic assays, or both.[6, 39-45] In general, these studies found that changes in therapy that were informed by resistance testing results produced better early virologic response to salvage regimens than regimen changes guided only by clinical judgment.

In addition, one observational cohort study found that performance of genotypic drug-resistance testing in ART-experienced patients with detectable plasma HIV RNA was independently associated with improved survival.[46] Thus, resistance testing is recommended as a tool in selecting active drugs when changing ARV regimens because of virologic failure in persons with HIV RNA >1,000 copies/mL **(AI)** (see Virologic and Immunologic Failure). In persons with HIV RNA >500 copies/mL but <1,000 copies/mL, testing may be unsuccessful but should still be considered **(BII)**. Drug-resistance testing in persons with a plasma viral load <500 copies/mL is not usually recommended because resistance assays cannot be consistently performed given low HIV RNA levels **(AIII)**.

Resistance testing also can help guide treatment decisions for patients with suboptimal viral load reduction **(AII)**. Virologic failure in the setting of combination ART is, for certain patients, associated with resistance to only one component of the regimen.[47-49] In this situation, substituting individual drugs in a failing regimen may be a possible option, but this concept will require clinical validation (see Virologic and Immunologic Failure).

In patients who are on a failing first or second ARV drug regimen and experiencing virologic failure or suboptimal viral load reduction, genotypic testing is generally preferred for resistance testing **(AII)**. This is based on the fact that, when compared with phenotypic testing, genotypic testing costs less to perform, has a faster turnaround time, and greater sensitivity for detecting mixtures of wild-type and resistant virus. In addition, observations show that the assays are comparable predictors of virologic response to subsequent ART regimens.[50]

Addition of phenotypic to genotypic testing is generally preferred for persons with known or suspected complex drug-resistance mutation patterns, particularly to PIs **(BIII)**.

In patients failing INSTI-based regimens, testing for INSTI resistance should be performed to determine whether to include drugs from this class in subsequent regimens **(AII)**; genotypic testing is preferred for this purpose.

When the use of a CCR5 antagonist is being considered, a co-receptor tropism assay should be performed **(AI)**. Phenotypic co-receptor tropism assays have been used in clinical practice. A genotypic assay to predict co-receptor use is now commercially available and is less expensive than phenotypic assays. Evaluation of genotypic assays is ongoing, but current data suggest that such testing should be considered as an alternative assay. The same principles regarding testing for co-receptor use also apply to testing when patients exhibit virologic failure on a CCR5 antagonist.[51] Resistance to CCR5 antagonists in the absence of detectable CXCR4-using virus has been reported, but such resistance is uncommon (see Co-receptor Tropism Assays).

Use of Resistance Assays in Pregnant Women

In pregnant women, the goal of ART is to maximally reduce plasma HIV RNA to provide optimal maternal therapy and to prevent perinatal transmission of HIV. Genotypic resistance testing is recommended for all pregnant women before initiation of therapy **(AIII)** and for those entering pregnancy with detectable HIV RNA levels while on therapy **(AI)**. Phenotypic testing in those found to have complex drug-resistance mutation patterns, particularly to PIs, may provide additional information **(BIII)**. Optimal prevention of perinatal transmission may require initiation of ART pending resistance testing results. Once the results are available, the ARV regimen can be changed as needed.

Table 4. Recommendations for Using Drug-Resistance Assays (page 1 of 2)

Clinical Setting/Recommendation	Rationale
Drug-resistance assay recommended	
In acute HIV infection: Drug-resistance testing is recommended regardless of whether antiretroviral therapy (ART) is initiated immediately or deferred **(AII)**. A genotypic assay is generally preferred **(AIII)**.	If ART is initiated immediately, drug-resistance testing can determine whether drug-resistant virus was transmitted. Test results will help in the design of initial regimens or to modify or change regimens if results are obtained after treatment initiation. Genotypic testing is preferred to phenotypic testing because of lower cost, faster turnaround time, and greater sensitivity for detecting mixtures of wild-type and resistant virus.
If ART is deferred, repeat resistance testing should be considered at the time therapy is initiated **(CIII)**. A genotypic assay generally is preferred **(AIII)**.	If ART is deferred, testing should still be performed because of the greater likelihood that transmitted resistance-associated mutations will be detected earlier in the course of HIV infection. Results of resistance testing may be important when treatment is initiated. Repeat testing at the time ART is initiated should be considered because the patient may have acquired a drug-resistant virus (i.e., superinfection).
In ART-naive patients with chronic HIV infection: Drug-resistance testing is recommended at entry into HIV care, regardless of whether therapy is initiated immediately or deferred **(AII)**. A genotypic assay is generally preferred **(AIII)**.	Transmitted HIV with baseline resistance to at least 1 drug is seen in 6% to 16% of patients, and suboptimal virologic responses may be seen in patients with baseline resistant mutations. Some drug-resistance mutations can remain detectable for years in untreated, chronically infected patients.
If therapy is deferred, repeat resistance testing should be considered before initiation of ART **(CIII)**. A genotypic assay is generally preferred **(AIII)**.	Repeat testing before initiation of ART should be considered because the patient may have acquired a drug-resistant virus (i.e., a superinfection). Genotypic testing is preferred to phenotypic testing because of lower cost, faster turnaround time, and greater sensitivity for detecting mixtures of wild-type and resistant virus.
If an INSTI is considered for an ART-naive patient and transmitted INSTI resistance is a concern, providers may supplement standard resistance testing with a specific INSTI genotypic resistance assay **(CIII)**.	Standard genotypic drug-resistance assays test only for mutations in the RT and PR genes.
If use of a CCR5 antagonist is being considered, a co-receptor tropism assay should be performed **(AI)** (see Co-receptor Tropism Assays)	(see Co-receptor Tropism Assays)
In patients with virologic failure: Drug-resistance testing is recommended in patients on combination ART with HIV RNA levels >1,000 copies/mL **(AI)**. In patients with HIV RNA levels >500 copies/mL but <1,000 copies/mL, testing may not be successful but should still be considered **(BII)**.	Testing can help determine the role of resistance in drug failure and maximize the clinician's ability to select active drugs for the new regimen. Drug-resistance testing should be performed while the patient is taking prescribed ARV drugs or, if not possible, within 4 weeks after discontinuing therapy.
A standard genotypic resistance assay is generally preferred for patients experiencing virologic failure on their first or second regimens **(AII)**.	Genotypic testing is preferred to phenotypic testing because of lower cost, faster turnaround time, and greater sensitivity for detecting mixtures of wild-type and resistant HIV.
In patients failing INSTI-based regimens, genotypic testing for INSTI resistance should be performed to determine whether to include drugs from this class in subsequent regimens **(AII)**.	Standard genotypic drug-resistance assays test only for mutations in the RT and PR genes.
If use of a CCR5 antagonist is being considered, a co-receptor tropism assay should be performed **(AI)** (see Co-receptor Tropism Assays).	
Addition of phenotypic assay to genotypic assay is generally preferred in patients with known or suspected complex drug-resistance patterns, particularly to protease inhibitors (PIs) **(BIII)**.	Phenotypic testing can provide additional useful information in patients with complex drug-resistance mutation patterns, particularly to PIs.

Table 4. Recommendations for Using Drug-Resistance Assays (page 2 of 2)

Clinical Setting/Recommendation	Rationale
Drug-resistance assay recommended	
In patients with suboptimal suppression of viral load: Drug-resistance testing is recommended in patients with suboptimal suppression of viral load after initiation of ART **(AII)**.	Testing can help determine the role of resistance and thus assist the clinician in identifying the number of active drugs available for a new regimen.
In HIV-infected pregnant women: Genotypic resistance testing is recommended for all pregnant women before initiation of ART **(AIII)** and for those entering pregnancy with detectable HIV RNA levels while on therapy **(AI)**.	The goal of ART in HIV-infected pregnant women is to achieve maximal viral suppression for treatment of maternal HIV infection and for prevention of perinatal transmission of HIV. Genotypic resistance testing will assist the clinician in selecting the optimal regimen for the patient.
Drug-resistance assay not usually recommended	
After therapy is discontinued: Drug-resistance testing is not usually recommended more than 4 weeks after discontinuation of ARV drugs **(BIII)**.	Drug-resistance mutations may become minor species in the absence of selective drug pressure, and available assays may not detect minor drug-resistant species. If testing is performed in this setting, the detection of drug resistance may be of value; however, the absence of resistance does not rule out the presence of minor drug-resistant species.
In patients with low HIV RNA levels: Drug-resistance testing is not usually recommended in patients with a plasma viral load <500 copies/mL **(AIII)**.	Resistance assays cannot be consistently performed given low HIV RNA levels.

References

1. Hirsch MS, Gunthard HF, Schapiro JM, et al. Antiretroviral drug-resistance testing in adult HIV-1 infection: 2008 recommendations of an International AIDS Society-USA panel. *Clin Infect Dis*. 2008;47(2):266-285. Available at http://www.ncbi.nlm.nih.gov/entrez/query.fcgi?cmd=Retrieve&db=PubMed&dopt=Citation&list_uids=18549313.

2. Flandre P, Costagliola D. On the comparison of artificial network and interpretation systems based on genotype resistance mutations in HIV-1-infected patients. *AIDS*. 2006;20(16):2118-2120. Available at http://www.ncbi.nlm.nih.gov/entrez/query.fcgi?cmd=Retrieve&db=PubMed&dopt=Citation&list_uids=17053360.

3. Vercauteren J, Vandamme AM. Algorithms for the interpretation of HIV-1 genotypic drug resistance information. *Antiviral Res*. 2006;71(2-3):335-342. Available at http://www.ncbi.nlm.nih.gov/entrez/query.fcgi?cmd=Retrieve&db=PubMed&dopt=Citation&list_uids=16782210.

4. Gianotti N, Mondino V, Rossi MC, et al. Comparison of a rule-based algorithm with a phenotype-based algorithm for the interpretation of HIV genotypes in guiding salvage regimens in HIV-infected patients by a randomized clinical trial: the mutations and salvage study. *Clin Infect Dis*. 2006;42(10):1470-1480. Available at http://www.ncbi.nlm.nih.gov/entrez/query.fcgi?cmd=Retrieve&db=PubMed&dopt=Citation&list_uids=16619162.

5. Torti C, Quiros-Roldan E, Regazzi M, et al. A randomized controlled trial to evaluate antiretroviral salvage therapy guided by rules-based or phenotype-driven HIV-1 genotypic drug-resistance interpretation with or without concentration-controlled intervention: the Resistance and Dosage Adapted Regimens (RADAR) study. *Clin Infect Dis*. 2005;40(12):1828-1836. Available at http://www.ncbi.nlm.nih.gov/entrez/query.fcgi?cmd=Retrieve&db=PubMed&dopt=Citation&list_uids=15909273.

6. Tural C, Ruiz L, Holtzer C, et al. Clinical utility of HIV-1 genotyping and expert advice: the Havana trial. *AIDS*. 2002;16(2):209-218. Available at http://www.ncbi.nlm.nih.gov/entrez/query.fcgi?cmd=Retrieve&db=PubMed&dopt=Citation&list_uids=11807305.

7. Lanier ER, Ait-Khaled M, Scott J, et al. Antiviral efficacy of abacavir in antiretroviral therapy-experienced adults harbouring HIV-1 with specific patterns of resistance to nucleoside reverse transcriptase inhibitors. *Antivir Ther.* 2004;9(1):37-45. Available at
http://www.ncbi.nlm.nih.gov/entrez/query.fcgi?cmd=Retrieve&db=PubMed&dopt=Citation&list_uids=15040535.

8. Miller MD, Margot N, Lu B, et al. Genotypic and phenotypic predictors of the magnitude of response to tenofovir disoproxil fumarate treatment in antiretroviral-experienced patients. *J Infect Dis.* 2004;189(5):837-846. Available at
http://www.ncbi.nlm.nih.gov/entrez/query.fcgi?cmd=Retrieve&db=PubMed&dopt=Citation&list_uids=14976601.

9. Flandre P, Chappey C, Marcelin AG, et al. Phenotypic susceptibility to didanosine is associated with antiviral activity in treatment-experienced patients with HIV-1 infection. *J Infect Dis.* 2007;195(3):392-398. Available at
http://www.ncbi.nlm.nih.gov/entrez/query.fcgi?cmd=Retrieve&db=PubMed&dopt=Citation&list_uids=17205478.

10. Naeger LK, Struble KA. Food and Drug Administration analysis of tipranavir clinical resistance in HIV-1-infected treatment-experienced patients. *AIDS.* 2007;21(2):179-185. Available at
http://www.ncbi.nlm.nih.gov/entrez/query.fcgi?cmd=Retrieve&db=PubMed&dopt=Citation&list_uids=17197808.

11. Naeger LK, Struble KA. Effect of baseline protease genotype and phenotype on HIV response to atazanavir/ritonavir in treatment-experienced patients. *AIDS.* 2006;20(6):847-853. Available at
http://www.ncbi.nlm.nih.gov/entrez/query.fcgi?cmd=Retrieve&db=PubMed&dopt=Citation&list_uids=16549968.

12. Verhofstede C, Wanzeele FV, Van Der Gucht B, De Cabooter N, Plum J. Interruption of reverse transcriptase inhibitors or a switch from reverse transcriptase to protease inhibitors resulted in a fast reappearance of virus strains with a reverse transcriptase inhibitor-sensitive genotype. *AIDS.* 1999;13(18):2541-2546. Available at
http://www.ncbi.nlm.nih.gov/entrez/query.fcgi?cmd=Retrieve&db=PubMed&dopt=Citation&list_uids=10630523.

13. Miller V, Sabin C, Hertogs K, et al. Virological and immunological effects of treatment interruptions in HIV-1 infected patients with treatment failure. *AIDS.* 2000;14(18):2857-2867. Available at
http://www.ncbi.nlm.nih.gov/entrez/query.fcgi?cmd=Retrieve&db=PubMed&dopt=Citation&list_uids=11153667.

14. Devereux HL, Youle M, Johnson MA, Loveday C. Rapid decline in detectability of HIV-1 drug resistance mutations after stopping therapy. *AIDS.* 1999;13(18):F123-127. Available at
http://www.ncbi.nlm.nih.gov/entrez/query.fcgi?cmd=Retrieve&db=PubMed&dopt=Citation&list_uids=10630517.

15. Benson CA, Vaida F, Havlir DV, et al. A randomized trial of treatment interruption before optimized antiretroviral therapy for persons with drug-resistant HIV: 48-week virologic results of ACTG A5086. *J Infect Dis.* 2006;194(9):1309-1318. Available at
http://www.ncbi.nlm.nih.gov/entrez/query.fcgi?cmd=Retrieve&db=PubMed&dopt=Citation&list_uids=17041858.

16. Little SJ, Holte S, Routy JP, et al. Antiretroviral-drug resistance among patients recently infected with HIV. *N Engl J Med.* 2002;347(6):385-394. Available at
http://www.ncbi.nlm.nih.gov/entrez/query.fcgi?cmd=Retrieve&db=PubMed&dopt=Citation&list_uids=12167680.

17. Borroto-Esoda K, Waters JM, Bae AS, et al. Baseline genotype as a predictor of virological failure to emtricitabine or stavudine in combination with didanosine and efavirenz. *AIDS Res Hum Retroviruses.* 2007;23(8):988-995. Available at
http://www.ncbi.nlm.nih.gov/entrez/query.fcgi?cmd=Retrieve&db=PubMed&dopt=Citation&list_uids=17725415.

18. Pozniak AL, Gallant JE, DeJesus E, et al. Tenofovir disoproxil fumarate, emtricitabine, and efavirenz versus fixed-dose zidovudine/lamivudine and efavirenz in antiretroviral-naive patients: virologic, immunologic, and morphologic changes—a 96-week analysis. *J Acquir Immune Defic Syndr.* 2006;43(5):535-540. Available at
http://www.ncbi.nlm.nih.gov/entrez/query.fcgi?cmd=Retrieve&db=PubMed&dopt=Citation&list_uids=17057609.

19. Kuritzkes DR, Lalama CM, Ribaudo HJ, et al. Preexisting resistance to nonnucleoside reverse-transcriptase inhibitors predicts virologic failure of an efavirenz-based regimen in treatment-naive HIV-1-infected subjects. *J Infect Dis.* 2008;197(6):867-870. Available at
http://www.ncbi.nlm.nih.gov/entrez/query.fcgi?cmd=Retrieve&db=PubMed&dopt=Citation&list_uids=18269317.

20. Weinstock HS, Zaidi I, Heneine W, et al. The epidemiology of antiretroviral drug resistance among drug-naive HIV-1-infected persons in 10 U.S. cities. *J Infect Dis*. 2004;189(12):2174-2180. Available at http://www.ncbi.nlm.nih.gov/entrez/query.fcgi?cmd=Retrieve&db=PubMed&dopt=Citation&list_uids=15181563.

21. Wensing AM, van de Vijver DA, Angarano G, et al. Prevalence of drug-resistant HIV-1 variants in untreated individuals in Europe: implications for clinical management. *J Infect Dis*. 2005;192(6):958-966. Available at http://www.ncbi.nlm.nih.gov/entrez/query.fcgi?cmd=Retrieve&db=PubMed&dopt=Citation&list_uids=16107947.

22. Cane P, Chrystie I, Dunn D, et al. Time trends in primary resistance to HIV drugs in the United Kingdom: multicentre observational study. *BMJ*. 2005;331(7529):1368. Available at http://www.ncbi.nlm.nih.gov/entrez/query.fcgi?cmd=Retrieve&db=PubMed&dopt=Citation&list_uids=16299012.

23. Bennett D, McCormick L, Kline R, et al. U.S. surveillance of HIV drug resistance at diagnosis using HIV diagnostic sera. Paper presented at: 12th Conference on Retroviruses and Opportunistic Infections. 2005. Boston, MA.

24. Wheeler WH, Ziebell RA, Zabina H, et al. Prevalence of transmitted drug resistance associated mutations and HIV-1 subtypes in new HIV-1 diagnoses, U.S.-2006. *AIDS*. 2010;24(8):1203-1212. Available at http://www.ncbi.nlm.nih.gov/entrez/query.fcgi?cmd=Retrieve&db=PubMed&dopt=Citation&list_uids=20395786.

25. Ross L, Lim ML, Liao Q, et al. Prevalence of antiretroviral drug resistance and resistance-associated mutations in antiretroviral therapy-naive HIV-infected individuals from 40 United States cities. *HIV Clin Trials*. 2007;8(1):1-8. Available at http://www.ncbi.nlm.nih.gov/entrez/query.fcgi?cmd=Retrieve&db=PubMed&dopt=Citation&list_uids=17434843.

26. Yanik EL, Napravnik S, Hurt CB, et al. Prevalence of transmitted antiretroviral drug resistance differs between acutely and chronically HIV-infected patients. *J Acquir Immune Defic Syndr*. 2012;61(2):258-262. Available at http://www.ncbi.nlm.nih.gov/pubmed/22692092.

27. Agwu AL, Bethel J, Hightow-Weidman LB, et al. Substantial multiclass transmitted drug resistance and drug-relevant polymorphisms among treatment-naive behaviorally HIV-infected youth. *AIDS Patient Care STDS*. 2012;26(4):193-196. Available at http://www.ncbi.nlm.nih.gov/pubmed/22563607.

28. Castor D, Low A, Evering T, et al. Transmitted drug resistance and phylogenetic relationships among acute and early HIV-1-infected individuals in New York City. *J Acquir Immune Defic Syndr*. 2012;61(1):1-8. Available at http://www.ncbi.nlm.nih.gov/pubmed/22592583.

29. Johnson JA, Li JF, Wei X, et al. Minority HIV-1 drug resistance mutations are present in antiretroviral treatment-naive populations and associate with reduced treatment efficacy. *PLoS Med*. 2008;5(7):e158. Available at http://www.ncbi.nlm.nih.gov/entrez/query.fcgi?cmd=Retrieve&db=PubMed&dopt=Citation&list_uids=18666824.

30. Simen BB, Simons JF, Hullsiek KH, et al. Low-abundance drug-resistant viral variants in chronically HIV-infected, antiretroviral treatment-naive patients significantly impact treatment outcomes. *J Infect Dis*. 2009;199(5):693-701. Available at http://www.ncbi.nlm.nih.gov/entrez/query.fcgi?cmd=Retrieve&db=PubMed&dopt=Citation&list_uids=19210162.

31. Paredes R, Lalama CM, Ribaudo HJ, et al. Pre-existing minority drug-resistant HIV-1 variants, adherence, and risk of antiretroviral treatment failure. *J Infect Dis*. 2010;201(5):662-671. Available at http://www.ncbi.nlm.nih.gov/entrez/query.fcgi?cmd=Retrieve&db=PubMed&dopt=Citation&list_uids=20102271.

32. Smith DM, Wong JK, Shao H, et al. Long-term persistence of transmitted HIV drug resistance in male genital tract secretions: implications for secondary transmission. *J Infect Dis*. 2007;196(3):356-360. Available at http://www.ncbi.nlm.nih.gov/entrez/query.fcgi?cmd=Retrieve&db=PubMed&dopt=Citation&list_uids=17597449.

33. Novak RM, Chen L, MacArthur RD, et al. Prevalence of antiretroviral drug resistance mutations in chronically HIV-infected, treatment-naive patients: implications for routine resistance screening before initiation of antiretroviral therapy. *Clin Infect Dis*. 2005;40(3):468-474. Available at http://www.ncbi.nlm.nih.gov/entrez/query.fcgi?cmd=Retrieve&db=PubMed&dopt=Citation&list_uids=15668873.

34. Little SJ, Frost SD, Wong JK, et al. Persistence of transmitted drug resistance among subjects with primary human immunodeficiency virus infection. *J Virol*. 2008;82(11):5510-5518. Available at http://www.ncbi.nlm.nih.gov/entrez/query.fcgi?cmd=Retrieve&db=PubMed&dopt=Citation&list_uids=18353964.

35. Saag MS, Cahn P, Raffi F, et al. Efficacy and safety of emtricitabine vs stavudine in combination therapy in antiretroviral-naive patients: a randomized trial. *JAMA*. 2004;292(2):180-189. Available at http://www.ncbi.nlm.nih.gov/entrez/query.fcgi?cmd=Retrieve&db=PubMed&dopt=Citation&list_uids=15249567.

36. Jourdain G, Ngo-Giang-Huong N, Le Coeur S, et al. Intrapartum exposure to nevirapine and subsequent maternal responses to nevirapine-based antiretroviral therapy. *N Engl J Med*. 2004;351(3):229-240. Available at http://www.ncbi.nlm.nih.gov/entrez/query.fcgi?cmd=Retrieve&db=PubMed&dopt=Citation&list_uids=15247339.

37. Pillay D, Bhaskaran K, Jurriaans S, et al. The impact of transmitted drug resistance on the natural history of HIV infection and response to first-line therapy. *AIDS*. 2006;20(1):21-28. Available at http://www.ncbi.nlm.nih.gov/entrez/query.fcgi?cmd=Retrieve&db=PubMed&dopt=Citation&list_uids=16327315.

38. Sax PE, Islam R, Walensky RP, et al. Should resistance testing be performed for treatment-naive HIV-infected patients? A cost-effectiveness analysis. *Clin Infect Dis*. 2005;41(9):1316-1323. Available at http://www.ncbi.nlm.nih.gov/entrez/query.fcgi?cmd=Retrieve&db=PubMed&dopt=Citation&list_uids=16206108.

39. Cingolani A, Antinori A, Rizzo MG, et al. Usefulness of monitoring HIV drug resistance and adherence in individuals failing highly active antiretroviral therapy: a randomized study (ARGENTA). *AIDS*. 2002;16(3):369-379. Available at http://www.ncbi.nlm.nih.gov/entrez/query.fcgi?cmd=Retrieve&db=PubMed&dopt=Citation&list_uids=11834948.

40. Durant J, Clevenbergh P, Halfon P, et al. Drug-resistance genotyping in HIV-1 therapy: the VIRADAPT randomised controlled trial. *Lancet*. 1999;353(9171):2195-2199. Available at http://www.ncbi.nlm.nih.gov/entrez/query.fcgi?cmd=Retrieve&db=PubMed&dopt=Citation&list_uids=10392984.

41. Baxter JD, Mayers DL, Wentworth DN, et all; for the CPCRA 046 Study Team for the Terry Beirn Community Programs for Clinical Research on AIDS. A randomized study of antiretroviral management based on plasma genotypic antiretroviral resistance testing in patients failing therapy. *AIDS*. 2000;14(9):F83-93. Available at http://www.ncbi.nlm.nih.gov/entrez/query.fcgi?cmd=Retrieve&db=PubMed&list_uids=10894268&dopt=Abstract.

42. Cohen CJ, Hunt S, Sension M, et al. A randomized trial assessing the impact of phenotypic resistance testing on antiretroviral therapy. *AIDS*. 2002;16(4):579-588. Available at http://www.ncbi.nlm.nih.gov/entrez/query.fcgi?cmd=Retrieve&db=PubMed&dopt=Citation&list_uids=11873001.

43. Meynard JL, Vray M, Morand-Joubert L, et al. Phenotypic or genotypic resistance testing for choosing antiretroviral therapy after treatment failure: a randomized trial. *AIDS*. 2002;16(5):727-736. Available at http://www.ncbi.nlm.nih.gov/entrez/query.fcgi?cmd=Retrieve&db=PubMed&dopt=Citation&list_uids=11964529.

44. Vray M, Meynard JL, Dalban C, et al. Predictors of the virological response to a change in the antiretroviral treatment regimen in HIV-1-infected patients enrolled in a randomized trial comparing genotyping, phenotyping and standard of care (Narval trial, ANRS 088). *Antivir Ther*. 2003;8(5):427-434. Available at http://www.ncbi.nlm.nih.gov/entrez/query.fcgi?cmd=Retrieve&db=PubMed&dopt=Citation&list_uids=14640390.

45. Wegner SA, Wallace MR, Aronson NE, et al. Long-term efficacy of routine access to antiretroviral-resistance testing in HIV type 1-infected patients: results of the clinical efficacy of resistance testing trial. *Clin Infect Dis*. 2004;38(5):723-730. Available at http://www.ncbi.nlm.nih.gov/entrez/query.fcgi?cmd=Retrieve&db=PubMed&dopt=Citation&list_uids=14986258.

46. Palella FJ, Jr., Armon C, Buchacz K, et al. The association of HIV susceptibility testing with survival among HIV-infected patients receiving antiretroviral therapy: a cohort study. *Ann Intern Med*. 2009;151(2):73-84. Available at http://www.ncbi.nlm.nih.gov/entrez/query.fcgi?cmd=Retrieve&db=PubMed&dopt=Citation&list_uids=19620160.

47. Havlir DV, Hellmann NS, Petropoulos CJ, et al. Drug susceptibility in HIV infection after viral rebound in patients receiving indinavir-containing regimens. *JAMA*. 2000;283(2):229-234. Available at

http://www.ncbi.nlm.nih.gov/entrez/query.fcgi?cmd=Retrieve&db=PubMed&dopt=Citation&list_uids=10634339.

48. Descamps D, Flandre P, Calvez V, et al. Mechanisms of virologic failure in previously untreated HIV-infected patients from a trial of induction-maintenance therapy. Trilege (Agence Nationale de Recherches sur le SIDA 072) Study Team). *JAMA*. 2000;283(2):205-211. Available at
http://www.ncbi.nlm.nih.gov/entrez/query.fcgi?cmd=Retrieve&db=PubMed&dopt=Citation&list_uids=10634336.

49. Machouf N, Thomas R, Nguyen VK, et al. Effects of drug resistance on viral load in patients failing antiretroviral therapy. *J Med Virol*. 2006;78(5):608-613. Available at
http://www.ncbi.nlm.nih.gov/entrez/query.fcgi?cmd=Retrieve&db=PubMed&dopt=Citation&list_uids=16555280.

50. Anderson JA, Jiang H, Ding X, et al. Genotypic susceptibility scores and HIV type 1 RNA responses in treatment-experienced subjects with HIV type 1 infection. *AIDS Res Hum Retroviruses*. 2008;24(5):685-694. Available at
http://www.ncbi.nlm.nih.gov/pubmed/18462083.

51. Lewis M MJ, Simpson P, et al. Changes in V3 loop sequence associated with failure of maraviroc treatment in patients enrolled in the MOTIVATE 1 and 2 trials. Paper presented at: 15th Conference on Retroviruses and Opportunistic Infections. 2008; Boston, MA.

Co-Receptor Tropism Assays (Last updated February 12, 2013; last reviewed February 12, 2013)

Panel's Recommendations

- A co-receptor tropism assay should be performed whenever the use of a CCR5 co-receptor antagonist is being considered **(AI)**.
- Co-receptor tropism testing is also recommended for patients who exhibit virologic failure on a CCR5 antagonist **(BIII)**.
- A phenotypic tropism assay is preferred to determine HIV-1 co-receptor usage **(AI)**.
- A genotypic tropism assay should be considered as an alternative test to predict HIV-1 co-receptor usage **(BII)**.

Rating of Recommendations: A = Strong; B = Moderate; C = Optional

Rating of Evidence: I = Data from randomized controlled trials; II = Data from well-designed nonrandomized trials or observational cohort studies with long-term clinical outcomes; III = Expert opinion

---

HIV enters cells by a complex process that involves sequential attachment to the CD4 receptor followed by binding to either the CCR5 or CXCR4 molecules and fusion of the viral and cellular membranes.[1] CCR5 co-receptor antagonists prevent HIV entry into target cells by binding to the CCR5 receptors.[2] Phenotypic and, to a lesser degree, genotypic assays have been developed that can determine or predict the co-receptor tropism (i.e., CCR5, CXCR4, or both) of the patient's dominant virus population. An older generation assay (*Trofile*, Monogram Biosciences, Inc., South San Francisco, CA) was used to screen patients who were participating in clinical trials that led to the approval of maraviroc (MVC), the only CCR5 antagonist currently available. The assay has been improved and is now available with enhanced sensitivity. In addition, a genotypic assay to predict co-receptor usage is now commercially available.

During acute/recent infection, the vast majority of patients harbor a CCR5-utilizing virus (R5 virus), which suggests that the R5 variant is preferentially transmitted. Viruses in many untreated patients eventually exhibit a shift in co-receptor tropism from CCR5 usage to either CXCR4 or both CCR5 and CXCR4 tropism (i.e., dual- or mixed-tropic; D/M-tropic). This shift is temporally associated with a more rapid decline in CD4 T-cell counts,[3, 4] but whether this tropism shift is a cause or a consequence of progressive immunodeficiency remains undetermined.[1] Antiretroviral (ARV)-treated patients with extensive drug resistance are more likely to harbor X4- or D/M-tropic variants than untreated patients with comparable CD4 counts.[5] The prevalence of X4- or D/M-tropic variants increases to more than 50% in treated patients who have CD4 counts <100 cells/mm^3.[5, 6]

Phenotypic Assays

Phenotypic assays characterize the co-receptor usage of plasma-derived virus. These assays involve the generation of laboratory viruses that express patient-derived envelope proteins (i.e., gp120 and gp41). These pseudoviruses, which are replication-defective, are used to infect target cell lines that express either CCR5 or CXCR4.[7, 8] Using the *Trofile* assay, the co-receptor tropism of the patient-derived virus is confirmed by testing the susceptibility of the virus to specific CCR5 or CXCR4 inhibitors *in vitro*. This assay takes about 2 weeks to perform and requires a plasma HIV RNA level ≥1,000 copies/mL.

The performance characteristics of these assays have evolved. Most, if not all, patients enrolled in pre-marketing clinical trials of MVC and other CCR5 antagonists were screened with an earlier, less sensitive version of the *Trofile* assay.[8] This earlier assay failed to routinely detect low levels of CXCR4-utilizing variants. As a consequence, some patients enrolled in these clinical trials harbored low levels of CXCR4-utilizing virus at baseline that were below the assay limit of detection and exhibited rapid virologic failure after initiation of a CCR5 antagonist.[9] The assay has been revised and is now able to detect lower levels of CXCR4-utlizing viruses. *In vitro*, the assay can detect CXCR4-utilizing clones with 100% sensitivity when those clones represent 0.3% or more of the virus population.[10] Although this more sensitive assay has had limited use in prospective clinical trials, it is now the only one that is commercially available. For unclear reasons, a minority of samples cannot be successfully phenotyped with either generation of the *Trofile* assay.

In patients with plasma HIV-1 RNA below the limit of detection, co-receptor usage can be determined from proviral DNA obtained from peripheral blood mononuclear cells; however, the clinical utility of this assay remains to be determined.[11]

Genotypic Assays

Genotypic determination of HIV-1 co-receptor usage is based on sequencing of the V3-coding region of HIV-1 *env*, the principal determinant of co-receptor usage. A variety of algorithms and bioinformatics programs can be used to predict co-receptor usage from the V3 sequence. When compared to the phenotypic assay, genotypic methods show high specificity (~90%) but only modest sensitivity (~50% 70%) for the presence of a CXCR4-utilizing virus. Given these performance characteristics, these assays may not be sufficiently robust to completely rule out the presence of an X4 or D/M variant.[12]

Studies in which V3 genotyping was performed on samples from patients screened for clinical trials of MVC suggest that genotyping performed as well as phenotyping in predicting the response to MVC.[13-15] On the basis of these data, accessibility, and cost, European guidelines currently favor genotypic testing to determine co-receptor usage.[16] An important caveat to these results is that the majority of patients who received MVC were first shown to have R5 virus by a phenotypic assay (*Trofile*). Consequently, the opportunity to assess treatment response to MVC in patients whose virus was considered R5 by genotype but D/M or X4 by phenotype was limited to a relatively small number of patients.

Use of Assays to Determine Co-Receptor Usage in Clinical Practice

An assay for HIV-1 co-receptor usage should be performed whenever the use of a CCR5 antagonist is being considered **(AI)**. In addition, because virologic failure may occur due to a shift from CCR5-using to CXCR4-using virus, testing for co-receptor usage is recommended in patients who exhibit virologic failure on a CCR5 antagonist **(BIII)**. Virologic failure also may be caused by resistance of a CCR5-using virus to a CCR5 antagonist, but such resistance is uncommon. Compared to genotypic testing, phenotypic testing has more evidence supporting its usefulness. Therefore, a phenotypic test for co-receptor usage is generally preferred **(AI)**. However, because phenotypic testing is more expensive and requires more time to perform, a genotypic test to predict HIV-1 co-receptor usage should be considered as an alternative test **(BII)**.

A tropism assay may potentially be used in clinical practice for prognostic purposes or to assess tropism before starting ART if future use of a CCR5 antagonist is anticipated (e.g., a regimen change for toxicity). Currently, sufficient data do not exist to support these uses.

References

1. Moore JP, Kitchen SG, Pugach P, Zack JA. The CCR5 and CXCR4 coreceptors—central to understanding the transmission and pathogenesis of human immunodeficiency virus type 1 infection. *AIDS Res Hum Retroviruses*. 2004;20(1):111-126. Available at http://www.ncbi.nlm.nih.gov/entrez/query.fcgi?cmd=Retrieve&db=PubMed&dopt=Citation&list_uids=15000703.

2. Fatkenheuer G, Pozniak AL, Johnson MA, et al. Efficacy of short-term monotherapy with maraviroc, a new CCR5 antagonist, in patients infected with HIV-1. *Nat Med*. 2005;11(11):1170-1172. Available at http://www.ncbi.nlm.nih.gov/entrez/query.fcgi?cmd=Retrieve&db=PubMed&dopt=Citation&list_uids=16205738.

3. Connor RI, Sheridan KE, Ceradini D, Choe S, Landau NR. Change in coreceptor use correlates with disease progression in HIV-1-infected individuals. *J Exp Med*. 1997;185(4):621-628. Available at http://www.ncbi.nlm.nih.gov/entrez/query.fcgi?cmd=Retrieve&db=PubMed&dopt=Citation&list_uids=9034141.

4. Koot M, Keet IP, Vos AH, et al. Prognostic value of HIV-1 syncytium-inducing phenotype for rate of CD4+ cell depletion and progression to AIDS. *Ann Intern Med.* 1993;118(9):681-688. Available at http://www.ncbi.nlm.nih.gov/entrez/query.fcgi?cmd=Retrieve&db=PubMed&dopt=Citation&list_uids=8096374.

5. Hunt PW, Harrigan PR, Huang W, et al. Prevalence of CXCR4 tropism among antiretroviral-treated HIV-1-infected patients with detectable viremia. *J Infect Dis.* 2006;194(7):926-930. Available at http://www.ncbi.nlm.nih.gov/entrez/query.fcgi?cmd=Retrieve&db=PubMed&dopt=Citation&list_uids=16960780.

6. Wilkin TJ, Su Z, Kuritzkes DR, et al. HIV type 1 chemokine coreceptor use among antiretroviral-experienced patients screened for a clinical trial of a CCR5 inhibitor: AIDS Clinical Trial Group A5211. *Clin Infect Dis.* 2007;44(4):591-595. Available at http://www.ncbi.nlm.nih.gov/entrez/query.fcgi?cmd=Retrieve&db=PubMed&dopt=Citation&list_uids=17243065.

7. Trouplin V, Salvatori F, Cappello F, et al. Determination of coreceptor usage of human immunodeficiency virus type 1 from patient plasma samples by using a recombinant phenotypic assay. *J Virol.* 2001;75(1):251-259. Available at http://www.ncbi.nlm.nih.gov/entrez/query.fcgi?cmd=Retrieve&db=PubMed&dopt=Citation&list_uids=11119595.

8. Whitcomb JM, Huang W, Fransen S, et al. Development and characterization of a novel single-cycle recombinant-virus assay to determine human immunodeficiency virus type 1 coreceptor tropism. *Antimicrob Agents Chemother.* 2007;51(2):566-575. Available at http://www.ncbi.nlm.nih.gov/entrez/query.fcgi?cmd=Retrieve&db=PubMed&dopt=Citation&list_uids=17116663.

9. Westby M, Lewis M, Whitcomb J, et al. Emergence of CXCR4-using human immunodeficiency virus type 1 (HIV-1) variants in a minority of HIV-1-infected patients following treatment with the CCR5 antagonist maraviroc is from a pretreatment CXCR4-using virus reservoir. *J Virol.* 2006;80(10):4909-4920. Available at http://www.ncbi.nlm.nih.gov/entrez/query.fcgi?cmd=Retrieve&db=PubMed&dopt=Citation&list_uids=16641282.

10. Trinh L, Han D, Huang W, et al. Technical validation of an enhanced sensitivity Trofile HIV coreceptor tropism assay for selecting patients for therapy with entry inhibitors targeting CCR5. *Antivir Ther.* 2008;13(Suppl 3):A128

11. Toma J, Frantzell A, Cook J, et al. Phenotypic determination of HIV-1 coreceptor tropism using cell-associated DNA derived from blood samples. Paper presented at: 17th Conference on Retroviruses and Opportunistic Infections; 2010; San Francisco, CA.

12. Lin NH, Kuritzkes DR. Tropism testing in the clinical management of HIV-1 infection. *Curr Opin HIV AIDS.* 2009;4(6):481-487. Available at http://www.ncbi.nlm.nih.gov/entrez/query.fcgi?cmd=Retrieve&db=PubMed&dopt=Citation&list_uids=20048714.

13. McGovern RA, Thielen A, Mo T, et al. Population-based V3 genotypic tropism assay: a retrospective analysis using screening samples from the A4001029 and MOTIVATE studies. *AIDS.* 2010;24(16):2517-2525. Available at http://www.ncbi.nlm.nih.gov/entrez/query.fcgi?cmd=Retrieve&db=PubMed&dopt=Citation&list_uids=20736814.

14. McGovern RA, Thielen A, Portsmouth S, et al. Population-based sequencing of the V3-loop can predict the virological response to maraviroc in treatment-naive patients of the MERIT trial. *J Acquir Immune Defic Syndr.* 2012;61(3):279-286. Available at http://www.ncbi.nlm.nih.gov/pubmed/23095934.

15. Archer J, Weber J, Henry K, et al. Use of four next-generationsequencing platforms to determine HIV-1 coreceptor tropism. *PLoS One.* 2012;7(11):e49602. Available at http://www.ncbi.nlm.nih.gov/pubmed/23166726.

16. Vandekerckhove LP, Wensing AM, Kaiser R, et al. European guidelines on the clinical management of HIV-1 tropism testing. *Lancet Infect Dis.* 2011;11(5):394-407. Available at http://www.ncbi.nlm.nih.gov/pubmed/21429803.

HLA-B*5701 Screening (Last updated December 1, 2007; last reviewed January 10, 2011)

Panel's Recommendations
• The Panel recommends screening for HLA-B*5701 before starting patients on an abacavir (ABC)-containing regimen to reduce the risk of hypersensitivity reaction (HSR) **(AI)**.
• HLA-B*5701-positive patients should not be prescribed ABC **(AI)**.
• The positive status should be recorded as an ABC allergy in the patient's medical record **(AII)**.
• When HLA-B*5701 screening is not readily available, it remains reasonable to initiate ABC with appropriate clinical counseling and monitoring for any signs of HSR **(CIII)**.

Rating of Recommendations: A = Strong; B = Moderate; C = Optional

Rating of Evidence: I = Data from randomized controlled trials; II = Data from well-designed nonrandomized trials or observational cohort studies with long-term clinical outcomes; III = Expert opinion

The ABC HSR is a multiorgan clinical syndrome typically seen within the initial 6 weeks of ABC treatment. This reaction has been reported in 5% 8% of patients participating in clinical trials when using clinical criteria for the diagnosis, and it is the major reason for early discontinuation of ABC. Discontinuing ABC usually promptly reverses HSR, whereas subsequent rechallenge can cause a rapid, severe, and even life-threatening recurrence.[1]

Studies that evaluated demographic risk factors for ABC HSR have shown racial background as a risk factor, with white patients generally having a higher risk (5% 8%) than black patients (2% 3%). Several groups reported a highly significant association between ABC HSR and the presence of the major histocompatibility complex (MHC) class I allele HLA-B*5701.[2-3] Because the clinical criteria used for ABC HSR are overly sensitive and may lead to false-positive ABC HSR diagnoses, an ABC skin patch test (SPT) was developed as a research tool to immunologically confirm ABC HSR.[4] A positive ABC SPT is an ABC-specific delayed HSR that results in redness and swelling at the skin site of application. All ABC SPT positive patients studied were also positive for the HLA-B*5701 allele.[5] The ABC SPT could be falsely negative for some patients with ABC HSR and, at this point, is not recommended for use as a clinical tool. The PREDICT-1 study randomized patients before starting ABC either to be prospectively screened for HLA-B*5701 (with HLA-B*5701 positive patients not offered ABC) or to standard of care at the time of the study (i.e., no HLA screening, with all patients receiving ABC).[6] The overall HLA-B*5701 prevalence in this predominately white population was 5.6%. In this cohort, screening for HLA-B*5701 eliminated immunologic ABC HSR (defined as ABC SPT positive) compared with standard of care (0% vs. 2.7%), yielding a 100% negative predictive value with respect to SPT and significantly decreasing the rate of clinically suspected ABC HSR (3.4% vs. 7.8%). The SHAPE study corroborated the low rate of immunologically validated ABC HSR in black patients and confirmed the utility of HLA-B*5701 screening for the risk of ABC HSR (100% sensitivity in black and white populations).[7]

On the basis of the results of these studies, the Panel recommends screening for HLA-B*5701 before starting patients on an ABC-containing regimen **(AI)**. HLA-B*5701 positive patients should not be prescribed ABC **(AI)**, and the positive status should be recorded as an ABC allergy in the patient's medical record **(AII)**. HLA-B*5701 testing is needed only once in a patient's lifetime; thus, efforts to carefully record and maintain the test result and to educate the patient about its implications are important. The specificity of the HLA-B*5701 test in predicting ABC HSR is lower than the sensitivity (i.e., 33% 50% of HLA-B*5701 positive patients would likely not develop confirmed ABC HSR if exposed to ABC). HLA-B*5701 should not be used as a substitute for clinical judgment or pharmacovigilance, because a negative HLA-B*5701 result does not absolutely rule out the possibility of some form of ABC HSR. When HLA-B*5701 screening is not readily available, it remains reasonable to initiate ABC with appropriate clinical counseling and monitoring for any signs of ABC HSR **(CIII)**.

References

1. Hetherington S, McGuirk S, Powell G, et al. Hypersensitivity reactions during therapy with the nucleoside reverse transcriptase inhibitor abacavir. *Clin Ther.* 2001;23(10):1603-1614.

2. Mallal S, Nolan D, Witt C, et al. Association between presence of HLA-B*5701, HLA-DR7, and HLA-DQ3 and hypersensitivity to HIV-1 reverse-transcriptase inhibitor abacavir. *Lancet.* 2002;359(9308):727-732.

3. Hetherington S, Hughes AR, Mosteller M, et al. Genetic variations in HLA-B region and hypersensitivity reactions to abacavir. *Lancet.* 2002;359(9312):1121-1122.

4. Phillips EJ, Sullivan JR, Knowles SR, et al. Utility of patch testing in patients with hypersensitivity syndromes associated with abacavir. *AIDS.* 2002;16(16):2223-2225.

5. Phillips E, Rauch A, Nolan D, et al. Pharmacogenetics and clinical characteristics of patch test confirmed patients with abacavir hypersensitivity. *Rev Antivir Ther.* 2006:3: Abstract 57.

6. Mallal S, Phillips E, Carosi G, et al. HLA-B*5701 screening for hypersensitivity to abacavir. *N Engl J Med.* 2008;358(6):568-579.

7. Saag M, Balu R, Phillips E, et al. High sensitivity of human leukocyte antigen-b*5701 as a marker for immunologically confirmed abacavir hypersensitivity in white and black patients. *Clin Infect Dis.* 2008;46(7):1111-1118.

Treatment Goals (Last updated March 27, 2012; last reviewed March 27, 2012)

Eradication of HIV infection cannot be achieved with available antiretroviral (ARV) regimens even when new, potent drugs are added to a regimen that is already suppressing plasma viral load below the limits of detection of commercially available assays.[1] This is chiefly because the pool of latently infected CD4 T cells is established during the earliest stages of acute HIV infection[2] and persists with a long half-life, despite prolonged suppression of plasma viremia.[3-7] Therefore the primary goals for initiating antiretroviral therapy (ART) are to:

- reduce HIV-associated morbidity and prolong the duration and quality of survival,
- restore and preserve immunologic function,
- maximally and durably suppress plasma HIV viral load (see Plasma HIV RNA Testing), and
- prevent HIV transmission.

ART has reduced HIV-related morbidity and mortality[8-11] and has reduced perinatal[12] and behavior-associated transmission of HIV.[13-17] HIV suppression with ART may also decrease inflammation and immune activation thought to contribute to higher rates of cardiovascular and other end-organ damage reported in HIV-infected cohorts. (See Initiating Antiretroviral Therapy.) Maximal and durable suppression of plasma viremia delays or prevents the selection of drug-resistance mutations, preserves CD4 T-cell numbers, and confers substantial clinical benefits, all of which are important treatment goals.[18-19]

Achieving viral suppression requires the use of ARV regimens with at least two, and preferably three, active drugs from two or more drug classes. Baseline resistance testing and patient characteristics should guide design of the specific regimen. (See What to Start: Initial Combination Regimens for the Antiretroviral-Naive Patient.) When initial suppression is not achieved or is lost, rapidly changing to a new regimen with at least two active drugs is required. (See Virologic and Immunologic Failure.) The increasing number of drugs and drug classes makes viral suppression below detection limits an appropriate goal in all patients.

Viral load reduction to below limits of assay detection in an ART-naive patient usually occurs within the first 12 24 weeks of therapy. Predictors of virologic success include:

- high potency of ARV regimen,
- excellent adherence to treatment regimen,[20]
- low baseline viremia,[21]
- higher baseline CD4 count (>200 cells/mm^3),[22] and
- rapid reduction of viremia in response to treatment.[21,23]

Successful outcomes are usually observed, although adherence difficulties may lower the success rate in clinical practice to below the 90% rate commonly seen in clinical trials.[24]

Strategies to Achieve Treatment Goals

Achieving treatment goals requires a balance of sometimes competing considerations, outlined below. Providers and patients must work together to define individualized strategies to achieve treatment goals.

Selection of Initial Combination Regimen

Several preferred and alternative ARV regimens are recommended for use. (See What to Start.) Many of these regimens have comparable efficacy but vary to some degree in dosing frequency and symmetry, pill burden, drug interactions, and potential side effects. Regimens should be tailored for the individual patient to enhance adherence and thus improve long-term treatment success. Individual regimen choice is based on such considerations as expected side effects, convenience, comorbidities, interactions with concomitant medications, and results of pretreatment genotypic drug-resistance testing.

Pretreatment Drug-Resistance Testing

Current studies suggest a 6% 16% prevalence of HIV drug resistance in ART-naive patients,[25-29] and some studies suggest that the presence of transmitted drug-resistant viruses may lead to suboptimal virologic responses.[30] Therefore, pretreatment genotypic resistance testing should be used to guide selection of the most optimal initial ARV regimen. (See Drug-Resistance Testing.)

Improving Adherence

Suboptimal adherence may result in reduced treatment response. Incomplete adherence can result from complex medication regimens; patient factors, such as active substance abuse and depression; and health system issues, including interruptions in patient access to medication and inadequate treatment education and support. Conditions that promote adherence should be maximized before and after initiation of ART. (See Adherence to Antiretroviral Therapy.)

References

1. Dinoso JB, Kim SY, Wiegand AM, et al. Treatment intensification does not reduce residual HIV-1 viremia in patients on highly active antiretroviral therapy. *Proc Natl Acad Sci U S A*. Jun 9 2009;106(23):9403-9408.

2. Chun TW, Engel D, Berrey MM, Shea T, Corey L, Fauci AS. Early establishment of a pool of latently infected, resting CD4(+) T cells during primary HIV-1 infection. *Proc Natl Acad Sci U S A*. Jul 21 1998;95(15):8869-8873.

3. Chun TW, Stuyver L, Mizell SB, et al. Presence of an inducible HIV-1 latent reservoir during highly active antiretroviral therapy. *Proc Natl Acad Sci U S A*. Nov 25 1997;94(24):13193-13197.

4. Finzi D, Hermankova M, Pierson T, et al. Identification of a reservoir for HIV-1 in patients on highly active antiretroviral therapy. *Science*. Nov 14 1997;278(5341):1295-1300.

5. Finzi D, Blankson J, Siliciano JD, et al. Latent infection of CD4+ T cells provides a mechanism for lifelong persistence of HIV-1, even in patients on effective combination therapy. *Nat Med*. May 1999;5(5):512-517.

6. Wong JK, Hezareh M, Gunthard HF, et al. Recovery of replication-competent HIV despite prolonged suppression of plasma viremia. *Science*. Nov 14 1997;278(5341):1291-1295.

7. Siliciano JD, Kajdas J, Finzi D, et al. Long-term follow-up studies confirm the stability of the latent reservoir for HIV-1 in resting CD4+ T cells. *Nat Med*. Jun 2003;9(6):727-728.

8. Mocroft A, Vella S, Benfield TL, et al. Changing patterns of mortality across Europe in patients infected with HIV-1. EuroSIDA Study Group. *Lancet*. Nov 28 1998;352(9142):1725-1730.

9. Palella FJ, Jr., Delaney KM, Moorman AC, et al. Declining morbidity and mortality among patients with advanced human immunodeficiency virus infection. HIV Outpatient Study Investigators. *N Engl J Med*. Mar 26 1998;338(13):853-860.

10. Vittinghoff E, Scheer S, O'Malley P, Colfax G, Holmberg SD, Buchbinder SP. Combination antiretroviral therapy and recent declines in AIDS incidence and mortality. *J Infect Dis*. Mar 1999;179(3):717-720.

11. ART CC AC. Life expectancy of individuals on combination antiretroviral therapy in high-income countries: a collaborative analysis of 14 cohort studies. *Lancet*. Jul 26 2008;372(9635):293-299.

12. Mofenson LM, Lambert JS, Stiehm ER, et al. Risk factors for perinatal transmission of human immunodeficiency virus type 1 in women treated with zidovudine. Pediatric AIDS Clinical Trials Group Study 185 Team. *N Engl J Med*. Aug 5 1999;341(6):385-393.

13. Wood E, Kerr T, Marshall BD, et al. Longitudinal community plasma HIV-1 RNA concentrations and incidence of HIV-1 among injecting drug users: prospective cohort study. *BMJ*. 2009;338:b1649.

14. Quinn TC, Wawer MJ, Sewankambo N, et al. Viral load and heterosexual transmission of human immunodeficiency virus type 1. Rakai Project Study Group. *N Engl J Med*. Mar 30 2000;342(13):921-929.

15. Dieffenbach CW, Fauci AS. Universal voluntary testing and treatment for prevention of HIV transmission. *JAMA*. Jun 10 2009;301(22):2380-2382.

16. Montaner JS, Hogg R, Wood E, et al. The case for expanding access to highly active antiretroviral therapy to curb the growth of the HIV epidemic. *Lancet*. Aug 5 2006;368(9534):531-536.

17. Cohen MS, Chen YQ, McCauley M, et al. Prevention of HIV-1 infection with early antiretroviral therapy. *N Engl J Med*. Aug 11 2011;365(6):493-505.

18. O'Brien WA, Hartigan PM, Martin D, et al. Changes in plasma HIV-1 RNA and CD4+ lymphocyte counts and the risk of progression to AIDS. Veterans Affairs Cooperative Study Group on AIDS. *N Engl J Med*. Feb 15 1996;334(7):426-431.

19. Garcia F, de Lazzari E, Plana M, et al. Long-term CD4+ T-cell response to highly active antiretroviral therapy according to baseline CD4+ T-cell count. *J Acquir Immune Defic Syndr*. Jun 1 2004;36(2):702-713.

20. Paterson DL, Swindells S, Mohr J, et al. Adherence to protease inhibitor therapy and outcomes in patients with HIV infection. *Ann Intern Med*. Jul 4 2000;133(1):21-30.

21. Powderly WG, Saag MS, Chapman S, Yu G, Quart B, Clendeninn NJ. Predictors of optimal virological response to potent antiretroviral therapy. *AIDS*. Oct 1 1999;13(14):1873-1880.

22. Yamashita TE, Phair JP, Munoz A, et al. Immunologic and virologic response to highly active antiretroviral therapy in the Multicenter AIDS Cohort Study. *AIDS*. Apr 13 2001;15(6):735-746.

23. Townsend D, Troya J, Maida I, et al. First HAART in HIV-infected patients with high viral load: value of HIV RNA levels at 12 weeks to predict virologic outcome. *J Int Assoc Physicians AIDS Care* (Chic Ill). Sep-Oct 2009;8(5):314-317.

24. Moore RD, Keruly JC, Gebo KA, Lucas GM. An improvement in virologic response to highly active antiretroviral therapy in clinical practice from 1996 through 2002. *J Acquir Immune Defic Syndr*. Jun 1 2005;39(2):195-198.

25. Weinstock HS, Zaidi I, Heneine W, et al. The epidemiology of antiretroviral drug resistance among drug-naive HIV-1-infected persons in 10 US cities. *J Infect Dis*. Jun 15 2004;189(12):2174-2180.

26. Bennett D, McCormick L, Kline R, et al. US surveillance of HIV drug resistance at diagnosis using HIV diagnostic sera. Paper presented at: 12th Conference on Retroviruses and Opportunistic Infections (CROI); February 22-25, 2005; Boston, MA.

27. Wheeler W, Mahle K, Bodnar U, et al. Antiretroviral drug-resistance mutations and subtypes in drug-naive persons newly diagnosed with HIV-1 infection, US, March 2003 to October 2006. Paper presented at: 14th Conference on Retroviruses and Opportunistic Infections (CROI); February 25-28, 2007; Los Angeles, CA.

28. Ross L, Lim ML, Liao Q, et al. Prevalence of antiretroviral drug resistance and resistance-associated mutations in antiretroviral therapy-naive HIV-infected individuals from 40 United States cities. *HIV Clin Trials*. Jan-Feb 2007;8(1):1-8.

29. Vercauteren J, Wensing AM, van de Vijver DA, et al. Transmission of drug-resistant HIV-1 is stabilizing in Europe. *J Infect Dis*. Nov 15 2009;200(10):1503-1508.

30. Borroto-Esoda K, Waters JM, Bae AS, et al. Baseline genotype as a predictor of virological failure to emtricitabine or stavudine in combination with didanosine and efavirenz. *AIDS Res Hum Retroviruses*. Aug 2007;23(8):988-995.

Initiating Antiretroviral Therapy in Treatment-Naive Patients (Last updated February 12, 2013; last reviewed February 12, 2013)

Panel's Recommendations

• Antiretroviral therapy (ART) is recommended for all HIV-infected individuals to reduce the risk of disease progression.
 	
    The strength and evidence for this recommendation vary by pretreatment CD4 cell count: CD4 count <350 cells/mm³ **(AI)**; CD4 count 350–500 cells/mm³ **(AII)**; CD4 count >500 cells/mm³ **(BIII)**.
 	
• ART also is recommended for HIV-infected individuals for the prevention of transmission of HIV.
 	
    The strength and evidence for this recommendation vary by transmission risks: perinatal transmission **(AI)**; heterosexual transmission **(AI)**; other transmission risk groups **(AIII)**.
 	
• Patients starting ART should be willing and able to commit to treatment and understand the benefits and risks of therapy and the importance of adherence **(AIII)**. Patients may choose to postpone therapy, and providers, on a case-by-case basis, may elect to defer therapy on the basis of clinical and/or psychosocial factors.

Rating of Recommendations: A = Strong; B = Moderate; C = Optional *Rating of Evidence:* I = Data from randomized controlled trials; II = Data from well-designed nonrandomized trials or observational cohort studies with long-term clinical outcomes; III = Expert opinion

Introduction

Without treatment, the vast majority of HIV-infected individuals will eventually develop progressive immunosuppression (as evident by CD4 count depletion), leading to AIDS-defining illnesses and premature death. The primary goal of antiretroviral therapy (ART) is to prevent HIV-associated morbidity and mortality. This goal is best accomplished by using effective ART to maximally inhibit HIV replication so that plasma HIV RNA levels (viral load) remain below that detectable by commercially available assays. Durable viral suppression improves immune function and quality of life, lowers the risk of both AIDS-defining and non-AIDS-defining complications, and prolongs life.

Furthermore, high plasma HIV RNA is a major risk factor for HIV transmission and use of effective ART can reduce viremia and transmission of HIV to sexual partners.[1, 2] Modelling studies suggest that the expanded use of ART may result in lower incidence and, eventually, prevalence of HIV on a community or population level.[3] Thus, a secondary goal of ART is to reduce the risk of HIV transmission.

Historically, HIV-infected individuals have presented for care with low CD4 counts,[4] but increasingly there have been concerted efforts to both increase testing of at-risk patients and to link HIV-infected patients to medical care soon after HIV diagnosis (and before they have advanced HIV diseases). For those with high CD4 cell counts, whose short-term risk for death may be low,[5] the recommendation to initiate ART is based on growing evidence that untreated HIV infection or uncontrolled viremia is associated with development of non-AIDS-defining diseases, including cardiovascular disease (CVD), kidney disease, liver disease, neurologic complications, and malignancies. Furthermore, newer ART regimens are more effective, more convenient, and better tolerated than regimens used in the past.

Regardless of CD4 count, the decision to initiate ART should always include consideration of any co-morbid conditions, the willingness and readiness of the patient to initiate therapy, and the availability of resources. In settings where resources are not available to initiate ART in all patients, treatment should be prioritized for patients with the lowest CD4 counts and those with the following clinical conditions: pregnancy, CD4 count <200 cells/mm³, or history of an AIDS-defining illness, including HIV-associated dementia, HIV-associated nephropathy (HIVAN), hepatitis B virus (HBV), and acute HIV infection.

Tempering the enthusiasm to treat all patients regardless of CD4 count is the absence of randomized data that definitively demonstrate a clear clinical benefit of ART in patients with CD4 count >350 cells/mm³ and mixed results from observational cohort studies on the definitive benefits of early ART. For some patients, the potential risks of short- or long-term, drug-related complications and non-adherence to long-term therapy in asymptomatic patients may offset possible benefits of earlier initiation of therapy. An ongoing randomized controlled trial to evaluate the role of immediate versus delayed ART in patients with CD4 count >500 cells/mm³ will help to further define the role of ART in this patient population (ClinicalTrials.gov identifier NCT00867048).

The known and potential benefits and limitations of ART overall, and in different patient populations are discussed below.

Benefits of Antiretroviral Therapy

Reduction in Mortality and/or AIDS-Related Morbidity According to Pretreatment CD4 Cell Count

Patients with a history of an AIDS-defining illness or CD4 count <350 cells/mm³

HIV-infected patients with CD4 counts <200 cells/mm³ are at higher risk of opportunistic diseases, non-AIDS morbidity, and death than HIV-infected patients with higher CD4 counts. Randomized controlled trials in patients with CD4 counts <200 cells/mm³ and/or a history of an AIDS-defining condition provide strong evidence that ART improves survival and delays disease progression in these patients.[6-8] Long-term data from multiple observational cohort studies comparing earlier ART (i.e., initiated at CD4 count >200 cells/mm³) with later treatment (i.e., initiated at CD4 count <200 cells/mm³) also have provided strong support for these findings.[9-14]

Few large, randomized controlled trials address when to start therapy in patients with CD4 counts >200 cells/mm³. CIPRA HT-001, a randomized clinical trial conducted in Haiti, enrolled 816 participants without AIDS. Participants were randomized to start ART with CD4 counts of 200 cells/mm³ to 350 cells/mm³ or to defer treatment until their CD4 counts dropped to <200 cells/mm³ or they developed an AIDS-defining condition. An interim analysis of the study showed that, when compared with participants who began ART with CD4 counts of 200 cells/mm³ to 350 cells/mm³, patients who deferred therapy had a higher mortality rate (23 versus 6 deaths; hazard ratio [HR]   4.0; 95% confidence interval [CI]: 1.6 9.8) and a higher rate of incident tuberculosis (TB) (HR   2.0, 95% CI: 1.2 3.6).[15]

Collectively, these studies support the Panel's recommendation that ART should be initiated in patients with a history of an AIDS-defining illness or with a CD4 count <350 cells/mm³ **(AI)**.

Patients with CD4 counts between 350 and 500 cells/mm³

Data supporting initiation of ART in patients with CD4 counts ranging from 350 cells/mm³ to 500 cells/mm³ are derived from large observational studies and secondary analysis of randomized controlled trials. Analysis of the findings from the observational studies involved use of advanced statistical methods that minimize the bias and confounding that arise when observational data are used to address the question of when to start ART. However, unmeasured confounders for which adjustment was not possible may have influenced the analysis.

The ART Cohort Collaboration (ART-CC) included 45,691 patients from 18 cohort studies conducted primarily in North America and Europe. Data from ART-CC showed that the rate of progression to AIDS and/or death was higher when therapy was deferred until a patient's CD4 count fell to the 251 cells/mm³ to 350 cells/mm³ range than when ART was initiated at the 351 cells/mm³ to 450 cells/mm³ range (risk ratio: 1.28, 95% CI: 1.04 1.57).[11] When analysis of the data was restricted to mortality alone, the difference between the 2 strategies was weaker and not statistically significant (risk ratio: 1.13, 95% CI: 0.80 1.60).

In a collaboration of North American cohort studies (NA-ACCORD) that evaluated patients regardless of whether they had started therapy, the 6,278 patients who deferred therapy until their CD4 counts were <350 cells/mm³ had greater risk of death than the 2,084 patients who initiated therapy with CD4 counts between 351 cells/mm³ and 500 cells/mm³ (risk ratio: 1.69, 95% CI: 1.26 2.26) after adjustment for other factors that differed between these 2 groups.[16]

Another collaboration of cohort studies from Europe and the United States (the HIV-CAUSAL Collaboration) included 8,392 ART-naive patients with initial CD4 counts >500 cells/mm³ who experienced declines in CD4 count to <500 cells/mm³.[14] The study estimated that delaying initiation of ART until CD4 count <350 cells/mm³ was associated with a greater risk of AIDS-defining illness or death than initating ART with CD4 count between 350 cells/mm³ and 500 cells/mm³ (HR: 1.38, 95% CI: 1.23 1.56). There was, however, no evidence of a difference in mortality (HR: 1.01, 95% CI: 0.84 1.22).

A collaboration of cohort studies from Europe, Australia, and Canada (the CASCADE Collaboration) included 5,527 ART-naive patients with CD4 counts in the 350 to 499 cells/mm³ range. Compared with patients who deferred therapy until their CD4 counts fell to <350 cells/mm³, patients who started ART immediately had a marginally lower risk of AIDS-defining illness or death (HR: 0.75, 95% CI: 0.49 1.14) and a lower risk of death (HR: 0.51, 95% CI: 0.33 0.80).[17]

Randomized data showing clinical evidence favoring ART in patients with higher CD4 cell counts came from two studies. First, in a small subgroup analysis of the SMART trial, undertaken primarily in North and South America, Europe, and Australia, which randomized participants with CD4 counts >350 cells/mm³ to continuous ART or to treatment interruption until CD4 count dropped to <250 cells/mm³. In the subgroup of 249 participants who were ART naive at enrollment (median CD4 count: 437 cells/mm³), participants who deferred therapy until CD4 count dropped to <250 cells/mm³ had a greater risk of serious AIDS- and non-AIDS-related events than those who initiated therapy immediately (7 vs. 2 events, HR: 4.6, 95% CI: 1.0 22.2).[18]

Second, the HPTN 052 was a large multinational, multicontinental (Africa, Asia, South America, and North America) randomized trial that examined whether treatment of HIV-infected individuals reduces transmission to their uninfected sexual partners.[2] A secondary objective of the study was to determine whether ART reduces clinical events in the HIV-infected participants. This trial enrolled 1,763 HIV-infected participants with CD4 counts between 350 cells/mm³ and 550 cells/mm³ and their HIV-uninfected partners. The infected participants were randomized to initiate ART immediately or to delay initiation until they had 2 consecutive CD4 counts <250 cells/mm³. At a median follow-up of 2.1 years, there were 77 primary events in the delayed arm versus 57 in the immediate therapy arm (adjusted HR: 1.39, 95% CI: 0.98 1.96). The most frequent event was tuberculosis (34 cases in the delayed therapy arm versus 17 in the immediate therapy arm); deaths were relatively rare (15 cases in the delayed therapy arm; 11 in the immediate therapy arm).[19]

Collectively, these studies suggest that initiating ART in patients with CD4 counts between 350 cells/mm³ and 500 cells/mm³ reduces HIV-related disease progression; whether there is a corresponding reduction in mortality is unclear. This benefit supports the Panel's recommendation that ART should be initiated in patients with CD4 counts 350 cells/mm³ to 500 cells/mm³ **(AII)**. Recent evidence demonstrating the public health benefit of earlier intervention further supports the strength of this recommendation (see Prevention of Sexual Transmission).

Patients with CD4 counts >500 cells/mm³

The NA-ACCORD study also observed patients who started ART with CD4 counts >500 cells/mm³ or after their CD4 counts dropped below this threshold. The adjusted mortality rates were significantly higher in the 6,935 patients who deferred therapy until their CD4 counts fell to <500 cells/mm³ than in the 2,200 patients who started therapy with CD4 counts >500 cells/mm³ (risk ratio: 1.94, 95% CI: 1.37 2.79).[16] Although large and generally representative of the HIV-infected patients in care in the United States, the study has several limitations, including the small number of deaths and the potential for unmeasured confounders that might have influenced outcomes independent of ART.

In contrast, results from 2 cohort studies did not identify a benefit of earlier initiation of therapy in reducing AIDS progression or death. In an analysis of the ART-CC cohort,[11] the rate of progression to AIDS/death associated with deferral of therapy until CD4 count is in the 351 to 450 cells/mm³ range was similar to the rate with initiation of therapy with CD4 count in the 451 to 550 cells/mm³ range (HR: 0.99, 95% CI: 0.76 1.29). There was no significant difference in rate of death identified between the two groups (HR: 0.93, 95% CI: 0.60 1.44). This study also found that the proportion of patients with CD4 counts between 451 and 550 cells/mm³ who would progress to AIDS or death before having a CD4 count <450 cells/mm³ was low (1.6%; 95% CI: 1.1% 2.1%). In the CASCADE Collaboration,[17] among the 5,162 patients with CD4 counts in the 500 to 799 cells/mm³ range, compared with patients who deferred therapy, those who started ART immediately did not experience a significant reduction in the composite outcome of progression to AIDS/death (HR: 1.10, 95% CI: 0.67 1.79) or death (HR: 1.02, 95% CI: 0.49 2.12).

While it was not a clinical endpoint study, a recent clinical trial (Setpoint Study) randomized patients within 6 months of HIV seroconversion to receive either immediate ART for 36 weeks or deferred treatment. More than 57% of the study participants had CD4 count >500 cells/mm³. The deferred treatment group had a statistically higher risk of meeting ART eligibility criteria than the immediate treatment group. The study was halted early and illustrated that the time from diagnosis of early infection to the need for initiation of ART was shorter than anticipated in the deferred therapy group.[20]

The expanded use of ART to treat individuals with CD4 counts >500 cells/mm³ has also demonstrated public health benefits. In 2010, a large, publicly-funded clinic in San Francisco adapted a universal ART approach to initiate ART in all HIV-infected persons and evaluated temporal trends in viral suppression. In 534 patients entering the clinic with CD4 counts >500 cells/mm³, the 1-year incidence of viral suppression increased from 9% to 14% before universal ART to >52% after the approach was adopted. After adjustment, this policy was associated with a six-fold increase in the probability of viral suppression six months after clinic entry.[21] Because the risk of HIV transmission is associated with level of viremia, from a public health standpoint, this reduction in community viral load can potentially reduce new HIV infections at the community level.

With a better understanding of the pathogenesis of HIV infection, the growing awareness that untreated HIV infection increases the risk of many non-AIDS-defining diseases (as discussed below), and the benefit of ART in reducing transmission of HIV, the Panel recommends initiation of ART in patients with CD4 counts >500 cells/mm³ **(BIII)**.

When discussing initiation of ART at high CD4 cell counts (i.e., >500 cells/mm³), clinicians should inform patients that data on the clinical benefit of starting treatment at such levels are not conclusive, especially for patients with very high CD4 counts. Clinicians should also inform patients that viral suppression from effective ART can reduce the risk of sexual transmission to others. Patients should also be told that untreated HIV infection will eventually lead to immunological deterioration and increased risk of clinical disease and death. Therefore, if therapy is not initiated, continued monitoring and close follow-up is necessary.

Further ongoing research (both randomized clinical trials and cohort studies) to assess the short- and long-term clinical and public health benefits and cost effectiveness of starting therapy at higher CD4 counts is needed. Findings from such research will provide the Panel with guidance to make future recommendations.

Effects of Viral Replication on HIV-Related Morbidity

Since the mid-1990s, it has been known that measures of viral replication are predictive of HIV disease progression. In untreated HIV-infected individuals, time to clinical progression and mortality is fastest in those with higher viral loads.[22] This finding is confirmed across the wide spectrum of HIV-infected patient populations, including injection drug users (IDUs),[23] women,[24] and individuals with hemophilia.[25] Several studies have shown the prognostic value of pre-treatment viral load for predicting post-therapy response.[26, 27] Once therapy has been initiated, failure to achieve viral suppression[28-30] and viral load at the time of treatment failure[31] are predictive of clinical disease progression.

More recent studies have examined the impact of ongoing viral replication for both longer durations and at higher CD4 cell counts. Using viremia copy-years, a novel metric for quantifying viral load over time, the Centers for AIDS Research Network of Integrated Clinical Systems (CNICS) cohort found that cumulative exposure to replicating virus is independently associated with mortality. Using viremia copy-years, the HR for mortality was 1.81 per $\log_{10}$ copy-year/mL (95% CI: 1.51 2.18), which was the only viral load-related variable that retained statistical significance in the multivariable model (HR 1.44 per $\log_{10}$ copy-year/mL; 95% CI: 1.07 1.94). These findings support the concept that unchecked viral replication, which occurs in the absence of effective ART, is a factor in disease progression and death independent of CD4 count.[32]

The EuroSIDA collaboration evaluated HIV-infected individuals with CD4 counts >350 cells/ mm^3 segregated by three viral load strata (<500 copies/mL, 500 9,999 copies/mL, and ≥10,000 copies/mL) to determine the impact of viral load on fatal and non-fatal AIDS-related and non-AIDS-related events. The lower viral load stratum included more subjects on ART (92%) than the middle (62%) and high (31%) viral load strata. After adjustment for age, region, and ART, the rates of non-AIDS events were 61% (P 0.001) and 66% (P 0.004) higher in participants with viral loads 500 to 9,999 copies/mL and >10,000 copies/mL, respectively, than in individuals with viral loads <500 copies/mL. These data further confirm that unchecked viral replication is associated with adverse clinical outcomes in individuals with CD4 counts >350 cells/mm^3.[33]

Collectively, these data show that the harm of ongoing viral replication affects both untreated patients and those who are on ART but continue to be viremic. The harm of ongoing viral replication in patients on ART is compounded by the risk of emergence of drug-resistant virus. Therefore, all patients on ART should be carefully monitored and counseled on the importance of adherence to therapy.

Effects of ART on HIV-Related Morbidity

HIV-associated immune deficiency, the direct effects of HIV on end organs, and the indirect effects of HIV-associated inflammation on these organs all most likely contribute to HIV-related morbidity and mortality. In general, the available data demonstrate that

- Untreated HIV infection may have detrimental effects at all stages of infection,
- Earlier treatment may prevent the damage associated with HIV replication during early stages of infection,
- ART is beneficial even when initiated later in infection; however, later therapy may not repair damage associated with viral replication that occurred during early stages of infection, and
- Sustaining viral suppression and maintaining higher CD4 count, mostly as a result of effective combination ART, may delay, prevent, or reverse some non-AIDS-defining complications, such as HIV-associated kidney disease, liver disease, CVD, neurologic complications, and malignancies, as discussed below.

HIV-associated nephropathy (HIVAN)

HIVAN is the most common cause of chronic kidney disease in HIV-infected individuals that may lead to end-stage kidney disease.[34] HIVAN is almost exclusively seen in black patients and can occur at any CD4 count. Ongoing viral replication appears to be directly involved in renal injury,[35] and HIVAN is extremely uncommon in virologically suppressed patients.[36] ART in patients with HIVAN has been associated with both preserved renal function and prolonged survival.[37-39] Therefore, ART should be started in all patients with HIVAN, regardless of CD4 count, at the earliest sign of renal dysfunction **(AII)**.

Coinfection with hepatitis B virus (HBV) and/or hepatitis C virus (HCV)

HIV infection is associated with more rapid progression of viral hepatitis-related liver disease, including cirrhosis, end-stage liver disease, hepatocellular carcinoma, and fatal hepatic failure.[40-42] The pathogenesis of accelerated liver disease in HIV-infected patients has not been fully elucidated, but HIV-related immunodeficiency and a direct interaction between HIV and hepatic stellate and Kupffer cells have been implicated.[43-46] In individuals co-infected with hepatitis B virus (HBV) and/or hepatitis C virus (HCV), ART may attenuate liver disease progression by preserving or restoring immune function and reducing HIV-related immune activation and inflammation.[47-49] ARV drugs active against both HIV and HBV (such as tenofovir disoproxil fumarate [TDF], lamivudine [3TC], and emtricitabine [FTC]) also may prevent development of significant liver disease by directly suppressing HBV replication.[50, 51] Although ARV drugs do not inhibit HCV replication directly, HCV treatment outcomes typically improve when HIV replication is controlled or CD4 counts are increased.[52] In one prospective cohort, after controlling for liver and HIV disease stage, HCV co-infected patients receiving ART were approximately 66% less likely to experience end-stage liver disease, hepatocellular carcinoma, and fatal hepatic failure than patients not receiving ART.[53] While some studies have shown that chronic viral hepatitis increases the risk of ART-induced liver injury, the majority of coinfected persons do not develop clinically significant liver injury[54-56] and the rate of hepatotoxicity may be greater in persons with more advanced HIV disease. Collectively, these data suggest that earlier treatment of HIV infection in persons coinfected with HBV (and likely HCV) may reduce the risk of liver disease progression. ART is recommended for patients coinfected with HBV; the ART regimen should include drugs with activity against both HIV and HBV **(AII)** (also see Hepatitis B Virus/HIV Co-Infection). ART also is recommended for most patients coinfected with HCV **(BII)**, including those with high CD4 counts and those with cirrhosis. This recommendation is based on findings from retrospective and prospective cohort studies that indicated that the receipt of ART is associated with slower progression of hepatic fibrosis and reduced risk of liver disease outcomes.[53, 57-59] Combined treatment of both HIV and HCV can be complicated by large pill burden, drug interactions, and overlapping toxicities. Although ART should be considered for HIV/HCV-co-infected patients regardless of CD4 cell count, for patients infected with HCV genotype 1, some clinicians may choose to defer ART in HIV treatment-naive patients with CD4 counts >500 cells/mm^3 until HCV treatment that includes the HCV NS3/4A protease inhibitors (PIs) is completed (also see HIV/Hepatitis C Virus Co-Infection).

Cardiovascular disease (CVD)

In HIV-infected patients, CVD is a major cause of morbidity and mortality, accounting for one-third of serious non-AIDS conditions and at least 10% of deaths.[60-62] A number of studies have found that, over time, HIV-infected persons are at greater risk for CVD events than age-matched uninfected individuals. In a meta-analysis and review of studies of CVD risk in HIV-infected individuals, the relative risk of CVD events was greater in untreated HIV-infected patients than in HIV-uninfected individuals (1.61: 95% CI 1.43 to 1.81).[63] It is important to note, however, that the selected studies made comparisons to the general population, did not control for smoking or other potential confounders that could be lead to excessive CVD in the HIV-infected individuals, and also did not attempt to account for competing risks.[64] Thus, questions remain regarding the relative contributions of host-, treatment-, and disease-related factors to excess number of CVD events in those with HIV infection.

Persons living with HIV infection have higher rates of established CVD risk factors, particularly smoking and dyslipidemia than HIV-uninfected individuals. In the Data Collection on Adverse Events of Anti-HIV Drugs (D:A:D) cohort study such factors, including age; male gender; obesity; smoking; family history of CVD; diabetes; and dyslipidemia, were each strongly and independently associated with risk of myocardial infarction (MI).[65] This study also found that the risk of CVD was greater with exposure to some ARV drugs, including certain PIs and abacavir, than with exposure to other ARV drugs.[65, 66]

In terms of preventing the progression to CVD events, it has not been determined whether delaying ART initiation is preferable to immediate treatment. In the meta-analysis mentioned above, the risk of CVD in HIV-infected individuals was 1.5 times higher in those being treated with ART than in those not being treated with ART.[63] These analyses were limited by concern that the treated individuals may have been infected for longer periods of time and had prior episodes of untreated HIV disease, as well as the fact that the untreated people were at higher risk for competing events, including death. Furthermore, there is evidence that untreated HIV infection also may be associated with an increased risk of CVD. In the SMART study, the risk of cardiovascular events was greater in participants randomized to CD4-guided treatment interruption than in participants who received continuous ART.[67] In other studies, ART resulted in marked improvement in parameters associated with CVD, including markers of inflammation (such as interleukin 6 [IL-6]), immune dysfunction (e.g., T cell activation, T cell senescence), monocyte activation (e.g., IL-6, CD163), hypercoagulation (e.g., D-dimers) and, most importantly, endothelial dysfunction.[68, 69] Low nadir and/or proximal on-therapy CD4 cell count has been linked to CVD (MI and/or stroke),[70-72] suggesting that low CD4 count might result in increased risk of CVD.

Collectively, the increased risk of cardiovascular events with treatment interruption, the effects of ART on markers of inflammation and endothelial dysfunction, and the association between CVD and CD4 cell depletion suggest that early control of HIV replication with ART can be used as a strategy to reduce risk of CVD, particularly if drugs with potential cardiovascular toxicity are avoided. However, at this time no study has demonstrated that initiation of ART prevents CVD. Therefore, a role for early ART in preventing CVD remains to be established. For HIV-infected individuals with a significant risk of CVD, as assessed by medical history and established estimated risk calculations, risk of CVD should be taken into consideration when selecting a specific ART regimen.

Malignancies

Population-based analyses suggest that the incidence of both AIDS-defining malignancies (i.e., Kaposi sarcoma, non-Hodgkin lymphoma, and cervical cancer) and non-AIDS-defining malignancies is increased in chronic HIV infection. The incidence of several malignancies (particularly liver, anal, oropharyngeal, and lung cancers, Hodgkin lymphoma, and melanoma) is higher in HIV-infected subjects than in matched HIV-uninfected controls,[73, 74] and the burden of these non-AIDS defining malignancies has continued to increase in the United States between 1996 and 2007.[75] Large cohort studies enrolling mainly patients receiving ART have reported a consistent link between low CD4 counts (<350 cells/mm^3 to 500 cells/mm^3) and the risk of AIDS- and/or non-AIDS-defining malignancies.[12, 72, 76-79] The ANRS C04 Study demonstrated a statistically significant relative risk of all cancers evaluated (except for anal carcinoma) in patients with CD4 counts <500 cells/mm^3 compared with patients with current CD4 counts >500 cells/mm^3, an increased risk of anal cancer based on time with CD4 counts <200 cells/mm^3, and, regardless of CD4 count, a protective effect of ART for HIV-associated malignancies.[76] This potential effect of HIV-associated immunodeficiency is striking particularly with regard to cancers associated with chronic viral infections such as HBV, HCV, human papilloma virus (HPV), Epstein-Barr virus (EBV), and human herpes virus-8 (HHV-8).[80, 81] Cumulative HIV viremia, independent of other factors, may also be associated with the risk of non-Hodgkin lymphoma and other AIDS-defining malignancies.[79, 82] From the early 1990s through 2000, incidence rates for many cancers, including Kaposi sarcoma, diffuse large B-cell lymphoma, and primary central nervous system (CNS) lymphoma, declined markedly in HIV-infected individuals in the United States, with more gradual declines noted after 2000.[83] However, for other AIDS-defining and non-AIDS defining cancers, such as Burkitt lymphoma, Hodgkin lymphoma, cervical cancer, and anal cancer, similar reductions in incidence have not been observed.[83, 84] Declines in overall mortality and aging of HIV-infected cohorts increase overall cancer incidence, which may confound a clear assessment of the impact of ART on preventing the development of malignancies.[75, 85] In the SMART study,[86] patients randomized to the drug conservation arm (i.e., those starting ART with CD4 count <250 cells/mm^3) had a higher incidence of AIDS-defining malignancies, but not non-AIDS defining malignancies, than patients in the viral suppression arm (i.e., those receiving continuous ART). In a pooled analysis of the ESPRIT and SMART studies,[87] history of an AIDS-defining event increased risk of any cancer. Taken together this evidence suggests that initiating ART to suppress HIV replication and maintain CD4 counts at levels >350 to 500 cells/mm^3 reduces the overall incidence of AIDS-defining malignancies and may also reduce the risk of non-AIDS-defining malignancies. The effect on incidence is most likely heterogeneous across various cancer types.

Neurological diseases

Although HIV RNA can be detected in the cerebrospinal fluid (CSF) of most untreated patients,[88, 89] these patients usually do not present with overt symptoms of HIV-associated neurological disease.[90] In some patients, CNS infection progresses to HIV encephalitis and can present as HIV-associated dementia (HAD).[91-93] This progression is usually in the context of more advanced untreated systemic HIV infection when severe CNS opportunistic infections (OIs) also cause high morbidity and mortality.[94]

Effective viral suppression resulting from ART has dramatically reduced the incidence of HAD and severe CNS OIs.[95-97] Suppressive ART usually reduces CSF HIV RNA to undetectable levels.[98, 99] Exceptional cases of symptomatic and asymptomatic CNS viral escape, in which HIV RNA is detectable in CSF despite viral suppression in plasma, have been documented.[100, 101] This suggests that in some settings it may be useful to monitor CSF HIV RNA.

Recent attention has turned to milder forms of CNS dysfunction, defined by impairment on formal neuropsychological testing.[93, 102] It is unclear whether this impairment is a consequence of injury sustained before treatment initiation or whether neurologic damage can continue or develop despite systemically effective ART.[103] The association between cognitive impairment and low nadir CD4 counts supports the hypothesis for pretreatment injury and bolsters the argument that earlier initiation of ART may prevent subsequent brain dysfunction.[104, 105]

The peripheral nervous system (PNS) also is a target in HIV infection, and several types of neuropathies have been identified.[106] Most common is HIV-associated polyneuropathy, a chronic, predominantly sensory and sometimes painful neuropathy. The impact of early treatment on this and other forms of neuropathy is not as clearly defined as that on HAD.[107, 108]

Age and treatment-related immune reconstitution (also see HIV and the Older Patient)

The CD4 cell response to ART is an important predictor of short- and long-term morbidity and mortality. Treatment initiation at an older age is consistently associated with a less robust CD4 count response; starting therapy at a younger age may result in better immunologic and perhaps clinical outcomes.[109-112]

T-cell activation and inflammation

Early untreated HIV infection is associated with sustained high-level inflammation and T-cell activation.[113-115] The degree of T-cell activation during untreated HIV disease is associated with risk of subsequent disease progression, independent of other factors such as plasma HIV RNA levels and peripheral CD4 T-cell count.[116, 117] ART results in a rapid, but often incomplete, decrease in most markers of HIV-associated immune activation.[87, 118-121] Persistent T-cell activation and/or T-cell dysfunction is particularly evident in patients who delay therapy until later stage disease (CD4 count <350 cells/mm^3).[119, 121, 122] The degree of persistent inflammation during treatment, as represented by the levels of IL-6, D-dimers, sCD14, and sCD163, may be independently associated with risk of morbidity and mortality.[123-125] Collectively, these observations support earlier use of ART for at least two reasons. First, treatment decreases the level of inflammation, which may be associated with reduced short-term risk of AIDS- and non-AIDS-related morbidity and mortality.[123, 126, 127] Second, because the degree of residual inflammation and/or T-cell dysfunction with ART appears to be higher in patients with lower CD4 cell nadirs,[119, 121, 122] earlier treatment may result in less residual immunological perturbations on therapy and, hence, less risk for AIDS- and non-AIDS-related complications **(CIII)**.

Antiretroviral Therapy for Prevention of HIV Transmission

Prevention of perinatal transmission

Effective ART reduces transmission of HIV. The most dramatic and well-established example of this effect is the use of ART in pregnant women to prevent perinatal transmission of HIV. Effective suppression of HIV replication, as reflected in plasma HIV RNA, is a key determinant in reducing perinatal transmission. In the setting of ART initiation before 28 weeks' gestation and an HIV RNA level <50 copies/mL near delivery, use of combination ART during pregnancy has reduced the rate of perinatal transmission of HIV from approximately 20% to 30% to <0.5%.[128] Thus, use of combination ART drug regimens is recommended for all HIV-infected pregnant women **(AI)**. Following delivery, in the absence of breastfeeding, considerations regarding continuation of the ARV regimen for maternal therapeutic indications are the same as those regarding ART for other non-pregnant individuals. For detailed recommendations, see the *Perinatal Guidelines*.[129]

Prevention of sexual transmission

Recent study results provide strong support for the premise that treatment of the HIV-infected individual can significantly reduce sexual transmission of HIV. Lower plasma HIV RNA levels are associated with decreases in the concentration of the virus in genital secretions.[130, 131] Studies of HIV-serodiscordant heterosexual couples have demonstrated a relationship between level of plasma viremia and risk of transmission of HIV: when plasma HIV RNA levels are lower, transmission events are less common.[1, 132-135]

HPTN 052 was a multicontinental trial that enrolled 1,763 HIV-serodiscordant couples in which the HIV-infected partner was ART naive with CD4 count 350 cells/mm^3 to 550 cells/mm^3 at enrollment. The study compared immediate ART with delayed therapy (i.e., not started until CD4 count <250 cells/mm^3) for the HIV-infected partner.[2] At study entry, 98% of the participants were in heterosexual monogamous relationships. All study participants were counseled on behavioral modification and condom use. Twenty-eight linked HIV transmission events were identified during the study period, but only 1 event occurred in the early therapy arm. This 96% reduction in transmission associated with early ART was statistically significant (HR 0.04, 95% CI: 0.01 0.27, *P* <0.001). These results show that early ART is more effective at preventing transmission of HIV than all other behavioral and biomedical prevention interventions studied to date, including condom use, male circumcision, vaginal microbicides, HIV vaccination, and pre-exposure prophylaxis. This study, as well as other observational studies and modeling analyses showing a decreased rate of HIV transmission in serodiscordant heterosexual couples following the introduction of ART, demonstrate that suppression of viremia in ART-adherent patients with no concomitant sexually transmitted diseases (STDs) substantially reduces the risk of transmission of HIV.[3, 134-138] HPTN 052 was conducted in heterosexual couples and not in populations at risk of transmission via homosexual exposure or needle sharing, but the prevention benefits of effective ART presumably apply to these populations as well. Therefore, the Panel recommends that ART be offered to patients who are at risk of transmitting HIV to sexual partners. (The strength of this recommendation varies according to mode of sexual transmission: **AI** for heterosexual transmission and **AIII** for male-to-male and other modes of sexual transmission.) Clinicians should discuss with patients the potential individual and public health benefits of therapy and the need for adherence to the prescribed regimen and counsel patients that ART is not a substitute for condom use and behavioral modification and that ART does not protect against other STDs (also see Preventing Secondary Transmission of HIV).

Concerns Regarding Earlier Initiation of Therapy

Despite increasing evidence for the benefits associated with earlier initiation of ART, three areas of concern have served as a rationale for deferral of HIV therapy:

ARV drug toxicities have an adverse affect on quality of life and adherence.

Earlier initiation of ART extends exposure to ARV agents by several years. The D:A:D study found an increased incidence of CVD associated with cumulative exposure to some drugs in the nucleoside reverse transcriptase inhibitor and PI drug classes.[65, 139] In the SMART study, when compared with interruption or deferral of therapy, continuous exposure to ART was associated with significantly greater loss of bone density.[67] There may be unknown complications related to cumulative use of ARV drugs for many decades. A list of known ARV-associated toxicities can be found in Adverse Effects of Antiretroviral Agents.

ART frequently improves quality of life for symptomatic patients. However, some side effects of ART may impair quality of life for some patients, especially those who are asymptomatic at initiation of therapy. For example, efavirenz (EFV) can cause neurocognitive or psychiatric side effects and PIs have been associated with gastrointestinal (GI) side effects. As noted above, it has been suggested that some therapies increase the risk of CVD. Some patients may find that the inconvenience of taking medication every day outweighs the overall benefit of early ART and may choose to delay therapy.

ARV non-adherence may have an impact on virologic efficacy.

At any CD4 count, adherence to therapy is essential to achieve viral suppression and prevent emergence of drug-resistance mutations. Several behavioral and social factors associated with poor adherence, such as untreated major psychiatric disorders, active substance abuse, unfavorable social circumstances, patient concerns about side effects, and poor adherence to clinic visits, have been identified. Clinicians should identify areas where additional intervention is needed to improve adherence both before and after initiation of therapy. Some strategies to improve adherence are discussed in Adherence to Antiretroviral Therapy.

Earlier development of resistance may reduce therapeutic options at a later time.

Despite concerns about the development of resistance to ARV drugs, the evidence thus far indicates that resistance occurs more frequently in individuals who initiate therapy later in the course of infection than in those who initiate ART earlier.[140] Furthermore, recent data have indicated a slight increase in the prevalence of 2-drug class resistance from 2000 to 2005.[141]

Cost.

In resource-rich countries, the cost of ART exceeds $10,000 per year (see Appendix B, Table 8). Several modeling studies support the cost effectiveness of HIV therapy initiated soon after diagnosis.[142-144] One study reported that the annual cost of care is 2.5 times higher for patients with CD4 counts <50 cells/mm^3 than for patients with CD4 counts >350 cells/mm^3.[145] A large proportion of the health care expenditure in patients with advanced infection is from non-ARV drugs and hospitalization. There are no cost comparisons for patients starting ART with CD4 count 350 to 500 cells/mm^3 and patients starting ART with CD4 count >500 cells/mm^3.

Conditions Favoring More Rapid Initiation of Therapy

Several conditions increase the urgency for therapy, including:

- Pregnancy **(AI)** (Clinicians should refer to the *Perinatal Guidelines* for more detailed recommendations on the management of HIV-infected pregnant women.)[129]

- AIDS-defining conditions, including HIV-associated dementia **(AI)**

- Acute opportunistic infections (OIs) (see discussion below)
- Lower CD4 counts (e.g., <200 cells/mm^3) **(AI)**
- HIVAN **(AII)**
- Acute/recent infection **(BII)** (see more discussion in the Acute and Recent (Early) Infection section)
- HIV/HBV coinfection **(AII)**
- HIV/HCV coinfection **(BII)**
- Rapidly declining CD4 counts (e.g., >100 cells/mm^3 decrease per year) **(AIII)**
- Higher viral loads (e.g., >100,000 copies/mL) **(BII)**

Acute opportunistic infections

In patients with opportunistic conditions for which no effective therapy exists (e.g., cryptosporidiosis, microsporidiosis, progressive multifocal leukoencephalopathy) but in whom ART may improve outcomes by improving immune responses, the benefits of ART outweigh any increased risk; therefore, treatment should be started as soon as possible **(AIII)**.

In the setting of some OIs for which immediate therapy may increase the risk of immune reconstitution inflammatory syndrome (IRIS) (e.g., cryptococcal meningitis or nontuberculous mycobacterial infections), a short delay before initiating ART may be warranted **(CIII)**.[146, 147] In the setting of other OIs, such as *Pneumocystis jiroveci* pneumonia (PCP), early initiation of ART is associated with increased survival;[8] therefore, therapy should not be delayed **(AI)**.

In patients who have active TB, initiating ART during treatment for TB confers a significant survival advantage;[148-152] therefore, ART should be initiated as recommended in *Mycobacterium Tuberculosis* Disease with HIV Coinfection.

Clinicians should refer to the *Guidelines for Prevention and Treatment of Opportunistic Infections in HIV-Infected Adults and Adolescents*[153] for more detailed discussion on when to initiate ART in the setting of a specific OI.

Conditions Where Deferral of Therapy May be Considered

Some patients and their clinicians may decide to defer therapy for a period of time on the basis of clinical or personal circumstances. Deferring therapy for the reasons discussed below may be reasonable in patients with high CD4 counts (e.g., >500 cells/mm^3) but deferring therapy in patients with much lower CD4 counts (e.g., <200 cells/mm^3) should be considered only in rare situations and should be undertaken with close clinical follow-up. Briefly delaying therapy to allow a patient more time to prepare for lifelong treatment may be considered.

When there are significant barriers to adherence (also see Adherence to Antiretroviral Therapy)

In patients with higher CD4 counts who are at risk of poor adherence, it may be prudent to defer treatment while addressing the barriers to adherence. However, in patients with conditions that require urgent initiation of ART (see above), therapy should be started while simultaneously addressing the barriers to adherence.

Several methodologies exist to help providers assess adherence. When the most feasible measure of adherence is self-report, this assessment should be completed at each clinic visit using one of the available reliable and valid instruments.[154, 155] If other objective measures (e.g., pharmacy refill data, pill count) are available, these methods should be used to assess adherence at each follow-up visit.[156-158] Continuous assessment and counseling make it possible for the clinician to intervene early to address barriers to adherence occurring at any point during treatment (see Adherence to Antiretroviral Therapy).

Presence of comorbidities that complicate or prohibit antiretroviral therapy

Deferral of ART may be considered when either the treatment or manifestations of other medical conditions may complicate the treatment of HIV infection or vice versa. Examples include:

- Surgery that may result in an extended interruption of ART
- Treatment with medications that have clinically significant drug interactions with ART and for which alternative medications are not available

In each of these circumstances, the assumption is that the situation is temporary and that ART will be initiated after the conflicting condition has resolved.

Some less common situations exist in which ART may not be indicated at any time while CD4 counts remain high. In particular, such situations include that of patients with a poor prognosis due to a concomitant medical condition who would not be expected to gain survival or quality-of-life benefits from ART. Examples include patients with incurable non-HIV-related malignancies or end-stage liver disease who are not being considered for liver transplantation. The decision to forego ART in such patients may be easier to make in those with higher CD4 counts; they are likely asymptomatic for HIV, and their survival is unlikely to be prolonged by ART. However, it should be noted that ART may improve outcomes, including survival, in patients with some HIV-associated malignancies (e.g., lymphoma or Kaposi sarcoma) and in patients with liver disease due to chronic HBV or HCV.

Long-term nonprogressors and elite HIV controllers

A small subset of HIV-infected individuals (~3% to 5%) maintain normal CD4 counts for many years in the absence of therapy (long-term nonprogressors), and an even smaller subset (~1%) maintain undetectable HIV RNA level for years ("elite" controllers).[159, 160] Many long-term non-progressors have detectable viremia while some elite controllers progress immunologically and/or clinically despite having no detectable viremia.

The evidence on how to manage these individuals is limited. Given the potential harm associated with uncontrolled HIV replication, many of the preceding arguments for early therapy most likely apply to non-progressors who have consistently detectable viremia (i.e., HIV RNA >200 to 1000 copies/mL). Also given that ongoing HIV replication occurs in elite controllers, ART is also recommended for those rare controllers who exhibit evidence of disease progression, as defined by declining CD4 counts or development of HIV-related complications. The Panel has no recommendations for the management of controllers with high CD4 counts, but the fact that these individuals have higher than normal levels of inflammation and immune activation provides at least some rationale for treatment. Clinical trials assessing the potential benefit of therapy in these individuals are ongoing.

The Need for Early Diagnosis of HIV

Fundamental to the earlier initiation of ART recommended in these guidelines is the assumption that patients will be diagnosed early in the course of HIV infection and linked to medical care, thereby, making earlier initiation of therapy an option. Unfortunately, most cases of HIV infection are not diagnosed until patients are at much later stages of disease,[161-164] although the mean CD4 count at initial presentation for care has increased in more recent years.[4] Despite the 2006 Centers for Disease Control and Prevention (CDC) recommendations for routine, opt-out HIV screening in the health care setting regardless of perceptions about a patient's risk of infection,[165] the median CD4 count of newly diagnosed patients remains below 350 cells/mm^3.[4] The exception is pregnant women whose infection was diagnosed during prenatal care; they have a much higher median initial CD4 count. Compared with other groups, diagnosis of HIV infection is more often delayed in nonwhites, IDUs, and older patients, and a substantial proportion of these individuals develop AIDS-defining illnesses within 1 year of diagnosis.[161-164] Thus, for the current treatment guidelines to have maximum impact, routine HIV screening per current CDC recommendations is essential. It is also critical to educate all newly diagnosed patients about HIV disease and link them to care for full evaluation, follow-up, and management. Once patients are in care, focused effort is required to retain them in the health care system so that both infected individuals and their sexual partners can accrue the full benefits of early diagnosis and treatment.

Conclusion

The current recommendations are based on greater evidence supporting earlier initiation of ART than was advocated in previous guidelines. The strength of the recommendations varies according to the quality and availability of existing evidence supporting each recommendation. In addition to benefitting the health of the HIV-infected individual, the evidence that effective ART reduces sexual transmission to HIV provides further reason for earlier initiation of ART. The Panel will continue to monitor and assess the results of ongoing and planned randomized clinical trials and observational studies. Findings from these studies will provide the Panel with additional guidance to form future recommendations.

References

1. Quinn TC, Wawer MJ, Sewankambo N, et al. Viral load and heterosexual transmission of human immunodeficiency virus type 1. Rakai Project Study Group. *N Engl J Med*. 2000;342(13):921-929. Available at http://www.ncbi.nlm.nih.gov/entrez/query.fcgi?cmd=Retrieve&db=PubMed&dopt=Citation&list_uids=10738050.

2. Cohen MS, Chen YQ, McCauley M, et al. Prevention of HIV-1 infection with early antiretroviral therapy. *N Engl J Med*. 2011;365(6):493-505. Available at http://www.ncbi.nlm.nih.gov/entrez/query.fcgi?cmd=Retrieve&db=PubMed&dopt=Citation&list_uids=21767103.

3. Granich RM, Gilks CF, Dye C, De Cock KM, Williams BG. Universal voluntary HIV testing with immediate antiretroviral therapy as a strategy for elimination of HIV transmission: a mathematical model. *Lancet*. 2009;373(9657):48-57. Available at http://www.ncbi.nlm.nih.gov/entrez/query.fcgi?cmd=Retrieve&db=PubMed&dopt=Citation&list_uids=19038438.

4. Althoff KN, Gange SJ, Klein MB, et al. Late presentation for human immunodeficiency virus care in the United States and Canada. *Clin Infect Dis*. 2010;50(11):1512-1520. Available at http://www.ncbi.nlm.nih.gov/pubmed/20415573.

5. Study Group on Death Rates at High CDCiANP, Lodwick RK, Sabin CA, et al. Death rates in HIV-positive antiretroviral-naive patients with CD4 count greater than 350 cells per microL in Europe and North America: a pooled cohort observational study. *Lancet*. 2010;376(9738):340-345. Available at http://www.ncbi.nlm.nih.gov/pubmed/20638118.

6. HIV Trialists' Collaborative Group. Zidovudine, didanosine, and zalcitabine in the treatment of HIV infection: meta-analyses of the randomised evidence. *Lancet*. 1999;353(9169):2014-2025. Available at http://www.ncbi.nlm.nih.gov/entrez/query.fcgi?cmd=Retrieve&db=PubMed&dopt=Citation&list_uids=10376616.

7. Hammer SM, Squires KE, Hughes MD, et al. A controlled trial of two nucleoside analogues plus indinavir in persons with human immunodeficiency virus infection and CD4 cell counts of 200 per cubic millimeter or less. AIDS Clinical Trials Group 320 Study Team. *N Engl J Med*. 1997;337(11):725-733. Available at http://www.ncbi.nlm.nih.gov/entrez/query.fcgi?cmd=Retrieve&db=PubMed&dopt=Citation&list_uids=9287227.

8. Zolopa A, Andersen J, Powderly W, et al. Early antiretroviral therapy reduces AIDS progression/death in individuals with acute opportunistic infections: a multicenter randomized strategy trial. *PLoS One*. 2009;4(5):e5575. Available at http://www.ncbi.nlm.nih.gov/entrez/query.fcgi?cmd=Retrieve&db=PubMed&dopt=Citation&list_uids=19440326.

9. Mocroft A, Vella S, Benfield TL, et al. Changing patterns of mortality across Europe in patients infected with HIV-1. EuroSIDA Study Group. *Lancet*. 1998;352(9142):1725-1730. Available at http://www.ncbi.nlm.nih.gov/entrez/query.fcgi?cmd=Retrieve&db=PubMed&dopt=Citation&list_uids=9848347.

10. Hogg RS, Yip B, Chan KJ, et al. Rates of disease progression by baseline CD4 cell count and viral load after initiating triple-drug therapy. *JAMA*. 2001;286(20):2568-2577. Available at http://www.ncbi.nlm.nih.gov/entrez/query.fcgi?cmd=Retrieve&db=PubMed&dopt=Citation&list_uids=11722271.

11. Sterne JA, May M, Costagliola D, et al. Timing of initiation of antiretroviral therapy in AIDS-free HIV-1-infected patients: a collaborative analysis of 18 HIV cohort studies. *Lancet*. 2009;373(9672):1352-1363. Available at http://www.ncbi.nlm.nih.gov/entrez/query.fcgi?cmd=Retrieve&db=PubMed&dopt=Citation&list_uids=19361855.

12. Baker JV, Peng G, Rapkin J, et al. CD4+ count and risk of non-AIDS diseases following initial treatment for HIV infection. *AIDS*. 2008;22(7):841-848. Available at http://www.ncbi.nlm.nih.gov/entrez/query.fcgi?cmd=Retrieve&db=PubMed&dopt=Citation&list_uids=18427202.

13. Palella FJ, Jr., Deloria-Knoll M, Chmiel JS, et al. Survival benefit of initiating antiretroviral therapy in HIV-infected persons in different CD4+ cell strata. *Ann Intern Med*. 2003;138(8):620-626. Available at http://www.ncbi.nlm.nih.gov/entrez/query.fcgi?cmd=Retrieve&db=PubMed&dopt=Citation&list_uids=12693883.

14. Cain LE, Logan R, Robins JM, et al. When to initiate combined antiretroviral therapy to reduce mortality and AIDS-defining illness in HIV-infected persons in developed countries: an observational study. *Ann Intern Med*. 2011;154(8):509-515. Available at http://www.ncbi.nlm.nih.gov/entrez/query.fcgi?cmd=Retrieve&db=PubMed&dopt=Citation&list_uids=21502648.

15. Severe P, Juste MA, Ambroise A, et al. Early versus standard antiretroviral therapy for HIV-infected adults in Haiti. *N Engl J Med*. 2010;363(3):257-265. Available at http://www.ncbi.nlm.nih.gov/entrez/query.fcgi?cmd=Retrieve&db=PubMed&dopt=Citation&list_uids=20647201.

16. Kitahata MM, Gange SJ, Abraham AG, et al. Effect of early versus deferred antiretroviral therapy for HIV on survival. *N Engl J Med*. 2009;360(18):1815-1826. Available at http://www.ncbi.nlm.nih.gov/entrez/query.fcgi?cmd=Retrieve&db=PubMed&dopt=Citation&list_uids=19339714.

17. Timing of HAART initiation and clinical outcomes in human immunodeficiency virus type 1 seroconverters. *Arch Intern Med*. 2011;171(17):1560-1569. Available at http://www.ncbi.nlm.nih.gov/entrez/query.fcgi?cmd=Retrieve&db=PubMed&dopt=Citation&list_uids=21949165.

18. Emery S, Neuhaus JA, Phillips AN, et al. Major clinical outcomes in antiretroviral therapy (ART)-naive participants and in those not receiving ART at baseline in the SMART study. *J Infect Dis*. 2008;197(8):1133-1144. Available at http://www.ncbi.nlm.nih.gov/entrez/query.fcgi?cmd=Retrieve&db=PubMed&dopt=Citation&list_uids=18476292.

19. Grinsztejn B HM, Swindells S, et al. Effect of early versus delayed initiation of antiretroviral therapy (ART) on clinical outcomes in the HPTN 052 randomized clinical trial. Paper presented at: AIDS 2012 Conference. 2012, Washington, DC. Abs ThLBB05.

20. Hogan CM, Degruttola V, Sun X, et al. The setpoint study (ACTG A5217): effect of immediate versus deferred antiretroviral therapy on virologic set point in recently HIV-1-infected individuals. *J Infect Dis*. 2012;205(1):87-96. Available at http://www.ncbi.nlm.nih.gov/pubmed/22180621.

21. Geng EH, Hare CB, Kahn JO, et al. The effect of a "universal antiretroviral therapy" recommendation on HIV RNA levels among HIV-infected patients entering care with a CD4 count greater than 500/muL in a public health setting. *Clin Infect Dis*. 2012;55(12):1690-1697. Available at http://www.ncbi.nlm.nih.gov/pubmed/22955429.

22. Mellors JW, Rinaldo CR, Jr., Gupta P, White RM, Todd JA, Kingsley LA. Prognosis in HIV-1 infection predicted by the quantity of virus in plasma. *Science*. 1996;272(5265):1167-1170. Available at http://www.ncbi.nlm.nih.gov/entrez/query.fcgi?cmd=Retrieve&db=PubMed&dopt=Citation&list_uids=8638160.

23. Vlahov D, Graham N, Hoover D, et al. Prognostic indicators for AIDS and infectious disease death in HIV-infected injection drug users: plasma viral load and CD4+ cell count. *JAMA*. 1998;279(1):35-40. Available at http://www.ncbi.nlm.nih.gov/entrez/query.fcgi?cmd=Retrieve&db=PubMed&dopt=Citation&list_uids=9424041.

24. Anastos K, Kalish LA, Hessol N, et al. The relative value of CD4 cell count and quantitative HIV-1 RNA in predicting

survival in HIV-1-infected women: results of the women's interagency HIV study. *AIDS*. 1999;13(13):1717-1726. Available at http://www.ncbi.nlm.nih.gov/entrez/query.fcgi?cmd=Retrieve&db=PubMed&dopt=Citation&list_uids=10509574.

25. O'Brien TR, Blattner WA, Waters D, et al. Serum HIV-1 RNA levels and time to development of AIDS in the Multicenter Hemophilia Cohort Study. *JAMA*. 1996;276(2):105-110. Available at http://www.ncbi.nlm.nih.gov/entrez/query.fcgi?cmd=Retrieve&db=PubMed&dopt=Citation&list_uids=8656501.

26. Egger M, May M, Chene G, et al. Prognosis of HIV-1-infected patients starting highly active antiretroviral therapy: a collaborative analysis of prospective studies. *Lancet*. 2002;360(9327):119-129. Available at http://www.ncbi.nlm.nih.gov/entrez/query.fcgi?cmd=Retrieve&db=PubMed&dopt=Citation&list_uids=12126821.

27. Anastos K, Barron Y, Cohen MH, et al. The prognostic importance of changes in CD4+ cell count and HIV-1 RNA level in women after initiating highly active antiretroviral therapy. *Ann Intern Med*. 2004;140(4):256-264. Available at http://www.ncbi.nlm.nih.gov/entrez/query.fcgi?cmd=Retrieve&db=PubMed&dopt=Citation&list_uids=14970148.

28. O'Brien WA, Hartigan PM, Martin D, et al. Changes in plasma HIV-1 RNA and CD4+ lymphocyte counts and the risk of progression to AIDS. Veterans Affairs Cooperative Study Group on AIDS. *N Engl J Med*. 1996;334(7):426-431. Available at http://www.ncbi.nlm.nih.gov/entrez/query.fcgi?cmd=Retrieve&db=PubMed&dopt=Citation&list_uids=8552144.

29. Hughes MD, Johnson VA, Hirsch MS, et al. Monitoring plasma HIV-1 RNA levels in addition to CD4+ lymphocyte count improves assessment of antiretroviral therapeutic response. ACTG 241 Protocol Virology Substudy Team. *Ann Intern Med*. 1997;126(12):929-938. Available at http://www.ncbi.nlm.nih.gov/entrez/query.fcgi?cmd=Retrieve&db=PubMed&dopt=Citation&list_uids=9182469.

30. Chene G, Sterne JA, May M, et al. Prognostic importance of initial response in HIV-1 infected patients starting potent antiretroviral therapy: analysis of prospective studies. *Lancet*. 2003;362(9385):679-686. Available at http://www.ncbi.nlm.nih.gov/entrez/query.fcgi?cmd=Retrieve&db=PubMed&dopt=Citation&list_uids=12957089.

31. Deeks SG, Gange SJ, Kitahata MM, et al. Trends in multidrug treatment failure and subsequent mortality among antiretroviral therapy-experienced patients with HIV infection in North America. *Clin Infect Dis*. 2009;49(10):1582-1590. Available at http://www.ncbi.nlm.nih.gov/entrez/query.fcgi?cmd=Retrieve&db=PubMed&dopt=Citation&list_uids=19845473.

32. Mugavero MJ, Napravnik S, Cole SR, et al. Viremia copy-years predicts mortality among treatment-naive HIV-infected patients initiating antiretroviral therapy. *Clin Infect Dis*. 2011;53(9):927-935. Available at http://www.ncbi.nlm.nih.gov/entrez/query.fcgi?cmd=Retrieve&db=PubMed&dopt=Citation&list_uids=21890751.

33. Reekie J, Gatell JM, Yust I, et al. Fatal and nonfatal AIDS and non-AIDS events in HIV-1-positive individuals with high CD4 cell counts according to viral load strata. *AIDS*. 2011;25(18):2259-2268. Available at http://www.ncbi.nlm.nih.gov/entrez/query.fcgi?cmd=Retrieve&db=PubMed&dopt=Citation&list_uids=21918422.

34. Szczech LA, Gupta SK, Habash R, et al. The clinical epidemiology and course of the spectrum of renal diseases associated with HIV infection. *Kidney Int*. 2004;66(3):1145-1152. Available at http://www.ncbi.nlm.nih.gov/entrez/query.fcgi?cmd=Retrieve&db=PubMed&dopt=Citation&list_uids=15327410.

35. Marras D, Bruggeman LA, Gao F, et al. Replication and compartmentalization of HIV-1 in kidney epithelium of patients with HIV-associated nephropathy. *Nat Med*. 2002;8(5):522-526. Available at http://www.ncbi.nlm.nih.gov/entrez/query.fcgi?cmd=Retrieve&db=PubMed&dopt=Citation&list_uids=11984599.

36. Estrella M, Fine DM, Gallant JE, et al. HIV type 1 RNA level as a clinical indicator of renal pathology in HIV-infected patients. *Clin Infect Dis*. 2006;43(3):377-380. Available at http://www.ncbi.nlm.nih.gov/entrez/query.fcgi?cmd=Retrieve&db=PubMed&dopt=Citation&list_uids=16804855.

37. Atta MG, Gallant JE, Rahman MH, et al. Antiretroviral therapy in the treatment of HIV-associated nephropathy. *Nephrol Dial Transplant*. 2006;21(10):2809-2813. Available at http://www.ncbi.nlm.nih.gov/entrez/query.fcgi?cmd=Retrieve&db=PubMed&dopt=Citation&list_uids=16864598.

38. Schwartz EJ, Szczech LA, Ross MJ, Klotman ME, Winston JA, Klotman PE. Highly active antiretroviral therapy and the epidemic of HIV+ end-stage renal disease. *J Am Soc Nephrol*. 2005;16(8):2412-2420. Available at

http://www.ncbi.nlm.nih.gov/entrez/query.fcgi?cmd=Retrieve&db=PubMed&dopt=Citation&list_uids=15987747.

39. Kalayjian RC, Franceschini N, Gupta SK, et al. Suppression of HIV-1 replication by antiretroviral therapy improves renal function in persons with low CD4 cell counts and chronic kidney disease. *AIDS*. 2008;22(4):481-487. Available at http://www.ncbi.nlm.nih.gov/entrez/query.fcgi?cmd=Retrieve&db=PubMed&dopt=Citation&list_uids=18301060.

40. Thein HH, Yi Q, Dore GJ, Krahn MD. Natural history of hepatitis C virus infection in HIV-infected individuals and the impact of HIV in the era of highly active antiretroviral therapy: a meta-analysis. *AIDS*. 2008;22(15):1979-1991. Available at http://www.ncbi.nlm.nih.gov/entrez/query.fcgi?cmd=Retrieve&db=PubMed&dopt=Citation&list_uids=18784461.

41. Thio CL, Seaberg EC, Skolasky R, Jr., et al. HIV-1, hepatitis B virus, and risk of liver-related mortality in the Multicenter Cohort Study (MACS). *Lancet*. 2002;360(9349):1921-1926. Available at http://www.ncbi.nlm.nih.gov/entrez/query.fcgi?cmd=Retrieve&db=PubMed&dopt=Citation&list_uids=12493258.

42. Ly KN, Xing J, Klevens RM, Jiles RB, Ward JW, Holmberg SD. The increasing burden of mortality from viral hepatitis in the United States between 1999 and 2007. *Ann Intern Med*. 2012;156(4):271-278. Available at http://www.ncbi.nlm.nih.gov/pubmed/22351712.

43. Weber R, Sabin CA, Friis-Moller N, et al. Liver-related deaths in persons infected with the human immunodeficiency virus: the D:A:D study. *Arch Intern Med*. Aug 14-28 2006;166(15):1632-1641. Available at http://www.ncbi.nlm.nih.gov/entrez/query.fcgi?cmd=Retrieve&db=PubMed&dopt=Citation&list_uids=16908797.

44. Balagopal A, Philp FH, Astemborski J, et al. Human immunodeficiency virus-related microbial translocation and progression of hepatitis C. *Gastroenterology*. 2008;135(1):226-233. Available at http://www.ncbi.nlm.nih.gov/entrez/query.fcgi?cmd=Retrieve&db=PubMed&dopt=Citation&list_uids=18457674.

45. Blackard JT, Kang M, St Clair JB, et al. Viral factors associated with cytokine expression during HCV/HIV co-infection. *J Interferon Cytokine Res*. 2007;27(4):263-269. Available at http://www.ncbi.nlm.nih.gov/entrez/query.fcgi?cmd=Retrieve&db=PubMed&dopt=Citation&list_uids=17477814.

46. Hong F, Tuyama A, Lee TF, et al. Hepatic stellate cells express functional CXCR4: role in stromal cell-derived factor-1alpha-mediated stellate cell activation. *Hepatology*. 2009;49(6):2055-2067. Available at http://www.ncbi.nlm.nih.gov/entrez/query.fcgi?cmd=Retrieve&db=PubMed&dopt=Citation&list_uids=19434726.

47. Macias J, Berenguer J, Japon MA, et al. Fast fibrosis progression between repeated liver biopsies in patients coinfected with human immunodeficiency virus/hepatitis C virus. *Hepatology*. 2009;50(4):1056-1063. Available at http://www.ncbi.nlm.nih.gov/entrez/query.fcgi?cmd=Retrieve&db=PubMed&dopt=Citation&list_uids=19670415.

48. Verma S, Goldin RD, Main J. Hepatic steatosis in patients with HIV-Hepatitis C Virus coinfection: is it associated with antiretroviral therapy and more advanced hepatic fibrosis? *BMC Res Notes*. 2008;1:46. Available at http://www.ncbi.nlm.nih.gov/entrez/query.fcgi?cmd=Retrieve&db=PubMed&dopt=Citation&list_uids=18710499.

49. Ragni MV, Nalesnik MA, Schillo R, Dang Q. Highly active antiretroviral therapy improves ESLD-free survival in HIV-HCV co-infection. *Haemophilia*. 2009;15(2):552-558. Available at http://www.ncbi.nlm.nih.gov/entrez/query.fcgi?cmd=Retrieve&db=PubMed&dopt=Citation&list_uids=19347994.

50. Matthews GV, Avihingsanon A, Lewin SR, et al. A randomized trial of combination hepatitis B therapy in HIV/HBV coinfected antiretroviral naive individuals in Thailand. *Hepatology*. 2008;48(4):1062-1069. Available at http://www.ncbi.nlm.nih.gov/entrez/query.fcgi?cmd=Retrieve&db=PubMed&dopt=Citation&list_uids=18697216.

51. Peters MG, Andersen J, Lynch P, et al. Randomized controlled study of tenofovir and adefovir in chronic hepatitis B virus and HIV infection: ACTG A5127. *Hepatology*. 2006;44(5):1110-1116. Available at http://www.ncbi.nlm.nih.gov/entrez/query.fcgi?cmd=Retrieve&db=PubMed&dopt=Citation&list_uids=17058225.

52. Avidan NU, Goldstein D, Rozenberg L, et al. Hepatitis C viral kinetics during treatment with peg IFN-alpha-2b in HIV/HCV coinfected patients as a function of baseline CD4+ T-cell counts. *J Acquir Immune Defic Syndr*. 2009;52(4):452-458. Available at http://www.ncbi.nlm.nih.gov/entrez/query.fcgi?cmd=Retrieve&db=PubMed&dopt=Citation&list_uids=19797971.

53. Limketkai BN, Mehta SH, Sutcliffe CG, et al. Relationship of liver disease stage and antiviral therapy with liver-related events and death in adults coinfected with HIV/HCV. *JAMA*. 2012;308(4):370-378. Available at http://www.ncbi.nlm.nih.gov/pubmed/22820790.

54. Clotet B, Bellos N, Molina JM, et al. Efficacy and safety of darunavir-ritonavir at week 48 in treatment-experienced patients with HIV-1 infection in POWER 1 and 2: a pooled subgroup analysis of data from two randomised trials. *Lancet*. 2007;369(9568):1169-1178. Available at http://www.ncbi.nlm.nih.gov/entrez/query.fcgi?cmd=Retrieve&db=PubMed&dopt=Citation&list_uids=17416261.

55. Steigbigel RT, Cooper DA, Kumar PN, et al. Raltegravir with optimized background therapy for resistant HIV-1 infection. *N Engl J Med*. 2008;359(4):339-354. Available at http://www.ncbi.nlm.nih.gov/entrez/query.fcgi?cmd=Retrieve&db=PubMed&dopt=Citation&list_uids=18650512.

56. Molina JM, Andrade-Villanueva J, Echevarria J, et al. Once-daily atazanavir/ritonavir compared with twice-daily lopinavir/ritonavir, each in combination with tenofovir and emtricitabine, for management of antiretroviral-naive HIV-1-infected patients: 96-week efficacy and safety results of the CASTLE study. *J Acquir Immune Defic Syndr*. 2010;53(3):323-332. Available at http://www.ncbi.nlm.nih.gov/entrez/query.fcgi?cmd=Retrieve&db=PubMed&dopt=Citation&list_uids=20032785.

57. Loko MA, Bani-Sadr F, Valantin MA, et al. Antiretroviral therapy and sustained virological response to HCV therapy are associated with slower liver fibrosis progression in HIV-HCV-coinfected patients: study from the ANRS CO 13 HEPAVIH cohort. *Antivir Ther*. 2012;17(7):1335-1343. Available at http://www.ncbi.nlm.nih.gov/pubmed/23052829.

58. Brau N, Salvatore M, Rios-Bedoya CF, et al. Slower fibrosis progression in HIV/HCV-coinfected patients with successful HIV suppression using antiretroviral therapy. *J Hepatol*. 2006;44(1):47-55. Available at http://www.ncbi.nlm.nih.gov/entrez/query.fcgi?cmd=Retrieve&db=PubMed&dopt=Citation&list_uids=16182404.

59. Thorpe J, Saeed S, Moodie EE, Klein MB, Canadian Co-infection Cohort S. Antiretroviral treatment interruption leads to progression of liver fibrosis in HIV-hepatitis C virus co-infection. *AIDS*. 24 2011;25(7):967-975. Available at http://www.ncbi.nlm.nih.gov/pubmed/21330904.

60. Smith C. Factors associated with specific causes of death amongst HIV-positive individuals in the D:A:D Study. *AIDS*. 2010;24(10):1537-1548. Available at http://www.ncbi.nlm.nih.gov/entrez/query.fcgi?cmd=Retrieve&db=PubMed&dopt=Citation&list_uids=20453631.

61. Mocroft A, Reiss P, Gasiorowski J, et al. Serious fatal and nonfatal non-AIDS-defining illnesses in Europe. *J Acquir Immune Defic Syndr*. 2010;55(2):262-270. Available at http://www.ncbi.nlm.nih.gov/entrez/query.fcgi?cmd=Retrieve&db=PubMed&dopt=Citation&list_uids=20700060.

62. Weber R SC, D:A:D Study Group. Trends over time in underlying causes of death in the D:A:D study from 1999 to 2011. Program and abstracts presented at: the XIX International AIDS Conference; 2012; Washington, DC. Abstract THAB0304.

63. Islam FM, Wu J, Jansson J, Wilson DP. Relative risk of cardiovascular disease among people living with HIV: a systematic review and meta-analysis. *HIV Med*. 2012;13(8):453-468. Available at http://www.ncbi.nlm.nih.gov/pubmed/22413967.

64. Althoff KA GS. A critical epidemiologic review of cardiovascular disease risk in HIV-infected adults: The importance of the HIV-uninfected comparison group, confounding, and competing risks. *HIV Medicine*. 2013;14(3):191-192. Available at http://www.ncbi.nlm.nih.gov/pubmed/23368691.

65. Friis-Moller N, Reiss P, Sabin CA, et al. Class of antiretroviral drugs and the risk of myocardial infarction. *N Engl J Med*. 2007;356(17):1723-1735. Available at http://www.ncbi.nlm.nih.gov/entrez/query.fcgi?cmd=Retrieve&db=PubMed&dopt=Citation&list_uids=17460226.

66. Sabin CA, Worm SW, Weber R, et al. Use of nucleoside reverse transcriptase inhibitors and risk of myocardial infarction in HIV-infected patients enrolled in the D:A:D study: a multi-cohort collaboration. *Lancet*. 2008;371(9622):1417-1426. Available at

http://www.ncbi.nlm.nih.gov/entrez/query.fcgi?cmd=Retrieve&db=PubMed&dopt=Citation&list_uids=18387667.

67. El-Sadr WM, Lundgren JD, Neaton JD, et al. CD4+ count-guided interruption of antiretroviral treatment. *N Engl J Med*. 2006;355(22):2283-2296. Available at http://www.ncbi.nlm.nih.gov/entrez/query.fcgi?cmd=Retrieve&db=PubMed&dopt=Citation&list_uids=17135583.

68. McComsey G, Smith K, Patel P, et al. Similar reductions in markers of inflammation and endothelial activation after initiation of abacavir/lamivudine or tenofovir/emtricitabine: The HEAT Study. Paper presented at: 16th Conference on Retroviruses and Opportunistic Infections. 2009. Montreal, Canada.

69. Torriani FJ, Komarow L, Parker RA, et al. Endothelial function in human immunodeficiency virus-infected antiretroviral-naive subjects before and after starting potent antiretroviral therapy: The ACTG (AIDS Clinical Trials Group) Study 5152s. *J Am Coll Cardiol*. 2008;52(7):569-576. Available at http://www.ncbi.nlm.nih.gov/entrez/query.fcgi?cmd=Retrieve&db=PubMed&dopt=Citation&list_uids=18687253.

70. Phillips AN, Neaton J, Lundgren JD. The role of HIV in serious diseases other than AIDS. *AIDS*. 2008;22(18):2409-2418. Available at http://www.ncbi.nlm.nih.gov/entrez/query.fcgi?cmd=Retrieve&db=PubMed&dopt=Citation&list_uids=19005264.

71. Baker JV, Duprez D, Rapkin J, et al. Untreated HIV infection and large and small artery elasticity. *J Acquir Immune Defic Syndr*. 2009;52(1):25-31. Available at http://www.ncbi.nlm.nih.gov/entrez/query.fcgi?cmd=Retrieve&db=PubMed&dopt=Citation&list_uids=19731451.

72. Marin B, Thiebaut R, Bucher HC, et al. Non-AIDS-defining deaths and immunodeficiency in the era of combination antiretroviral therapy. *AIDS*. 2009;23(13):1743-1753. Available at http://www.ncbi.nlm.nih.gov/entrez/query.fcgi?cmd=Retrieve&db=PubMed&dopt=Citation&list_uids=19571723.

73. Bedimo RJ, McGinnis KA, Dunlap M, Rodriguez-Barradas MC, Justice AC. Incidence of non-AIDS-defining malignancies in HIV-infected versus noninfected patients in the HAART era: impact of immunosuppression. *J Acquir Immune Defic Syndr*. 2009. Available at http://www.ncbi.nlm.nih.gov/entrez/query.fcgi?cmd=Retrieve&db=PubMed&dopt=Citation&list_uids=19617846.

74. Silverberg MJ, Chao C, Leyden WA, et al. HIV infection, immunodeficiency, viral replication, and the risk of cancer. *Cancer Epidemiol Biomarkers Prev*. 2011;20(12):2551-2559. Available at http://www.ncbi.nlm.nih.gov/pubmed/22109347.

75. Shiels MS, Pfeiffer RM, Gail MH, et al. Cancer burden in the HIV-infected population in the United States. *J Natl Cancer Inst*. 2011;103(9):753-762. Available at http://www.ncbi.nlm.nih.gov/entrez/query.fcgi?cmd=Retrieve&db=PubMed&dopt=Citation&list_uids=21483021.

76. Guiguet M, Boue F, Cadranel J, Lang JM, Rosenthal E, Costagliola D. Effect of immunodeficiency, HIV viral load, and antiretroviral therapy on the risk of individual malignancies (FHDH-ANRS CO4): a prospective cohort study. *Lancet Oncol*. 2009. Available at http://www.ncbi.nlm.nih.gov/entrez/query.fcgi?cmd=Retrieve&db=PubMed&dopt=Citation&list_uids=19818686.

77. Monforte A, Abrams D, Pradier C, et al. HIV-induced immunodeficiency and mortality from AIDS-defining and non-AIDS-defining malignancies. *AIDS*. 2008;22(16):2143-2153. Available at http://www.ncbi.nlm.nih.gov/entrez/query.fcgi?cmd=Retrieve&db=PubMed&dopt=Citation&list_uids=18832878.

78. Reekie J, Kosa C, Engsig F, et al. Relationship between current level of immunodeficiency and non-acquired immunodeficiency syndrome-defining malignancies. *Cancer*. 2010;116(22):5306-5315. Available at http://www.ncbi.nlm.nih.gov/entrez/query.fcgi?cmd=Retrieve&db=PubMed&dopt=Citation&list_uids=20661911.

79. Bruyand M, Thiebaut R, Lawson-Ayayi S, et al. Role of uncontrolled HIV RNA level and immunodeficiency in the occurrence of malignancy in HIV-infected patients during the combination antiretroviral therapy era: Agence Nationale de Recherche sur le Sida (ANRS) CO3 Aquitaine Cohort. *Clin Infect Dis*. 2009;49(7):1109-1116. Available at http://www.ncbi.nlm.nih.gov/entrez/query.fcgi?cmd=Retrieve&db=PubMed&dopt=Citation&list_uids=19705973.

80. Silverberg MJ, Chao C, Leyden WA, et al. HIV infection and the risk of cancers with and without a known infectious cause. *AIDS*. 2009;23(17):2337-2345. Available at

http://www.ncbi.nlm.nih.gov/entrez/query.fcgi?cmd=Retrieve&db=PubMed&dopt=Citation&list_uids=19741479.

81. Grulich AE, van Leeuwen MT, Falster MO, Vajdic CM. Incidence of cancers in people with HIV/AIDS compared with immunosuppressed transplant recipients: a meta-analysis. *Lancet*. 2007;370(9581):59-67. Available at http://www.ncbi.nlm.nih.gov/entrez/query.fcgi?cmd=Retrieve&db=PubMed&dopt=Citation&list_uids=17617273.

82. Zoufaly A, Stellbrink HJ, Heiden MA, et al. Cumulative HIV viremia during highly active antiretroviral therapy is a strong predictor of AIDS-related lymphoma. *J Infect Dis*. 2009;200(1):79-87. Available at http://www.ncbi.nlm.nih.gov/entrez/query.fcgi?cmd=Retrieve&db=PubMed&dopt=Citation&list_uids=19476437.

83. Shiels MS, Pfeiffer RM, Hall HI, et al. Proportions of Kaposi sarcoma, selected non-Hodgkin lymphomas, and cervical cancer in the United States occurring in persons with AIDS, 1980-2007. *JAMA*. 2011;305(14):1450-1459. Available at http://www.ncbi.nlm.nih.gov/entrez/query.fcgi?cmd=Retrieve&db=PubMed&dopt=Citation&list_uids=21486978.

84. Patel P, Hanson DL, Sullivan PS, et al. Incidence of types of cancer among HIV-infected persons compared with the general population in the United States, 1992–2003. *Ann Intern Med*. 2008;148(10):728-736. Available at http://www.ncbi.nlm.nih.gov/entrez/query.fcgi?cmd=Retrieve&db=PubMed&dopt=Citation&list_uids=18490686.

85. Simard EP, Pfeiffer RM, Engels EA. Cumulative incidence of cancer among individuals with acquired immunodeficiency syndrome in the United States. *Cancer*. 2011;117(5):1089-1096. Available at http://www.ncbi.nlm.nih.gov/entrez/query.fcgi?cmd=Retrieve&db=PubMed&dopt=Citation&list_uids=20960504.

86. Silverberg MJ, Neuhaus J, Bower M, et al. Risk of cancers during interrupted antiretroviral therapy in the SMART study. *AIDS*. 2007;21(14):1957-1963. Available at http://www.ncbi.nlm.nih.gov/pubmed/17721103.

87. Neuhaus J, Jacobs DR, Jr., Baker JV, et al. Markers of inflammation, coagulation, and renal function are elevated in adults with HIV infection. *J Infect Dis*. 2010;201(12):1788-1795. Available at http://www.ncbi.nlm.nih.gov/entrez/query.fcgi?cmd=Retrieve&db=PubMed&dopt=Citation&list_uids=20446848.

88. Ellis RJ, Hsia K, Spector SA, et al, for the HIV Neurobehavioral Research Center Group. Cerebrospinal fluid human immunodeficiency virus type 1 RNA levels are elevated in neurocognitively impaired individuals with acquired immunodeficiency syndrome. *Ann Neurol*. 1997;42(5):679-688. Available at http://www.ncbi.nlm.nih.gov/entrez/query.fcgi?cmd=Retrieve&db=PubMed&dopt=Citation&list_uids=9392566.

89. McArthur JC, McClernon DR, Cronin MF, et al. Relationship between human immunodeficiency virus-associated dementia and viral load in cerebrospinal fluid and brain. *Ann Neurol*. 1997;42(5):689-698. Available at http://www.ncbi.nlm.nih.gov/entrez/query.fcgi?cmd=Retrieve&db=PubMed&dopt=Citation&list_uids=9392567.

90. Spudich SS, Huang W, Nilsson AC, et al. HIV-1 chemokine coreceptor utilization in paired cerebrospinal fluid and plasma samples: a survey of subjects with viremia. *J Infect Dis*. 2005;191(6):890-898. Available at http://www.ncbi.nlm.nih.gov/entrez/query.fcgi?cmd=Retrieve&db=PubMed&dopt=Citation&list_uids=15717264.

91. Navia BA, Jordan BD, Price RW. The AIDS dementia complex: I. Clinical features. *Ann Neurol*. 1986;19(6):517-524. Available at http://www.ncbi.nlm.nih.gov/entrez/query.fcgi?cmd=Retrieve&db=PubMed&dopt=Citation&list_uids=3729308.

92. Price RW, Brew BJ. The AIDS dementia complex. *J Infect Dis*. 1988;158(5):1079-1083. Available at http://www.ncbi.nlm.nih.gov/entrez/query.fcgi?cmd=Retrieve&db=PubMed&dopt=Citation&list_uids=3053922.

93. Antinori A, Arendt G, Becker JT, et al. Updated research nosology for HIV-associated neurocognitive disorders. *Neurology*. 2007;69(18):1789-1799. Available at http://www.ncbi.nlm.nih.gov/entrez/query.fcgi?cmd=Retrieve&db=PubMed&dopt=Citation&list_uids=17914061.

94. Snider WD, Simpson DM, Nielsen S, Gold JW, Metroka CE, Posner JB. Neurological complications of acquired immune deficiency syndrome: analysis of 50 patients. *Ann Neurol*. 1983;14(4):403-418. Available at http://www.ncbi.nlm.nih.gov/entrez/query.fcgi?cmd=Retrieve&db=PubMed&dopt=Citation&list_uids=6314874.

95. d'Arminio Monforte A, Cinque P, Mocroft A, et al. Changing incidence of central nervous system diseases in the EuroSIDA cohort. *Ann Neurol*. 2004;55(3):320-328. Available at

http://www.ncbi.nlm.nih.gov/entrez/query.fcgi?cmd=Retrieve&db=PubMed&dopt=Citation&list_uids=14991809.

96. Bhaskaran K, Mussini C, Antinori A, et al. Changes in the incidence and predictors of human immunodeficiency virus-associated dementia in the era of highly active antiretroviral therapy. *Ann Neurol*. 2008;63(2):213-221. Available at http://www.ncbi.nlm.nih.gov/entrez/query.fcgi?cmd=Retrieve&db=PubMed&dopt=Citation&list_uids=17894380.

97. Lescure FX, Omland LH, Engsig FN, et al. Incidence and impact on mortality of severe neurocognitive disorders in persons with and without HIV infection: a Danish nationwide cohort study. *Clin Infect Dis*. Jan 15 2011;52(2):235-243. Available at http://www.ncbi.nlm.nih.gov/entrez/query.fcgi?cmd=Retrieve&db=PubMed&dopt=Citation&list_uids=21288850.

98. Mellgren A, Antinori A, Cinque P, et al. Cerebrospinal fluid HIV-1 infection usually responds well to antiretroviral treatment. *Antivir Ther*. 2005;10(6):701-707. Available at http://www.ncbi.nlm.nih.gov/entrez/query.fcgi?cmd=Retrieve&db=PubMed&dopt=Citation&list_uids=16218168.

99. Spudich S, Lollo N, Liegler T, Deeks SG, Price RW. Treatment benefit on cerebrospinal fluid HIV-1 levels in the setting of systemic virological suppression and failure. *J Infect Dis*. 2006;194(12):1686-1696. Available at http://www.ncbi.nlm.nih.gov/entrez/query.fcgi?cmd=Retrieve&db=PubMed&dopt=Citation&list_uids=17109340.

100. Canestri A, Lescure FX, Jaureguiberry S, et al. Discordance Between Cerebral Spinal Fluid and Plasma HIV Replication in Patients with Neurological Symptoms Who Are Receiving Suppressive Antiretroviral Therapy. *Clin Infect Dis*. 2010. Available at http://www.ncbi.nlm.nih.gov/entrez/query.fcgi?cmd=Retrieve&db=PubMed&dopt=Citation&list_uids=20100092.

101. Eden A, Fuchs D, Hagberg L, et al. HIV-1 viral escape in cerebrospinal fluid of subjects on suppressive antiretroviral treatment. *J Infect Dis*. 2010;202(12):1819-1825. Available at http://www.ncbi.nlm.nih.gov/pubmed/21050119.

102. Simioni S, Cavassini M, Annoni JM, et al. Cognitive dysfunction in HIV patients despite long-standing suppression of viremia. *AIDS*. 2010;24(9):1243-1250. Available at http://www.ncbi.nlm.nih.gov/entrez/query.fcgi?cmd=Retrieve&db=PubMed&dopt=Citation&list_uids=19996937.

103. Smurzynski M, Wu K, Letendre S, et al. Effects of central nervous system antiretroviral penetration on cognitive functioning in the ALLRT cohort. *AIDS*. 2011;25(3):357-365. Available at http://www.ncbi.nlm.nih.gov/entrez/query.fcgi?cmd=Retrieve&db=PubMed&dopt=Citation&list_uids=21124201.

104. Munoz-Moreno JA, Fumaz CR, Ferrer MJ, et al. Nadir CD4 cell count predicts neurocognitive impairment in HIV-infected patients. *AIDS Res Hum Retroviruses*. 2008;24(10):1301-1307. Available at http://www.ncbi.nlm.nih.gov/pubmed/18844464.

105. Heaton RK, Clifford DB, Franklin DR, Jr., et al. HIV-associated neurocognitive disorders persist in the era of potent antiretroviral therapy: CHARTER Study. *Neurology*. 2010;75(23):2087-2096. Available at http://www.ncbi.nlm.nih.gov/entrez/query.fcgi?cmd=Retrieve&db=PubMed&dopt=Citation&list_uids=21135382.

106. Cornblath DR, McArthur JC. Predominantly sensory neuropathy in patients with AIDS and AIDS-related complex. *Neurology*. 1988;38(5):794-796. Available at http://www.ncbi.nlm.nih.gov/entrez/query.fcgi?cmd=Retrieve&db=PubMed&dopt=Citation&list_uids=2834669.

107. Ellis RJ, Rosario D, Clifford DB, et al. Continued high prevalence and adverse clinical impact of human immunodeficiency virus-associated sensory neuropathy in the era of combination antiretroviral therapy: the CHARTER Study. *Arch Neurol*. 2010;67(5):552-558. Available at http://www.ncbi.nlm.nih.gov/entrez/query.fcgi?cmd=Retrieve&db=PubMed&dopt=Citation&list_uids=20457954.

108. Evans SR, Ellis RJ, Chen H, et al. Peripheral neuropathy in HIV: prevalence and risk factors. *AIDS*. 2011;25(7):919-928. Available at http://www.ncbi.nlm.nih.gov/entrez/query.fcgi?cmd=Retrieve&db=PubMed&dopt=Citation&list_uids=21330902.

109. The Collaboration of Observational HIV Epidemiological Research Europe (COHERE) study group. Response to combination antiretroviral therapy: variation by age. *AIDS*. 2008;22(12):1463-1473. Available at http://www.ncbi.nlm.nih.gov/entrez/query.fcgi?cmd=Retrieve&db=PubMed&dopt=Citation&list_uids=18614870.

110. Nogueras M, Navarro G, Anton E, et al. Epidemiological and clinical features, response to HAART, and survival in HIV-

infected patients diagnosed at the age of 50 or more. *BMC Infect Dis*. 2006;6:159. Available at http://www.ncbi.nlm.nih.gov/entrez/query.fcgi?cmd=Retrieve&db=PubMed&dopt=Citation&list_uids=17087819.

111. Bosch RJ, Bennett K, Collier AC, Zackin R, Benson CA. Pretreatment factors associated with 3-year (144-week) virologic and immunologic responses to potent antiretroviral therapy. *J Acquir Immune Defic Syndr*. 2007;44(3):268-277. Available at http://www.ncbi.nlm.nih.gov/entrez/query.fcgi?cmd=Retrieve&db=PubMed&dopt=Citation&list_uids=17146370.

112. Althoff KN, Justice AC, Gange SJ, et al. Virologic and immunologic response to HAART, by age and regimen class. *AIDS*. 2010;24(16):2469-2479. Available at http://www.ncbi.nlm.nih.gov/entrez/query.fcgi?cmd=Retrieve&db=PubMed&dopt=Citation&list_uids=20829678.

113. Fahey JL, Taylor JM, Detels R, et al. The prognostic value of cellular and serologic markers in infection with human immunodeficiency virus type 1. *N Engl J Med*. 1990;322(3):166-172. Available at http://www.ncbi.nlm.nih.gov/entrez/query.fcgi?cmd=Retrieve&db=PubMed&dopt=Citation&list_uids=1967191.

114. Giorgi JV, Lyles RH, Matud JL, et al. Predictive value of immunologic and virologic markers after long or short duration of HIV-1 infection. *J Acquir Immune Defic Syndr*. 2002;29(4):346-355. Available at http://www.ncbi.nlm.nih.gov/entrez/query.fcgi?cmd=Retrieve&db=PubMed&dopt=Citation&list_uids=11917238.

115. Deeks SG, Kitchen CM, Liu L, et al. Immune activation set point during early HIV infection predicts subsequent CD4+ T-cell changes independent of viral load. *Blood*. 2004;104(4):942-947. Available at http://www.ncbi.nlm.nih.gov/entrez/query.fcgi?cmd=Retrieve&db=PubMed&dopt=Citation&list_uids=15117761.

116. Giorgi JV, Hultin LE, McKeating JA, et al. Shorter survival in advanced human immunodeficiency virus type 1 infection is more closely associated with T lymphocyte activation than with plasma virus burden or virus chemokine coreceptor usage. *J Infect Dis*. 1999;179(4):859-870. Available at http://www.ncbi.nlm.nih.gov/entrez/query.fcgi?cmd=Retrieve&db=PubMed&dopt=Citation&list_uids=10068581.

117. Hazenberg MD, Otto SA, van Benthem BH, et al. Persistent immune activation in HIV-1 infection is associated with progression to AIDS. *AIDS*. 2003;17(13):1881-1888. Available at http://www.ncbi.nlm.nih.gov/entrez/query.fcgi?cmd=Retrieve&db=PubMed&dopt=Citation&list_uids=12960820.

118. Gandhi RT, Spritzler J, Chan E, et al. Effect of baseline- and treatment-related factors on immunologic recovery after initiation of antiretroviral therapy in HIV-1-positive subjects: results from ACTG 384. *J Acquir Immune Defic Syndr*. 2006;42(4):426-434. Available at http://www.ncbi.nlm.nih.gov/entrez/query.fcgi?cmd=Retrieve&db=PubMed&dopt=Citation&list_uids=16810109.

119. Hunt PW, Martin JN, Sinclair E, et al. T cell activation is associated with lower CD4+ T cell gains in human immunodeficiency virus-infected patients with sustained viral suppression during antiretroviral therapy. *J Infect Dis*. 2003;187(10):1534-1543. Available at http://www.ncbi.nlm.nih.gov/entrez/query.fcgi?cmd=Retrieve&db=PubMed&dopt=Citation&list_uids=12721933.

120. Valdez H, Connick E, Smith KY, et al. Limited immune restoration after 3 years' suppression of HIV-1 replication in patients with moderately advanced disease. *AIDS*. 2002;16(14):1859-1866. Available at http://www.ncbi.nlm.nih.gov/entrez/query.fcgi?cmd=Retrieve&db=PubMed&dopt=Citation&list_uids=12351945.

121. Robbins GK, Spritzler JG, Chan ES, et al. Incomplete reconstitution of T cell subsets on combination antiretroviral therapy in the AIDS Clinical Trials Group protocol 384. *Clin Infect Dis*. 2009;48(3):350-361. Available at http://www.ncbi.nlm.nih.gov/entrez/query.fcgi?cmd=Retrieve&db=PubMed&dopt=Citation&list_uids=19123865.

122. Lange CG, Lederman MM, Medvik K, et al. Nadir CD4+ T-cell count and numbers of CD28+ CD4+ T-cells predict functional responses to immunizations in chronic HIV-1 infection. *AIDS*. 2003;17(14):2015-2023. Available at http://www.ncbi.nlm.nih.gov/entrez/query.fcgi?cmd=Retrieve&db=PubMed&dopt=Citation&list_uids=14502004.

123. Kuller LH, Tracy R, Belloso W, et al. Inflammatory and coagulation biomarkers and mortality in patients with HIV infection. *PLoS Med*. 2008;5(10):e203. Available at http://www.ncbi.nlm.nih.gov/entrez/query.fcgi?cmd=Retrieve&db=PubMed&dopt=Citation&list_uids=18942885.

124. Sandler NG, Wand H, Roque A, et al. Plasma levels of soluble CD14 independently predict mortality in HIV infection. *J Infect Dis*. 2011;203(6):780-790. Available at http://www.ncbi.nlm.nih.gov/pubmed/21252259.

125. Burdo TH, Lentz MR, Autissier P, et al. Soluble CD163 made by monocyte/macrophages is a novel marker of HIV activity in early and chronic infection prior to and after anti-retroviral therapy. *J Infect Dis*. 2011;204(1):154-163. Available at http://www.ncbi.nlm.nih.gov/pubmed/21628670.

126. Palella FJ, Jr., Gange SJ, Benning L, et al. Inflammatory biomarkers and abacavir use in the Women's Interagency HIV Study and the Multicenter AIDS Cohort Study. *AIDS*. 2010;24(11):1657-1665. Available at http://www.ncbi.nlm.nih.gov/entrez/query.fcgi?cmd=Retrieve&db=PubMed&dopt=Citation&list_uids=20588104.

127. Rodger AJ, Fox Z, Lundgren JD, et al. Activation and coagulation biomarkers are independent predictors of the development of opportunistic disease in patients with HIV infection. *J Infect Dis*. 2009;200(6):973-983. Available at http://www.ncbi.nlm.nih.gov/entrez/query.fcgi?cmd=Retrieve&db=PubMed&dopt=Citation&list_uids=19678756.

128. Tubiana R, Le Chenadec J, Rouzioux C, et al. Factors associated with mother-to-child transmission of HIV-1 despite a maternal viral load <500 copies/ml at delivery: a case-control study nested in the French perinatal cohort (EPF-ANRS CO1). *Clin Infect Dis*. 2010;50(4):585-596. Available at http://www.ncbi.nlm.nih.gov/pubmed/20070234.

129. Panel on Treatment of HIV-Infected Pregnant Women and Prevention of Perinatal Transmission. *Recommendations for Use of Antiretroviral Drugs in Pregnant HIV-1-Infected Women for Maternal Health and Interventions to Reduce Perinatal HIV Transmission in the United States*. Available at http://aidsinfo.nih.gov/contentfiles/lvguidelines/PerinatalGL.pdf.

130. Vernazza PL, Troiani L, Flepp MJ, et al. Potent antiretroviral treatment of HIV-infection results in suppression of the seminal shedding of HIV. The Swiss HIV Cohort Study. *AIDS*. 2000;14(2):117-121. Available at http://www.ncbi.nlm.nih.gov/entrez/query.fcgi?cmd=Retrieve&db=PubMed&dopt=Citation&list_uids=10708281.

131. Coombs RW, Reichelderfer PS, Landay AL. Recent observations on HIV type-1 infection in the genital tract of men and women. *AIDS*. 2003;17(4):455-480. Available at http://www.ncbi.nlm.nih.gov/entrez/query.fcgi?cmd=Retrieve&db=PubMed&dopt=Citation&list_uids=12598766.

132. Tovanabutra S, Robison V, Wongtrakul J, et al. Male viral load and heterosexual transmission of HIV-1 subtype E in northern Thailand. *J Acquir Immune Defic Syndr*. 2002;29(3):275-283. Available at http://www.ncbi.nlm.nih.gov/entrez/query.fcgi?cmd=Retrieve&db=PubMed&dopt=Citation&list_uids=11873077.

133. Kayitenkore K, Bekan B, Rufagari J, et al. The impact of ART on HIV transmission among HIV serodiscordant couples. Paper presented at: XVI International AIDS Conference. 2006. Toronto, Canada.

134. Reynolds S, Makumbi F, Kagaayi J, al. e. ART reduced the rate of sexual transmission of HIV among HIV-discordant couples in rural Rakai, Uganda. Paper presented at:16th Conference on Retroviruses and Opportunistic Infections. 2009. Montreal, Canada.

135. Sullivan P, Kayitenkore K, Chomba E, al. e. Reduction of HIV transmission risk and high risk sex while prescribed ART: Results from discordant couples in Rwanda and Zambia. Paper presented at: 16th Conference on Retroviruses and Opportunistic Infections. 2009. Montreal, Canada.

136. Bunnell R, Ekwaru JP, Solberg P, et al. Changes in sexual behavior and risk of HIV transmission after antiretroviral therapy and prevention interventions in rural Uganda. *AIDS*. 2006;20(1):85-92. Available at http://www.ncbi.nlm.nih.gov/entrez/query.fcgi?cmd=Retrieve&db=PubMed&dopt=Citation&list_uids=16327323.

137. Castilla J, Del Romero J, Hernando V, Marincovich B, Garcia S, Rodriguez C. Effectiveness of highly active antiretroviral therapy in reducing heterosexual transmission of HIV. *J Acquir Immune Defic Syndr*. 2005;40(1):96-101. Available at http://www.ncbi.nlm.nih.gov/entrez/query.fcgi?cmd=Retrieve&db=PubMed&dopt=Citation&list_uids=16123689.

138. Wilson DP, Law MG, Grulich AE, Cooper DA, Kaldor JM. Relation between HIV viral load and infectiousness: a model-based analysis. *Lancet*. 2008;372(9635):314-320. Available at http://www.ncbi.nlm.nih.gov/entrez/query.fcgi?cmd=Retrieve&db=PubMed&dopt=Citation&list_uids=18657710.

139. Worm SW, Sabin C, Weber R, et al. Risk of myocardial infarction in patients with HIV infection exposed to specific individual antiretroviral drugs from the 3 major drug classes: the data collection on adverse events of anti-HIV drugs (D:A:D) study. *J Infect Dis*. 2010;201(3):318-330. Available at http://www.ncbi.nlm.nih.gov/entrez/query.fcgi?cmd=Retrieve&db=PubMed&dopt=Citation&list_uids=20039804.

140. Uy J, Armon C, Buchacz K, Wood K, Brooks JT. Initiation of HAART at higher CD4 cell counts is associated with a lower frequency of antiretroviral drug resistance mutations at virologic failure. *J Acquir Immune Defic Syndr*. 2009;51(4):450-453. Available at http://www.ncbi.nlm.nih.gov/entrez/query.fcgi?cmd=Retrieve&db=PubMed&dopt=Citation&list_uids=19474757.

141. Abraham AG, Lau B, Deeks S, et al. Missing data on the estimation of the prevalence of accumulated human immunodeficiency virus drug resistance in patients treated with antiretroviral drugs in north america. *Am J Epidemiol*. 2011;174(6):727-735. Available at http://www.ncbi.nlm.nih.gov/pubmed/21813792.

142. Freedberg KA, Losina E, Weinstein MC, et al. The cost effectiveness of combination antiretroviral therapy for HIV disease. *N Engl J Med*. 2001;344(11):824-831. Available at http://www.ncbi.nlm.nih.gov/entrez/query.fcgi?cmd=Retrieve&db=PubMed&dopt=Citation&list_uids=11248160.

143. Schackman BR, Goldie SJ, Weinstein MC, Losina E, Zhang H, Freedberg KA. Cost-effectiveness of earlier initiation of antiretroviral therapy for uninsured HIV-infected adults. *Am J Public Health*. 2001;91(9):1456-1463. Available at http://www.ncbi.nlm.nih.gov/entrez/query.fcgi?cmd=Retrieve&db=PubMed&dopt=Citation&list_uids=11527782.

144. Mauskopf J, Kitahata M, Kauf T, Richter A, Tolson J. HIV antiretroviral treatment: early versus later. *J Acquir Immune Defic Syndr*. 2005;39(5):562-569. Available at http://www.ncbi.nlm.nih.gov/entrez/query.fcgi?cmd=Retrieve&db=PubMed&dopt=Citation&list_uids=16044008.

145. Chen RY, Accortt NA, Westfall AO, et al. Distribution of health care expenditures for HIV-infected patients. *Clin Infect Dis*. 2006;42(7):1003-1010. Available at http://www.ncbi.nlm.nih.gov/entrez/query.fcgi?cmd=Retrieve&db=PubMed&dopt=Citation&list_uids=16511767.

146. Bicanic T, Meintjes G, Rebe K, et al. Immune reconstitution inflammatory syndrome in HIV-associated cryptococcal meningitis: a prospective study. *J Acquir Immune Defic Syndr*. 2009;51(2):130-134. Available at http://www.ncbi.nlm.nih.gov/entrez/query.fcgi?cmd=Retrieve&db=PubMed&dopt=Citation&list_uids=19365271.

147. Phillips P, Bonner S, Gataric N, et al. Nontuberculous mycobacterial immune reconstitution syndrome in HIV-infected patients: spectrum of disease and long-term follow-up. *Clin Infect Dis*. 2005;41(10):1483-1497. Available at http://www.ncbi.nlm.nih.gov/entrez/query.fcgi?cmd=Retrieve&db=PubMed&dopt=Citation&list_uids=16231262.

148. Velasco M, Castilla V, Sanz J, et al. Effect of simultaneous use of highly active antiretroviral therapy on survival of HIV patients with tuberculosis. *J Acquir Immune Defic Syndr*. 2009;50(2):148-152. Available at http://www.ncbi.nlm.nih.gov/entrez/query.fcgi?cmd=Retrieve&db=PubMed&dopt=Citation&list_uids=19131895.

149. Abdool Karim SS, Naidoo K, Grobler A, et al. Timing of initiation of antiretroviral drugs during tuberculosis therapy. *N Engl J Med*. 2010;362(8):697-706. Available at http://www.ncbi.nlm.nih.gov/entrez/query.fcgi?cmd=Retrieve&db=PubMed&dopt=Citation&list_uids=20181971.

150. Abdool Karim SS, Naidoo K, Grobler A, et al. Integration of antiretroviral therapy with tuberculosis treatment. *N Engl J Med*. 2011;365(16):1492-1501. Available at http://www.ncbi.nlm.nih.gov/entrez/query.fcgi?cmd=Retrieve&db=PubMed&dopt=Citation&list_uids=22010915.

151. Blanc FX, Sok T, Laureillard D, et al. Earlier versus later start of antiretroviral therapy in HIV-infected adults with tuberculosis. *N Engl J Med*. 2011;365(16):1471-1481. Available at http://www.ncbi.nlm.nih.gov/entrez/query.fcgi?cmd=Retrieve&db=PubMed&dopt=Citation&list_uids=22010913.

152. Havlir DV, Kendall MA, Ive P, et al. Timing of antiretroviral therapy for HIV-1 infection and tuberculosis. *N Engl J Med*. 2011;365(16):1482-1491. Available at http://www.ncbi.nlm.nih.gov/entrez/query.fcgi?cmd=Retrieve&db=PubMed&dopt=Citation&list_uids=22010914.

153. Centers for Disease Control and Prevention (CDC). Guidelines for prevention and treatment of opportunistic infections in HIV-infected adults and adolescents: recommendations from CDC, the National Institutes of Health, and the HIV Medicine Association of the Infectious Diseases Society of America. *MMWR Recomm Rep.* 2009;58(RR-4):1-207. Available at http://www.ncbi.nlm.nih.gov/entrez/query.fcgi?cmd=Retrieve&db=PubMed&dopt=Citation&list_uids=19357635.

154. Lu M, Safren SA, Skolnik PR, et al. Optimal recall period and response task for self-reported HIV medication adherence. *AIDS Behav.* 2008;12(1):86-94. Available at http://www.ncbi.nlm.nih.gov/entrez/query.fcgi?cmd=Retrieve&db=PubMed&dopt=Citation&list_uids=17577653.

155. Simoni JM, Kurth AE, Pearson CR, Pantalone DW, Merrill JO, Frick PA. Self-report measures of antiretroviral therapy adherence: A review with recommendations for HIV research and clinical management. *AIDS Behav.* 2006;10(3):227-245. Available at http://www.ncbi.nlm.nih.gov/entrez/query.fcgi?cmd=Retrieve&db=PubMed&dopt=Citation&list_uids=16783535.

156. Bisson GP, Gross R, Bellamy S, et al. Pharmacy refill adherence compared with CD4 count changes for monitoring HIV-infected adults on antiretroviral therapy. *PLoS Med.* 20 2008;5(5):e109. Available at http://www.ncbi.nlm.nih.gov/entrez/query.fcgi?cmd=Retrieve&db=PubMed&dopt=Citation&list_uids=18494555.

157. Kalichman SC, Amaral CM, Cherry C, et al. Monitoring medication adherence by unannounced pill counts conducted by telephone: reliability and criterion-related validity. *HIV Clin Trials.* 2008;9(5):298-308. Available at http://www.ncbi.nlm.nih.gov/entrez/query.fcgi?cmd=Retrieve&db=PubMed&dopt=Citation&list_uids=18977718.

158. Moss AR, Hahn JA, Perry S, et al. Adherence to highly active antiretroviral therapy in the homeless population in San Francisco: a prospective study. *Clin Infect Dis.* 2004;39(8):1190-1198. Available at http://www.ncbi.nlm.nih.gov/entrez/query.fcgi?cmd=Retrieve&db=PubMed&dopt=Citation&list_uids=15486844.

159. Hunt PW, Brenchley J, Sinclair E, et al. Relationship between T cell activation and CD4+ T cell count in HIV-seropositive individuals with undetectable plasma HIV RNA levels in the absence of therapy. *J Infect Dis.* 2008;197(1):126-133. Available at http://www.ncbi.nlm.nih.gov/entrez/query.fcgi?cmd=Retrieve&db=PubMed&dopt=Citation&list_uids=18171295.

160. Choudhary SK, Vrisekoop N, Jansen CA, et al. Low immune activation despite high levels of pathogenic human immunodeficiency virus type 1 results in long-term asymptomatic disease. *J Virol.* 2007;81(16):8838-8842. Available at http://www.ncbi.nlm.nih.gov/entrez/query.fcgi?cmd=Retrieve&db=PubMed&dopt=Citation&list_uids=17537849.

161. Egger M. Outcomes of ART in resource-limited and industrialized countries. Paper presented at:14th Conference on Retroviruses and Opportunistic Infections. 2007. Los Angeles, CA.

162. Wolbers M, Bucher HC, Furrer H, et al. Delayed diagnosis of HIV infection and late initiation of antiretroviral therapy in the Swiss HIV Cohort Study. *HIV Med.* 2008;9(6):397-405. Available at http://www.ncbi.nlm.nih.gov/entrez/query.fcgi?cmd=Retrieve&db=PubMed&dopt=Citation&list_uids=18410354.

163. Grigoryan A, Hall HI, Durant T, Wei X. Late HIV diagnosis and determinants of progression to AIDS or death after HIV diagnosis among injection drug users, 33 US States, 1996-2004. *PLoS One.* 2009;4(2):e4445. Available at http://www.ncbi.nlm.nih.gov/entrez/query.fcgi?cmd=Retrieve&db=PubMed&dopt=Citation&list_uids=19214229.

164. Centers for Disease Control and Prevention (CDC). Late HIV testing - 34 states, 1996-2005. *MMWR Morb Mortal Wkly Rep.* 2009;58(24):661-665. Available at http://www.ncbi.nlm.nih.gov/entrez/query.fcgi?cmd=Retrieve&db=PubMed&dopt=Citation&list_uids=19553901.

165. Branson BM, Handsfield HH, Lampe MA, et al. Revised recommendations for HIV testing of adults, adolescents, and pregnant women in health-care settings. *MMWR Recomm Rep.* 2006;55(RR-14):1-17. Available at http://www.ncbi.nlm.nih.gov/entrez/query.fcgi?cmd=Retrieve&db=PubMed&dopt=Citation&list_uids=16988643.

What to Start: Initial Combination Regimens for the Antiretroviral-Naive Patient (Last updated February 12, 2013; last reviewed February 12, 2013)

Panel's Recommendations

- The Panel recommends the following as preferred regimens (listed in order of FDA approval) for antiretroviral (ARV)-naive patients:

  - efavirenz/tenofovir disoproxil fumarate/emtricitabine (EFV/TDF/FTC) **(AI)**
  - ritonavir-boosted atazanavir + tenofovir disoproxil fumarate/emtricitabine (ATV/r + TDF/FTC) **(AI)**
  - ritonavir-boosted darunavir + tenofovir disoproxil fumarate/emtricitabine (DRV/r + TDF/FTC) **(AI)**
  - raltegravir + tenofovir disoproxil fumarate/emtricitabine (RAL + TDF/FTC) **(AI)**

- Panel-recommended alternative and other regimens can be found in Table 5a and Table 5b.

- Selection of a regimen should be individualized on the basis of virologic efficacy, toxicity, pill burden, dosing frequency, drug-drug interaction potential, resistance testing results, and comorbid conditions.

- Based on individual patient characteristics and needs, in some instances, an alternative or other regimen may be a preferred regimen for a specific patient.

Rating of Recommendations: A = Strong; B = Moderate; C = Optional

Rating of Evidence: I = Data from randomized controlled trials; II = Data from well-designed nonrandomized trials or observational cohort studies with long-term clinical outcomes; III = Expert opinion

---

More than 20 approved antiretroviral (ARV) drugs in 6 mechanistic classes are available to design combination regimens. These 6 classes include the nucleoside/nucleotide reverse transcriptase inhibitors (NRTIs), non-nucleoside reverse transcriptase inhibitors (NNRTIs), protease inhibitors (PIs), fusion inhibitors (FIs), CCR5 antagonists, and integrase strand transfer inhibitors (INSTIs).

An initial ARV regimen generally consists of two NRTIs in combination with an NNRTI, a PI (preferably boosted with ritonavir [RTV]), an INSTI, or a CCR5 antagonist (namely maraviroc [MVC]). In clinical trials, NNRTI-, PI-, INSTI-, or CCR5 antagonist-based regimens have all resulted in HIV RNA decreases and CD4 cell increases in a large majority of patients.[1-7]

Data Used for Making Recommendations

The Panel's recommendations are primarily based on clinical trial data published in peer-reviewed journals and data prepared by manufacturers for Food and Drug Administration (FDA) review. In select cases, the Panel considers data presented in abstract format at major scientific meetings. The first criterion for selection of evidence on which to base recommendations is published information from a randomized, prospective clinical trial with an adequate sample size that demonstrates that an ARV regimen has shown durable viral suppression and immunologic enhancement (as evidenced by increase in CD4 count). Few of these trials include clinical endpoints, such as development of AIDS-defining illness or death. Thus, assessment of regimen efficacy and potency is primarily based on surrogate marker endpoints (HIV RNA and CD4 responses).

The Panel reviewed data from randomized clinical trials and other reports to arrive at "preferred," "alternative," or "other" ratings for each regimen noted in Tables 5a and 5b. "Preferred regimens" are those regimens studied in randomized controlled trials and shown to have optimal and durable virologic efficacy, favorable tolerability and toxicity profiles, and ease of use. "Alternative regimens" are those regimens that are effective but have potential disadvantages when compared with preferred regimens. In certain situations and based on individual patient characteristics and needs, a regimen listed as an alternative may actually be the preferred regimen for a specific patient. Some regimens are classified as "other regimens" because of reduced virologic activity, lack of efficacy data from large clinical trials, or other factors (such as greater toxicities, pill burden, drug interaction potential, or need for additional testing before use) when compared with preferred or alternative regimens.

Considerations When Selecting a First Antiretroviral Regimen for Antiretroviral Therapy-Naive Patients

Factors to Consider When Selecting an Initial Regimen

Regimen selection should be individualized on the basis of several factors, including the following:

- the patient's comorbid conditions (e.g., cardiovascular disease [CVD], chemical dependency, liver or renal disease, psychiatric illnesses, or tuberculosis [TB]);
- potential adverse drug effects;
- known or potential drug interactions with other medications;
- pregnancy or pregnancy potential;
- results of genotypic drug-resistance testing;
- pre-treatment HIV viral load;
- gender and pretreatment CD4 count if considering nevirapine (NVP);
- HLA-B*5701 testing if considering abacavir (ABC);
- coreceptor tropism assay if considering MVC;
- patient preferences (when possible) and adherence potential; and
- convenience (e.g., factors such as pill burden, dosing frequency, availability of fixed dose combination products, and food and fluid requirements).

Potential advantages and disadvantages of the components recommended as initial therapy for ARV-naive patients are listed in Table 6 to guide prescribers in choosing the optimal regimen for an individual patient. Table 7 provides a list of agents or components not recommended for initial treatment. Appendix B, Tables 1 6 list characteristics of individual ARV agents, such as formulations, dosing recommendations, pharmacokinetics (PKs), and common adverse effects. Appendix B, Table 7 provides clinicians with ARV dosing recommendations for patients who have renal or hepatic insufficiency.

Choosing Between Preferred Initial Regimens

Each of the four preferred initial regimens listed in Table 5a has shown potent virologic efficacy as measured by the proportion of subjects achieving and maintaining viral suppression in comparative clinical trials. Given the comparable efficacy of the preferred regimens, selection of an optimal regimen for a specific patient will depend on other factors, including characteristics of the regimen (e.g., adverse event profile, barrier to resistance, dosing frequency, pill burden, food restrictions, the availability of fixed-dose combination formulations, the potential for drug-drug interactions), the patient's pre-treatment resistance testing results, and whether the patient is a woman who may become pregnant. A complete description of the advantages and disadvantages of the preferred and alternative options for therapy are listed in Table 6.

Currently, all of the preferred initial regimens include the NRTI combination of tenofovir disoproxil fumarate/emtricitabine (TDF/FTC), which is available as a fixed-dose combination tablet. In two comparative clinical trials, this NRTI combination was more effective than the alternative NRTI pair, abacavir/lamivudine (ABC/3TC),[8, 9] but in a third study, the NRTI combinations showed comparable efficacy.[10] TDF may cause kidney injury in some patients, particularly in those who have pre-existing renal disease or are receiving concomitant nephrotoxic drugs. In addition, TDF induces a greater decline in bone mineral density than other ARV drugs.[11]

Of the four preferred regimens, efavirenz (EFV) in combination with TDF/FTC has been studied in the greatest number of clinical trials.[6, 12-15] This regimen is available in a single tablet, once-daily formulation, and is generally well tolerated. Disadvantages of the regimen include central nervous system (CNS) side effects that resolve over time in some (but not all) patients, a higher incidence of rash (including severe skin reactions) than with other preferred regimens, and dyslipidemia. Owing to concerns related to potential teratogenicity emerging from animal studies and some human case reports, ARV regimens that do not include EFV should be strongly considered in women who wish to conceive or are sexually active and not using effective contraception, assuming these alternative regimens are not thought to compromise the woman's health.

Initial treatment with ritonavir (RTV) boosted PI-containing regimens is unique from the resistance perspective, as virologic failure rarely selects for PI-resistance and NRTI resistance is uncommon. As a result, some clinicians consider these the initial regimens of choice for patients at higher risk for virologic failure due to suboptimal adherence, inconsistent follow-up, or other factors. A disadvantage of RTV-boosted PI-based regimens is the large number of drug-drug interactions, in particular with medications metabolized through the cytochrome p450 pathway. As a result, RTV-boosted PI-based regimens may be difficult to use in patients who are taking many other medications.

RTV-boosted atazanavir (ATV/r) is as effective as EFV, but causes less rash and has a more favorable lipid profile.[13] ATV induces reversible indirect hyperbilirubinemia, which may result in visible jaundice or scleral icterus in a small proportion of patients; ATV has also been associated with nephrolithiasis and cholelithiasis. Optimal absorption of ATV depends on presence of food and low gastric pH; if acid-reducing agents are needed, co-administration should be done according to the dosing guidelines shown in Table 15a. RTV-boosted darunavir (DRV/r) shares many of the characteristics of boosted ATV, but does not cause hyperbilirubinemia and can be given with acid-reducing agents. There are no fully-powered clinical trials that compare the virologic efficacy of DRV/r and ATV/r. One small study found that these boosted-PIs had comparable effects on lipids.[16] Both ATV/r and DRV/r can be given once daily.

Raltegravir (RAL) plus TDF/FTC demonstrated comparable antiviral efficacy to EFV/TDF/FTC, with fewer drug-related adverse effects and a more favorable lipid profile.[6] RAL has fewer drug-drug interactions than both boosted-PI and EFV-based regimens, and is therefore easier to add to a patient's complex medication regimen. Rare but severe side effects (e.g., rhabdomyolysis, severe skin, systemic hypersensitivity reactions) have been reported with RAL. RAL plus TDF/FTC is the only preferred regimen that requires twice-daily dosing.

There are clinical scenarios in which options for initial therapy should be chosen from the list of alternative and other regimens rather than from the preferred list. Tables 5a and 5b provide a list of alternative and other regimens that may be prescribed for select patients. Table 6 lists the advantages and disadvantages of the individual ARV components of the regimens.

Acute symptomatic HIV infection may be diagnosed while an individual is receiving TDF/FTC for pre-exposure prophylaxis (PrEP) (see Acute and Recent [Early] HIV Infection). As with all newly diagnosed cases of HIV-infection, genotype testing should be performed. In most cases, HIV infection in this setting is secondary to suboptimal adherence[17] to the prescribed daily TDF/FTC regimen, hence resistance in the setting of PrEP failure in clinical trials has been uncommon. Pending genotype testing results, a regimen consisting of a boosted PI (ATV/r or DRV/r) plus TDF/FTC **(AIII)** can be initiated. ARV drugs should be modified as needed based on the results of baseline resistance testing.

Table 5a. Preferred and Alternative Antiretroviral Regimens for Antiretroviral Therapy-Naive Patients

A combination antiretroviral therapy (ART) regimen generally consists of two NRTIs plus one active drug from one of the following classes: NNRTI, PI (generally boosted with RTV), INSTI, or a CCR5 antagonist. Selection of a regimen should be individualized on the basis of virologic efficacy, toxicity, pill burden, dosing frequency, drug-drug interaction potential, and the patient's resistance testing results and comorbid conditions. Refer to Table 6 for a list of advantages and disadvantages of the individual ARV agents listed below and to Appendix B, Tables 1–6 for dosing information. The regimens in each category are listed in alphabetical order. For more detailed recommendations on ARV use in HIV-infected pregnant women, refer to the latest perinatal guidelines available at http://aidsinfo.nih.gov/guidelines.

Preferred Regimens
Regimens with optimal and durable efficacy, favorable tolerability and toxicity profile, and ease of use.

The preferred regimens for non-pregnant patients are arranged by chronological order of FDA approval of components other than nucleosides and, thus, by duration of clinical experience.

	Comments
NNRTI-Based Regimen • EFV/TDF/FTC[a] **(AI)** **PI-Based Regimens** *(in alphabetical order)* • ATV/r + TDF/FTC[a] **(AI)** • DRV/r (once daily) + TDF/FTC[a] **(AI)** **INSTI-Based Regimen** • RAL + TDF/FTC[a] **(AI)**	• **EFV** is teratogenic in non-human primates. A regimen that does not include EFV should be strongly considered in women who are planning to become pregnant or who are sexually active and not using effective contraception. • **TDF** should be used with caution in patients with renal insufficiency. • **ATV/r should not be used** in patients who require >20 mg omeprazole equivalent per day. Refer to Table 15a for dosing recommendations regarding interactions between ATV/r and acid-lowering agents.

Alternative Regimens
Regimens that are effective and tolerable, but have potential disadvantages when compared with preferred regimens. An alternative regimen may be the preferred regimen for some patients.

	Comments
NNRTI-Based Regimens *(in alphabetical order)* • EFV + ABC/3TC[a] **(BI)** • RPV/TDF/FTC[a] **(BI)** • RPV + ABC/3TC[a] **(BIII)** **PI-Based Regimens** *(in alphabetical order)* • ATV/r + ABC/3TC[a] **(BI)** • DRV/r + ABC/3TC[a] **(BII)** • FPV/r (once or twice daily) + ABC/3TC[a] or TDF/FTC[a] **(BI)** • LPV/r (once or twice daily) + ABC/3TC[a] or TDF/FTC[a] **(BI)** **INSTI-Based Regimen** • EVG/COBI/TDF/FTC[a] **(BI)** • RAL + ABC/3TC[a] **(BIII)**	• **RPV is not recommended** in patients with pretreatment HIV RNA >100,000 copies/mL. • Higher rate of virologic failures reported in patients with pre-ART CD4 count <200 cells/mm^3 who are treated with RPV + 2NRTI • Use of PPIs with **RPV** is contraindicated. • **ABC should not be used** in patients who test positive for HLA-B*5701. • Use **ABC** with caution in patients with known high risk of CVD or with pretreatment HIV RNA >100,000 copies/mL (see text). • **Once-daily LPV/r is not recommended** for use in pregnant women. • **EVG/COBI/TDF/FTC** should not be started in patients with an estimated CrCl <70 ml/min, and should be changed to an alternative regimen if the patient's CrCl falls below 50 mL/min • **COBI** is a potent CYP 3A inhibitor. It can increase the concentration of other drugs metabolized by this pathway. Refer to Tables 15d and 16c for drug interaction information for concomitantly administered drugs. • **EVG/COBI/TDF/FTC** should not be used with other ARV drugs or with nephrotoxic drugs.

[a] 3TC may substitute for FTC or vice versa. The following combinations in the recommended list above are available as coformulated fixed-dose combinations: ABC/3TC, EFV/TDF/FTC, EVG/COBI/TDF/FTC, LPV/r, RPV/TDF/FTC, TDF/FTC, and ZDV/3TC.

Key to Abbreviations: 3TC = lamivudine, ABC = abacavir, ART = antiretroviral therapy, ARV = antiretroviral, ATV/r = atazanavir/ritonavir, COBI = cobicistat, CrCl = creatinine clearance, CVD = cardiovascular disease, DRV/r = darunavir/ritonavir, EFV = efavirenz, EVG = elvitegravir, FDA = Food and Drug Administration, FPV/r = fosamprenavir/ritonavir, FTC = emtricitabine, INSTI = integrase strand transfer inhibitor, LPV/r = lopinavir/ritonavir, NNRTI = non-nucleoside reverse transcriptase inhibitor, NRTI = nucleoside reverse transcriptase inhibitor, PI = protease inhibitor, PPI = proton pump inhibitor, RAL = raltegravir, RPV = rilpivirine, RTV = ritonavir, TDF = tenofovir disoproxil fumarate, ZDV = zidovudine

Rating of Recommendations: A = Strong; B = Moderate; C = Optional

Rating of Evidence: I = Data from randomized controlled trials; II = Data from well-designed nonrandomized trials or observational cohort studies with long-term clinical outcomes; III = Expert opinion

Guidelines for the Use of Antiretroviral Agents in HIV-1-Infected Adults and Adolescents

Table 5b. Other Antiretroviral Regimens for Antiretroviral Therapy-Naive Patients

Regimens that may be selected for some patients but are less satisfactory than preferred or alternative regimens listed in Table 5a.	

NNRTI-Based Regimen
• EFV + ZDV/3TC[a]
• NVP + (ABC/3TC[a] or TDF/FTC[a] or ZDV/3TC[a])
• RPV + ZDV/3TC[a]
 	
PI-Based Regimens
• (ATV or ATV/r or DRV/r or FPV/r or LPV/r or SQV/r) + ZDV/3TC[a]
• ATV + ABC/3TC[a]
• SQV/r + (ABC/3TC[a] or TDF/FTC[a])
 	
INSTI-Based Regimen
• RAL + ZDV/3TC[a]
 	
CCR5 Antagonist-Based Regimens
• MVC + (ABC/3TC or TDF/FTC or ZDV/3TC[a])
	Comments
	• **NVP** should not be used in patients with moderate to severe hepatic impairment (Child-Pugh B or C).[b]
	• **NVP** should not be used in women with pre-ART CD4 count >250 cells/mm^3 or in men with pre-ART CD4 count >400 cells/mm^3.
	• Use **NVP** and **ABC** together with caution; both can cause HSRs within the first few weeks after initiation of therapy.
	• **ZDV** can cause bone marrow suppression, myopathy, lipoatrophy, and rarely lactic acidosis with hepatic steatosis.
	• **ATV/r** is generally preferred over **unboosted ATV**.
	• Perform tropism testing before initiation of therapy with **MVC**. **MVC** may be considered in patients who have only CCR5-tropic virus.
	• **SQV/r** was associated with PR and QT prolongation in a healthy volunteer study. Baseline ECG is recommended before initiation of **SQV/r**.
	• **SQV/r** is not recommended in patients with:
	  • pretreatment QT interval >450 msec
	  • refractory hypokalemia or hypomagnesemia
	  • concomitant therapy with other drugs that prolong QT interval
	  • complete AV block without implanted pacemaker,
	  • risk of complete AV block

[a] 3TC may be substituted with FTC or vice versa.

[b] Refer to Appendix B, Table 7 for the criteria for Child-Pugh classification.

Key to Abbreviations: 3TC = lamivudine, ABC = abacavir, ART = antiretroviral therapy, ATV = atazanavir, ATV/r = atazanavir/ritonavir, AV = atrioventricular, DRV/r = darunavir/ritonavir, ECG = electrocardiogram, EFV = efavirenz, FPV/r = fosamprenavir/ritonavir, FTC = emtricitabine, HSR = hypersensitivity reaction, INSTI = integrase strand transfer inhibitor, LPV/r = lopinavir/ritonavir, msec = millisecond, MVC = maraviroc, NNRTI = non-nucleoside reverse transcriptase inhibitor, NVP = nevirapine, PI = protease inhibitor, RAL = raltegravir, RPV = rilpivirine, RTV = ritonavir, SQV/r = saquinavir/ritonavir, TDF = tenofovir disoproxil fumarate, ZDV = zidovudine

The discussions below focus on the rationale for the Panel's recommendations, which are based on the efficacy, safety, and other characteristics of different agents within the individual drug classes.

Non-Nucleoside Reverse Transcriptase Inhibitor-Based Regimens

Summary: Non-Nucleoside Reverse Transcriptase Inhibitor-Based Regimens

Five NNRTIs (delavirdine [DLV], EFV, etravirine [ETR], NVP, and rilpivirine [RPV]) are currently FDA approved.

NNRTI-based regimens have demonstrated virologic potency and durability. The major disadvantages of currently available NNRTIs involve the prevalence of NNRTI-resistant viral strains in ART-naive patients[18-21] and the NNRTIs' low genetic barrier for the development of resistance. Resistance testing should be performed to guide therapy selection for ART-naive patients (see Drug-Resistance Testing). High level resistance to all NNRTIs (except ETR) may occur with a single mutation; cross resistance is common. ETR has *in vitro* activity against some viruses with mutations that confer resistance to DLV, EFV, and NVP.[22] In RPV-treated patients, the presence of RPV-resistant mutations at virologic failure is common and may confer cross resistance to other NNRTIs including ETR.[14, 23]

The Panel recommends that EFV, RPV, or NVP may be used as part of an initial regimen. EFV is preferred on the basis of its potency (as discussed below). RPV may be used as an alternative NNRTI option in patients with pre-treatment HIV RNA < 100,000 copies/mL; NVP may be another NNRTI option in women with pretreatment CD4 counts $\leq$250 cells/mm^3 or in men with pretreatment CD4 counts $\leq$400 cells/mm^3 (see discussions below).

Compared with the other NNRTIs, DLV has the highest dosing frequency (three times daily), the least supportive clinical trial data, and the least antiviral activity. Therefore, DLV is **not recommended** as part of an initial regimen **(BIII)**. ETR at a dose of 200 mg twice daily is approved for use in treatment-experienced patients with virologic failure.[24] In a small, randomized, double-blinded, placebo-controlled trial, ETR 400 mg once daily was compared with EFV 600 mg once daily (both in combination with two NRTIs) in treatment-naive subjects (79 and 78 subjects in the ETR and EFV arms, respectively). Virologic responses were comparable at 48 weeks.[25] However, pending results from larger clinical trials, the panel cannot recommend ETR as initial therapy at this time.

Following is a more detailed discussion of individual NNRTI-based regimens for initial therapy.

Preferred Non-Nucleoside Reverse Transcriptase Inhibitor-Based Regimens

Efavirenz (EFV). Large randomized, controlled trials and cohort studies of ART-naive patients have demonstrated potent viral suppression in patients treated with EFV plus two NRTIs; a substantial proportion of these patients had HIV RNA <50 copies/mL at up to 7 years of follow-up.[1, 2, 26] Studies that compared EFV-based regimens with other regimens demonstrated that the combination of EFV with two NRTIs was superior or non-inferior virologically to ritonavir-boosted lopinavir (LPV/r),[4] NVP-,[27, 28] RPV-,[14] ATV-,[5] elvitegravir (EVG)-,[15] RAL-,[6] and MVC-based[7] regimens.

EFV can cause CNS adverse effects, such as abnormal dreams, dizziness, headache, and depression, which usually resolve over a few weeks in some (but not all) patients. In animal reproductive studies, EFV at drug exposure levels similar to those achieved in humans caused major congenital anomalies in the CNS of nonhuman primates.[29] In humans, several cases of neural tube defects in newborns of mothers exposed to EFV during the first trimester of pregnancy have been reported.[30, 31] Although emerging information about the use of EFV in pregnancy is reassuring,[32, 33] data remain insufficient to rule out a potential 2 to 3 fold increase in neural tube birth defects with first-trimester exposure to EFV. Therefore, alternative ARV regimens that do not include EFV should be strongly considered in women who are planning to become pregnant or who are sexually active and not using effective contraception, assuming these alternative regimens are acceptable to the provider and are not thought to compromise the woman's health. Because the risk of neural tube defects is restricted to the first 5 to 6 weeks of pregnancy (before pregnancy is usually recognized), and because unnecessary ARV changes during pregnancy may be associated with loss of viral control and increased risk of perinatal transmission, EFV can be continued in pregnant women receiving an EFV-based regimen who present for antenatal care in the first trimester, provided the regimen produces virologic suppression.[34]

In studies using EFV and dual-NRTI combinations (ABC, didanosine [ddI], stavudine [d4T], TDF, or zidovudine [ZDV] together with FTC or 3TC), the regimens show durable virologic activity, although responses vary depending on the dual-NRTI combination chosen (see Dual-Nucleoside Reverse Transcriptase Inhibitor Options). EFV is formulated both as a single-drug tablet and in a fixed-dose combination tablet of EFV/TDF/FTC that allows for once daily dosing. EFV/TDF/FTC is currently a preferred initial treatment regimen **(AI)**.

Alternative Non-Nucleoside Reverse Transcriptase Inhibitor-Based Regimens

Rilpivirine (RPV). In two large, multinational, randomized, double-blind clinical trials, RPV (25 mg once daily) was compared with EFV (600 mg once daily), each agent in combination with two NRTIs. In a pooled analysis of the 2 studies, 76% of RPV-treated subjects and 77% of EFV-treated subjects had plasma HIV RNA <50 copies/mL at 96 weeks.[23] Although RPV demonstrated non-inferiority to EFV overall, in participants with higher pretreatment HIV RNA (>100,000 copies/mL), virologic failure occurred more frequently in those randomized to receive RPV. Moreover, more subjects with pre-treatment CD4 count <200 cells/mm[3], regardless of baseline HIV RNA, experienced virologic failure than those with pre-ART CD4 count ≥200 cells/mm[3]. Subjects with virologic failure on RPV were also more likely to have genotypic resistance to other NNRTIs (i.e., EFV, ETR, and NVP) and to have TDF- and/or 3TC/FTC-associated genotypic resistance.

Drug discontinuations because of adverse effects were more common with EFV than with RPV. The frequency of depressive disorders and discontinuations due to depressive disorders were similar between the two arms, whereas dizziness, abnormal dreams, rash, and hyperlipidemia were more frequent with EFV than with RPV.

At higher than the approved dose of 25 mg, RPV (75 mg once daily or 300 mg once daily) may prolong the QTc interval. As a result, RPV should be used cautiously when co-administered with a drug that has a known risk of torsades de pointes. Although RPV has shown no teratogenicity in animal studies, data on PKs and safety of RPV in pregnant HIV-infected women are insufficient at this time.

RPV is formulated both as an individual tablet and in a fixed-dose combination tablet of RPV/TDF/FTC. The latter allows for one-tablet once-daily dosing. RPV must be administered with a meal. Because the oral bioavailability of RPV may be significantly reduced in the presence of acid-lowering agents, RPV should be used with caution with antacids and H2-receptor antagonists. RPV use with proton pump inhibitors (PPIs) is contraindicated. Table 15b provides guidance on the timing of RPV administration when the agent is used with antacids or H2 receptor antagonists.

In patients with high pretreatment viral load (HIV RNA >100,000 copies/mL) or low CD4 cell count (<200 cells/mm[3]), RPV has less virologic activity and a higher rate of resistance at virologic failure than EFV. The panel recommends RPV/TDF/FTC as an alternative regimen for initial therapy, which should only be used in patients with pre-treatment HIV RNA < 100,000 copies/mL **(BI)**. RPV should not be used in patients with plasma HIV RNA >100,000 copies/mL.

Other Non-Nucleoside Reverse Transcriptase Inhibitor-Based Regimens

Nevirapine (NVP). The 2NN trial compared NVP with EFV, both given d4T and 3TC, in ART-naive patients. In this trial, 65% of participants in the twice-daily NVP arm and 70% in the EFV arm achieved virologic suppression (defined as HIV RNA <50 copies/mL) at 48 weeks. This difference did not reach criteria necessary to demonstrate non-inferiority of NVP.[27] Two deaths were attributed to NVP use: one from fulminant hepatitis and one from staphylococcal sepsis as a complication of Stevens-Johnson syndrome (SJS).

In the ARTEN trial, ART-naive participants were randomized to NVP 200 mg twice daily or 400 mg once daily, or to RTV-boosted ATV (ATV/r), all in combination with TDF/FTC. The proportion of participants in each arm who achieved the primary endpoint of having at least two consecutive plasma HIV RNA levels <50 copies/mL before Week 48 was similar (66.8% of NVP participants vs. 65.3% of ATV/r participants). However, more participants in the NVP arms than in the ATV/r arm discontinued study drugs before Week 48 because of adverse events (13.6% on NVP vs. 2.6% on ATV/r) or lack of efficacy (8.4% on NVP vs. 1.6% on ATV/r). NNRTI- and/or NRTI-resistance mutations were selected in 29 of 44 (65.9%) participants who experienced virologic failure while on NVP, whereas resistance mutations were not detected in any of the 28 participants who had virologic failure on ATV/r.[35]

Serious hepatic events have been observed when NVP was initiated in ART-naive patients. These events generally occur within the first few weeks of treatment. In addition to experiencing elevated serum transaminases, approximately half of the patients also develop skin rash, with or without fever or flu-like symptoms. Some events, particularly those with rash and other systemic symptoms, have progressed to liver failure. Retrospective analysis of reported events suggests that women with higher CD4 counts appear to be at highest risk for serious hepatic events.[36, 37] A 12-fold higher incidence of symptomatic hepatic events was seen in women with CD4 counts >250 cells/mm^3 at the time of NVP initiation than in women with CD4 counts ≤250 cells/mm^3 at NVP initiation (11.0% vs. 0.9%, respectively). The risk was also greater in men with pre-treatment CD4 counts >400 cells/mm^3 than in with men with pre-treatment CD4 counts ≤400 cells/mm^3 (6.3% vs. 1.2%, respectively). Most of these patients had no identifiable underlying hepatic abnormalities. In some cases, hepatic injuries continued to progress despite discontinuation of NVP.[37, 38] In contrast, other studies have not shown an association between baseline CD4 counts and severe NVP hepatotoxicity.[39, 40] Symptomatic hepatic events have not been reported in mothers or infants given single-dose NVP to prevent perinatal HIV infection.

On the basis of the safety and efficacy data discussed above, the Panel classifies NVP-based combinations in the Other NNRTI-Based Regimens category as initial therapy in women with pretreatment CD4 counts ≤250 cells/mm^3 or in men with pretreatment CD4 counts ≤400 cells/mm^3 **(C)**. Patients whose CD4 count increases to levels above these thresholds as a result of NVP-containing therapy can safely continue therapy without an increased risk of adverse hepatic events.[41]

NVP should be initiated at a dosage of 200 mg once daily for a 14-day lead-in period before being increased to the maintenance dosage of 400 mg per day (as an extended-release 400 mg tablet once daily or 200 mg immediate-release tablet twice daily). The lead-in period has been observed to decrease the incidence of rash. Some experts recommend monitoring serum transaminases at baseline, at 2 weeks, again 2 weeks after dose escalation, and then monthly for the first 18 weeks. Clinical and laboratory parameters should be assessed at each patient visit.

Protease Inhibitor-Based Regimens

Summary: Protease Inhibitor-Based Regimens

PI-based regimens (particularly with RTV-boosting) have demonstrated virologic potency and durability in treatment-naive subjects. In contrast to NNRTI- and INSTI-based regimens, few or no PI mutations are detected in patients who developed virologic failure on their first PI-based regimen.[35, 42] Each PI has its own virologic potency, adverse effect profile, and pharmacokinetic (PK) properties. The characteristics, advantages, and disadvantages of each PI are listed in Table 6 and Appendix B, Table 3. When selecting a boosted PI-based regimen for an ART-naive patient, clinicians should consider factors such as dosing frequency, food requirements, pill burden, daily RTV dose, drug interaction potential, toxicity profile of the individual PI, and baseline lipid profile and pregnancy status of the patient. See the *Perinatal Guidelines* for specific recommendations in pregnancy.[34]

A number of metabolic abnormalities, including dyslipidemia and insulin resistance, have been associated with PI use. The currently available PIs differ in their propensity to cause these metabolic complications, which also depends on the dose of RTV used as a PK boosting agent. Two large observational cohort studies suggest that LPV/r, indinavir (IDV), fosamprenavir (FPV), or RTV-boosted FPV (FPV/r) may be associated with increased rates of myocardial infarction (MI) or stroke.[43, 44] This association was not seen with ATV.[45] These studies had too few patients receiving DRV/r to be included in the analysis.

RTV-boosted saquinavir (SQV/r) can prolong the PR and QT intervals on electrocardiogram (ECG). The degree of QT prolongation seen with SQV/r is greater than that seen with some other boosted PIs. Therefore, SQV/r should be used with caution in patients with underlying heart conditions such as heart rate or rhythm problems, or who use concomitant drugs that may increase the risk of developing these ECG abnormalities.[46] SQV/r is rarely used for initial therapy for this reason, and because, when compared with other PI-based regimens, the regimen has a higher pill burden and no clear advantages.

The potent inhibitory effect of RTV on the cytochrome P (CYP) 450 3A isoenzyme allows the addition of low-dose RTV to other PIs as a PK enhancer to increase drug exposure and prolong the plasma half-life of the active PI. The drawbacks associated with this strategy are the potential for increased risk of hyperlipidemia and a greater potential of drug-drug interactions from the addition of RTV. RTV boosting is recommended in all PI-based regimens whenever possible; when boosting is not possible and a PI-based regimen is desired, only ATV should be used. In patients without pre-existing PI resistance, once-daily boosted PI regimens that use only 100 mg of RTV per day are preferred. These regimens tend to cause fewer gastrointestinal (GI) side effects and less metabolic toxicity than regimens that use RTV at a dose of 200 mg per day.

The Panel uses the following criteria to distinguish between preferred, alternative, and other PIs for use in ART-naive patients:

*   Demonstrated superior or non-inferior virologic efficacy when compared with at least one other PI-based regimen, based on, at least, published 48-week data
*   RTV-boosted PI using no more than 100 mg of RTV per day
*   Once-daily dosing
*   Low pill count
*   Good tolerability.

Using these criteria, the Panel recommends once-daily ATV/r and DRV/r as preferred PIs.

Preferred Protease Inhibitor-Based Regimens

In alphabetical order, by active PI component

Ritonavir-Boosted Atazanavir (ATV/r). In a clinical trial, ATV/r enhanced ATV concentrations and improved virologic activity more than unboosted ATV.[47] The CASTLE study compared once-daily ATV/r with twice-daily LPV/r, each in combination with TDF/FTC, in 883 ARV-naive participants. In this open-label, noninferiority study, the two regimens showed similar virologic and CD4 responses at 48 weeks[48] and at 96 weeks.[49] More hyperbilirubinemia and less GI toxicity were seen in the ATV/r arm than in the LPV/r arm. This study supports the designation of ATV/r + TDF/FTC as a preferred PI-based regimen (**AI**).

The main adverse effect associated with ATV/r is indirect hyperbilirubinemia, with or without jaundice or scleral icterus, but without concomitant hepatic transaminase elevations. Nephrolithiasis[50-52] and cholelithiasis[53] also have been reported in patients who received ATV. ATV/r requires acidic gastric pH for dissolution. Thus, concomitant use of drugs that raise gastric pH (e.g., antacids, H2 antagonists, and particularly PPIs), may impair absorption of ATV. Table 15a provides recommendations for use of ATV/r with these agents.

Ritonavir-Boosted Darunavir (DRV/r). The ARTEMIS study compared DRV/r (800/100 mg once daily) with LPV/r (once or twice daily), both in combination with TDF/FTC, in a randomized, open-label, non-inferiority trial. The study enrolled 689 ART-naive participants. DRV/r was non-inferior to LPV/r at 48 weeks[54], and superior at week 192.[55] In participants with baseline HIV RNA levels >100,000 copies/mL, virologic response rates were lower in the LPV/r arm than in the DRV/r arm. Grades 2 to 4 adverse events, primarily diarrhea, were seen more frequently in LPV/r recipients than in DRV/r recipients. At virologic failure, no major PI mutations were detected in participants randomized to either arm.[42, 55] Based on these data, the Panel recommends DRV/r + TDF/FTC as a preferred PI-based regimen (**AI**). No randomized controlled trial to evaluate the efficacy of DRV/r with other 2-NRTI combinations exists. A small retrospective study suggested that DRV/r plus ABC/3TC may be effective in treatment-naive patients for up to 48 weeks.[56] Based on this preliminary information, the Panel recommends this combination as an alternative PI-based regimen **(BIII)**.

Alternative Protease Inhibitor-Based Regimens

In alphabetical order, by active PI component

Ritonavir-Boosted Fosamprenavir (FPV/r, once or twice daily). FPV/r is an alternative PI. The KLEAN trial compared twice-daily FPV/r with LPV/r, each in combination with ABC and 3TC, in ART-naive patients. At Weeks 48 and 144, similar percentages of subjects achieved viral loads <400 copies/mL.[57, 58] The frequency and severity of adverse events did not differ between the regimens. Twice-daily FPV/r was non-inferior to twice-daily LPV/r. Based on the preference for once-daily regimens with no more than 100 mg/day of RTV, twice-daily FPV is considered an alternative choice.

A comparative trial of once-daily FPV/r (1400/100 mg) and once-daily ATV/r, both in combination with TDF/FTC, was conducted in 106 ARV-naive participants.[59] The regimens showed similar virologic and CD4 benefits. The study's small sample size precludes the assessment of superior or non-inferior virologic efficacy required for a preferred PI. Collectively, FPV/r regimens, with once- or twice-daily dosing, are recommended as alternative PI-based regimens.

Ritonavir-Boosted Lopinavir (LPV/r, coformulated). LPV/r is the only available coformulated boosted PI. It can be given once or twice daily. However, because LPV/r must be boosted with 200 mg/day of RTV and is associated with higher rates of GI side effects and hyperlipidemia than other PIs boosted with 100 mg of RTV, LPV/r is recommended as an alternative PI for ART-naive patients. A 7-year follow-up study of LPV/r and 2 NRTIs showed sustained virologic suppression in patients who were maintained on the originally assigned regimen.[60] Results of clinical trials that compared LPV/r with ATV/r, DRV/r, FPV/r, or SQV/r are discussed in the related sections of this document. The ACTG 5142 study showed that, when compared with EFV plus 2 NRTIs, the regimen of twice-daily LPV/r plus 2 NRTIs had decreased virologic efficacy. However, the CD4 response was greater with LPV/r, and there was less drug resistance associated with virologic failure.[4]

In addition to diarrhea, major adverse effects of LPV/r include insulin resistance and hyperlipidemia, especially hypertriglyceridemia; these required pharmacologic management in some patients. In the D:A:D and French observational cohorts, cumulative use of LPV/r was associated with a slightly increased risk of MI.[43, 44] Once-daily LPV/r should not be used in patients who have HIV mutations associated with PI resistance, because higher LPV trough levels may be required to suppress resistant virus. Once-daily dosing should not be used in pregnant women, especially during the third trimester, when LPV levels are expected to decline. For more detailed information regarding ART drug choices and related issues in pregnancy, see the *Perinatal Guidelines*.[34]

Other Protease Inhibitor-Based Regimens

Atazanavir (ATV). In a clinical trial, ATV concentrations were enhanced with the addition of RTV 100 mg when compared to once-daily unboosted ATV, as a result, better virologic activity was seen with ATV/r.[47] Nevertheless, unboosted ATV may be selected for some patients because it has fewer GI adverse effects including less hyperbilirubinemia and less impact on lipid profiles than ATV/r. Three studies compared unboosted ATV-based combination regimens with either NFV- or EFV-based regimens. These studies established that ATV 400 mg once daily and both comparator treatments had similar virologic efficacy in ARV-naive patients after 48 weeks of therapy.[5, 47, 61, 62] In a multinational randomized trial comparing three initial treatment strategies, unboosted ATV + ddI + FTC was inferior to both EFV + TDF/FTC and EFV + ZDV/3TC.[63]

Unboosted ATV may be used as initial therapy when a once-daily regimen without RTV is desired and in patients with underlying risk factors that indicate that hyperlipidemia may be particularly undesirable (C). However, in these situations, other NNRTI- and INSTI-based regimens should generally be used instead of unboosted ATV. When ATV is co-administered with TDF or EFV, it should be boosted with RTV because ATV concentrations are reduced in the presence of these drugs. ATV requires acidic gastric pH for dissolution. Thus, concomitant use of drugs that raise gastric pH (such as antacids, H2 antagonists, and PPIs) may significantly impair ATV absorption. PPIs should not be used in patients who are taking unboosted ATV. H2 antagonists and antacids should be used with caution and with careful dose separation (see Tables 14 and 15a).

Ritonavir-Boosted Saquinavir (SQV/r). The GEMINI study compared SQV/r (1000/100 mg twice daily) and LPV/r, both given twice daily, in combination with TDF/FTC given once daily, in 337 ART-naive participants who were monitored over 48 weeks. Levels of viral suppression and increases in CD4 counts were similar in both arms of the study.[64] Triglyceride (TG) levels were higher in the LPV/r arm than in the SQV/r arm. The SQV/r regimen has a higher pill burden and requires twice-daily dosing and 200 mg of RTV. In a healthy volunteer study, SQV/r use at the recommended dose was associated with increases in both QT and PR intervals. The degree of QT prolongation with SQV/r was greater than that seen with some other boosted PIs used at their recommended doses. Rare cases of torsades de pointes and complete heart block have been reported in post-marketing surveillance. Based on these findings, an ECG before initiation of SQV/r is recommended. SQV/r is not recommended for patients with any of the following conditions: documented congenital or acquired QT prolongation, pretreatment QT interval of >450 milliseconds (msec), refractory hypokalemia or hypomagnesemia, complete atrioventricular (AV) block without implanted pacemakers, at risk of complete AV block, or receiving other drugs that prolong QT interval.[46] On the basis of these restrictions, and because several other preferred or alternative PI options are available, the Panel recommends that, although SQV/r may be acceptable, it should be used with caution in select ARV-naive patients (C).

Integrase Strand Transfer Inhibitor (INSTI)-Based Regimens

Preferred Integrase Strand Transfer Inhibitor-Based Regimen

Raltegravir (RAL). RAL is an INSTI that is approved for use in ART-naive patients on the basis of results of STARTMRK, a Phase III study that compared RAL (400 mg twice daily) and EFV (600 mg once daily), each in combination with TDF/FTC, in ART-naive subjects. This multinational, double-blind, placebo-controlled study enrolled 563 subjects with plasma viral loads >5,000 copies/mL. At Week 48, similar percentages of subjects in both groups achieved viral loads <50 copies/mL (86.1% and 81.9% for RAL and EFV, respectively, P <0.001 for non-inferiority). CD4 counts rose by 189 cells/mm^3 in the RAL group and 163 cells/mm^3 in the EFV group. The frequency of serious adverse events was similar in both groups.[6] At 156 weeks, virologic and immunologic responses remained similar in both groups with no new safety concerns identified.[65] On the basis of these data, the Panel recommends RAL + TDF/FTC as a preferred regimen in ART-naive patients (AI). In a small single-arm pilot study of 35 subjects who received a regimen of RAL + ABC/3TC, 91% of subjects had viral loads <50 copies/mL at Week 48.[66] On the basis of these preliminary data, RAL + ABC/3TC may be used as an alternative INSTI-based regimen (BIII). RAL use has been associated with creatine kinase elevations. Myositis and rhabdomyolysis have been reported. Rare cases of severe skin reactions and systemic hypersensitivity reactions (HSRs) in patients who received RAL have been reported during post-marketing surveillance.[67]

Comparisons of RAL-based regimens and boosted PI-based regimens in ART-naive subjects have not been reported. RAL must be administered twice daily a potential disadvantage when comparing RAL-based treatment with some other regimens. RAL, like EFV, has a lower genetic barrier to resistance than RTV-boosted PIs. In the STARTMRK comparative trial, resistance mutations were observed with approximately the same frequency in RAL- and EFV-treated participants.

Alternative Integrase Strand Transfer Inhibitor-Based Regimen

Elvitegravir (EVG). EVG is an INSTI available as a fixed-dose combination product with cobicistat (COBI), TDF, and FTC (EVG/COBI/TDF/FTC), and is approved as a single-tablet, once-daily regimen for ART-naive patients. EVG is metabolized primarily by CYP3A enzymes; as a result, CYP3A inducers or inhibitors may alter EVG concentrations. COBI is a specific, potent CYP3A inhibitor with no activity against HIV. It acts as a PK enhancer of EVG, which allows for once daily dosing of the combination product.[68] EVG/COBI/TDF/FTC is not recommended for patients with pre-treatment estimated creatinine clearance less than 70 mL/min.[69] For more information on PK enhancement with RTV or COBI, see Drug-Drug Interactions   Pharmacokinetic Enhancing.

In two Phase 3 randomized clinical studies, the safety and efficacy of this combination regimen in ART-naive HIV-infected subjects was compared to that of two currently recommended first-line regimens. Co-formulated EVG/COBI/TDF/FTC was non-inferior to co-formulated EFV/TDF/FTC: 87.6% of the EVG/COBI/TDF/FTC-treated subjects versus 84.1% of the EFV/TDF/FTC-treated subjects achieved virologic suppression <50 copies/mL at 48 weeks (difference 3.5%, 95% CI -1.6, 8.8).[15] Similarly, EVG/COBI/TDF/FTC was non-inferior to ATV/r plus co-formulated TDF/FTC: 89.5% versus 86.8% of subjects achieved virologic suppression <50 copies/mL at 48 weeks, respectively (difference 3%, 95% CI - 1.9, 7.8).[70] Rates of virologic failure were low and comparable across study arms, with non-inferior results for treatment arms maintained at 96 weeks.[71, 72] At virologic failure, INSTI-associated mutations were detected in some EVG/COBI/TDF/FTC-treated patients who failed therapy.[15, 70] These mutations conferred varying degrees of cross-resistance to RAL. The most common adverse events reported with EVG/COBI/TDF/FTC were diarrhea, nausea, and headache.

COBI inhibits active tubular secretion of creatinine, resulting in increases in serum creatinine and a reduction in estimated creatinine clearance (CrCl) without reducing glomerular function.[73] Although the overall incidence of study drug discontinuation due to adverse events was lower in the EVG/COBI/TDF/FTC arms (3.7%) than in either comparator arm (5.1% each), more subjects in the EVG/COBI/TDF/FTC arms (8 subjects) discontinued study drugs because of renal adverse events than in the comparator arms (one in the ATV/r + TDF/FTC arm). Four of the eight subjects in the EVG/COBI/TDF/FTC arms who discontinued study drug had evidence of proximal tubular dysfunction; after drug discontinuation, abnormal lab values in these four patients improved but did not completely resolve. CrCl, urine glucose and urine protein should be assessed before starting therapy and monitored during therapy. Consideration should be given to periodic monitoring of serum phosphorus in patients at risk for renal impairment. Although COBI may cause modest increases in serum creatinine and modest declines in CrCl, patients who experience a confirmed increase in serum creatinine of greater than 0.4 mg/dL from baseline should be closely monitored and evaluated for evidence of tubulopathy. Proteinuria, normoglycemic glycosuria, and increased fractional excretion of phosphorous may represent the first signs of tubulopathy and precede any decline in renal function. Patients on EVG/COBI/TDF/FTC should be switched to an alternative ARV regimen if estimated CrCl decreases to less than 50 mL/min. Concomitant use of nephrotoxic drugs should be avoided.

In summary, EVG/COBI/FTC/TDF has rates of virologic suppression comparable to two currently preferred regimens. As a co-formulated tablet, it can be given as one tablet, once daily. Limitations of this combination include a possible increased risk of proximal renal tubulopathy in addition to inhibition of active tubular secretion of creatinine, significant drug-drug interactions, limited data in patients with advanced HIV disease and in women, and food requirement. On the basis of these factors, the Panel recommends EVG/COBI/FTC/TDF as an alternative regimen in ART-naive patients **(BI)**.

CCR5 Antagonist-Based Regimens

Maraviroc (MVC). The MERIT study compared the CCR5 antagonist MVC with EFV, both in combination with ZDV/3TC, in a randomized, double-blind trial in ART-naive participants.[7] Only participants who had

CCR5-tropic virus and no evidence of resistance to any drugs used in the study were enrolled (n 721). At 48 weeks, HIV RNA level <50 copies/mL was observed in 65.3% of MVC recipients and 69.3% of EFV recipients. The HIV RNA <50 copies/mL results did not meet the criteria set by the investigators to demonstrate noninferiority for MVC in this study. CD4 count increased by an average of 170 cells/mm^3 in the MVC arm and by 144 cells/mm^3 in the EFV arm. Through 48 weeks, compared with participants receiving EFV, more participants discontinued MVC because of lack of efficacy (11.9% vs. 4.2%), whereas fewer participants discontinued MVC because of toxicity (4.2% vs. 13.6%). Follow-up results at 96 weeks demonstrated durable responses for both ARVs.[74] In a post-hoc reanalysis using a more sensitive viral tropism assay, 15% of patients with dual/mixed tropic virus at screening virus were excluded from analysis. Their retrospective exclusion resulted in similar virologic suppression in both arms. Because MVC requires twice-daily dosing and requires a tropism assay before use, and experience with regimens other than ZDV/3TC is limited, the Panel recommends MVC + ZDV/3TC as another option for use in ART-naive patients **(CI)**. Although ZDV/3TC was used as the NRTI backbone in the MERIT trial, pending further data, many clinicians favor the combination of MVC with TDF/FTC or ABC/3TC **(CIII)**.

Dual-Nucleoside Reverse Transcriptase Inhibitor Options as Part of Initial Combination Therapy

Summary: Dual-Nucleoside Reverse Transcriptase Inhibitor Components

Dual NRTIs are commonly used in combination with an NNRTI, a PI (usually boosted with RTV), an INSTI, or a CCR5 antagonist. Most dual-NRTI combinations used in clinical practice consist of a primary NRTI plus 3TC or FTC. Both 3TC and FTC have few adverse effects but may select for the M184V resistance mutation, which confers high-level resistance to both drugs; a modest decrease in susceptibility to ddI and ABC; and improved susceptibility to ZDV, d4T, and TDF.[75]

All NRTIs except ddI can be taken with or without food. Adherence may be additionally improved with once-daily dosing (available for all NRTIs except d4T and ZDV) and with fixed-dosage combinations, such as ABC/3TC, TDF/FTC (with or without EFV, RPV, or EVG/COBI), or ZDV/3TC.

The Panel's recommendations on specific dual-NRTI options are made on the basis of virologic potency and durability, short- and long-term toxicities, the propensity to select for resistance mutations, and dosing convenience.

Preferred Dual-Nucleoside Reverse Transcriptase Inhibitors

Tenofovir/Emtricitabine (TDF/FTC, co-formulated). TDF is a nucleotide analog with potent activity against both HIV and hepatitis B virus (HBV) and a long intracellular half-life that allows for once-daily dosing. The fixed-dose combinations of TDF/FTC, EFV/TDF/FTC, RPV/TDF/FTC, and EVG/COBI/TDF/FTC are administered as one tablet, once daily and are designed to improve adherence.

TDF, when used with either 3TC or FTC as part of an EFV-based regimen in ART-naive patients, demonstrated potent virologic suppression[26] and was superior to ZDV/3TC in virologic efficacy up to 144 weeks.[76] In the 934 study, more participants in the ZDV/3TC arm than in the TDF/FTC arm developed loss of limb fat (as assessed by dual-energy x-ray absorptiometry [DXA]) and anemia at 96 and 144 weeks.[76] Emergence of the M184V mutation was less frequent with TDF/FTC than with ZDV/3TC, and by 144 weeks of therapy no participant had developed the K65R mutation. TDF + FTC or 3TC has also been studied in combination with RPV, several boosted PIs, EVG/COBI, and RAL in randomized clinical trials; all trials demonstrate good virologic benefit.[6, 15, 48, 54, 59, 70, 77]

TDF/FTC was compared with ABC/3TC in the ACTG 5202 study[8] and the HEAT trial.[10] In the ACTG 5202 trial, inferior virologic responses were observed in participants randomized to ABC/3TC who had a pretreatment HIV RNA >100,000 copies/mL. This was not observed in the HEAT trial or in other trials (see the ABC/3TC section below for more detailed discussion).

Renal impairment, manifested by increases in serum creatinine, proteinuria, glycosuria, hypophosphatemia, proximal renal tubulopathy, and acute tubular necrosis, has been associated with TDF use.[78, 79] Risk factors may include advanced HIV disease, longer treatment history, and pre-existing renal impairment.[80] In the HEAT trial, 15% of subjects receiving TDF/FTC versus 10% of those receiving ABC/3TC progressed to a more advanced stage of chronic kidney disease (CKD) on treatment.[10] Renal function, urinalysis, and electrolytes should be monitored in patients who are on TDF. In patients who have some degree of pre-existing renal insufficiency (CrCl <50 mL/min), TDF dosage adjustment is required (see Appendix B, Table 7 for dosage recommendations). However, in this setting, the use of alternative NRTIs (for example, ABC) may be preferred over dose-adjusted TDF because available dosage adjustment guidelines for renal dysfunction are based on PK studies only and not on safety and efficacy data.

Concomitant use of boosted PIs and COBI can increase TDF concentrations, and studies have suggested a greater risk of renal dysfunction when TDF is used in PI- and COBI-based regimens.[69, 78, 81-84] TDF has been used in combination with PIs without significant renal toxicity in several clinical trials that involved patients who had CrCl >50 mL/min to 60 mL/min.[49, 85] Furthermore, in two randomized studies comparing TDF/FTC with ABC/3TC, participants receiving TDF/FTC experienced a significantly greater decline in bone mineral density than ABC/3TC-treated participants.[11, 86]

TDF plus FTC is the preferred NRTI combination, especially in HIV/HBV-coinfected patients because these drugs have activity against both viruses. The use of a single HBV-active NRTI (e.g., 3TC or FTC) can lead to HBV resistance and is not recommended (see HIV/Hepatitis B Co-infection).

Alternative Dual Nucleoside Reverse Transcriptase Inhibitors

Abacavir/Lamivudine (ABC/3TC, co-formulated) for patients who test negative for HLA-B*5701. In a comparative trial of ABC/3TC and ZDV/3TC (both given twice daily and combined with EFV), participants in both arms achieved similar virologic responses. CD4 T-cell increase at 48 weeks was greater in the ABC-treated participants than in the ZDV-treated participants.[87] The ACTG 5202 study, a randomized controlled trial in more than 1,800 participants, evaluated the efficacy and safety of ABC/3TC and TDF/FTC when used in combination with either EFV or RTV-boosted ATV. Treatment randomization was stratified on the basis of a screening HIV RNA of <100,000 copies/mL or ≥100,000 copies/mL. HLA-B*5701 testing was not required before study entry, which may have influenced the results of the trial with respect to some of the safety and tolerability endpoints. A Data Safety Monitoring Board recommended early termination of the ≥100,000 copies/mL stratification group because of a significantly shorter time to study-defined virologic failure in the ABC/3TC arm than in the TDF/FTC arm.[8] This difference in time to virologic failure between arms was observed regardless of whether the third active drug was EFV or ATV/r. There was no difference between ABC/3TC and TDF/FTC in time to virologic failure for participants who had plasma HIV RNA <100,000 copies/mL at screening.[88]

In the HEAT study, 688 participants received ABC/3TC or TDF/FTC in combination with once-daily LPV/r. A subgroup analysis according to baseline HIV RNA <100,000 copies/mL or ≥100,000 copies/mL yielded similar percentages of participants with HIV RNA <50 copies/mL at 96 weeks in the two regimens (63% vs. 58% in those with HIV RNA <100,000 copies/mL and 56% vs. 58% in those with ≥100,000 copies/mL).[10] The ASSERT study compared open label ABC/3TC with TDF/FTC in 385 HLA-B*5701-negative, ART-naive patients; all study subjects also received EFV. At 48 weeks, the proportion of participants with HIV RNA <50 copies/mL was lower among ABC/3TC-treated subjects (59%) than among TDF/FTC subjects (71%) (difference 11.6%, 95% confidence interval [CI], 2.2–21.1).[9]

Clinically suspected HSRs have been observed in 5% to 8% of patients who start ABC. The risk of this reaction is highly associated with the presence of the HLA-B*5701 allele (see HLA-B*5701 Screening).[89, 90] HLA-B*5701 testing should precede use of ABC. ABC should not be given to patients who test positive for HLA-B*5701 and, on the basis of test results, ABC hypersensitivity should be noted on the patient's allergy list. Patients who test HLA-B*5701 negative are less likely to experience an HSR, but they should be counseled about the symptoms of the reaction. Patients who discontinue ABC for suspected HSR should never be rechallenged, regardless of HLA-B*5701 status.

An association between ABC use and MI was first reported in the D:A:D study. This large, multinational observational study group found that recent (within 6 months) or current use of ABC, but not TDF, was associated with an increased risk of MI, particularly in participants with pre-existing cardiac risk factors.[43, 91] Since the report of this study, multiple studies have explored this association. Some studies have found an association;[92-95] others have found a weak association or no association.[44, 96-99] Several studies have also been conducted to evaluate potential mechanistic pathways that may underlie the association between ABC use and an increased risk of MI, including endothelial dysfunction, increased platelet reactivity, leukocyte adhesion, inflammation, and hypercoagulability.[100-107] However, to date, no consensus on the association between ABC use and MI risk or the mechanism for such an association has been reached.

The fixed-dose combination of ABC/3TC allows for once-daily dosing. Pending additional data, ABC/3TC should be used with caution in individuals who have plasma HIV RNA levels ≥100,000 copies/mL and in persons at high risk of CVD. However, the combination of ABC/3TC remains an alternative dual-NRTI option for some ART-naive patients **(BI)**.

Other Dual Nucleoside Reverse Transcriptase Inhibitors

Zidovudine/Lamivudine (ZDV/3TC, coformulated). The dual-NRTI combination of ZDV/3TC has extensive durability, safety, and tolerability experience.[3, 5, 108-112] In a multinational, randomized trial comparing three initial treatment strategies, EFV/ZDV/3TC and EFV/TDF/FTC showed similar virologic efficacy; both regimens were superior to ATV/ddI/FTC.[63]

A fixed-dose combination of ZDV/3TC is available for one-tablet, twice-daily dosing. Selection of the 3TC-associated M184V mutation has been associated with increased susceptibility to ZDV. In a comparative trial of ABC/3TC and ZDV/3TC (both given twice daily and combined with EFV), the CD4 count increase was greater in the ABC/3TC-treated patients than in the ZDV/3TC-treated patients,[87] even though virologic responses were similar in both arms.

Bone marrow suppression, manifested by macrocytic anemia and/or neutropenia, is seen in some patients. ZDV also is associated with GI toxicity, fatigue, and possibly mitochondrial toxicity, including lactic acidosis/hepatic steatosis and lipoatrophy. Because ZDV/3TC has greater toxicity than TDF/FTC or ABC/3TC and requires twice-daily dosing, the Panel classifies ZDV/3TC in the Other Dual-NRTI category, rather than as a preferred or alternative, dual-NRTI option **(CI)**.

ZDV/3TC remains as a preferred NRTI option in pregnant women because the two drugs have the most PK, safety, and efficacy data for both mother and newborn of any other ARVs. For more detailed information regarding ARV drug choices and related issues in pregnancy, see the *Perinatal Guidelines*.[34]

Nucleoside Reverse Transcriptase Inhibitors (NRTIs) and Hepatitis B Virus (HBV). Three of the currently approved NRTIs   FTC, 3TC, and TDF   have activity against HBV. Most HIV/HBV-coinfected patients should use coformulated TDF/FTC (or TDF + 3TC) as their NRTI backbone to provide additional activity against HBV and to avoid selection of HBV mutation that confers resistance to 3TC and FTC. Importantly, patients who have HIV/HBV coinfection may be at risk of acute exacerbation of hepatitis after initiation or discontinuation of TDF, 3TC, or FTC.[113-115] Thus, these patients should be monitored closely for clinical or chemical hepatitis if these drugs are initiated or discontinued (see HIV/Hepatitis B Coinfection and Initiating Antiretroviral Therapy).

Table 6. Advantages and Disadvantages of Antiretroviral Components Recommended as Initial Antiretroviral Therapy (page 1 of 4)

ARV Class	ARV Agent(s)	Advantages	Disadvantages
NNRTIs (in alphabetical order)		**NNRTI Class Advantages:** • Long half-lives	**NNRTI Class Disadvantages:** • Greater risk of resistance at the time of treatment failure than with PIs • Potential for cross resistance • Skin rash • Potential for CYP450 drug interactions (see Tables 14, 15b, and 16b) • Transmitted resistance more common than with PIs.
	EFV	• Virologic responses non-inferior or superior to most comparators to date • Once-daily dosing • Coformulated with TDF/FTC	• Neuropsychiatric side effects • Teratogenic in nonhuman primates. Several cases of neural tube defect in infants born to women who were exposed to EFV in the first trimester of pregnancy have been reported. • Dyslipidemia
	NVP	• No food requirement • Fewer lipid effects than EFV • Once-daily dosing with extended-release tablet formulation	• Higher incidence of rash, including rare but serious HSRs (SJS or TEN), than with other NNRTIs • Higher incidence of hepatotoxicity, including serious and even fatal cases of hepatic necrosis, than with other NNRTIs • Contraindicated in patients with moderate or severe (Child-Pugh B or C) hepatic impairment • ART-naive patients with high pre-treatment CD4 counts (>250 cells/mm^3 for females, >400 cells/mm^3 for males) are at higher risk of symptomatic hepatic events. NVP is not recommended in these patients unless the benefit clearly outweighs the risk. • Early virologic failure of NVP + TDF + (FTC or 3TC) in small clinical trials

	RPV	• Once-daily dosing
		• Co-formulated with TDF/FTC
		• Smaller pill size than co-formulated TDF/FTC/EFV or TDF/FTC/EVG/COBI
		• Compared with EFV:
		  • Fewer discontinuations for CNS adverse effects
		  • Fewer lipid effects
		  • Fewer rashes
		  • Smaller pill size
			• Not recommended for use in patients with pre-ART HIV RNA >100,000 copies/mL because the rate of virologic failures is higher in these patients
			• Higher rate of virologic failures observed in patients with pre-ART CD4 count < 200 cells/mm^3
			• More NNRTI-, TDF-, and 3TC-associated mutations at virological failure than with regimen containing EFV + two NRTIs
			• Meal requirement
			• Absorption depends on lower gastric pH (see Table 15a for detailed information regarding interactions with H2 antagonists and antacids).
			• Contraindicated with PPIs
			• RPV-associated depression reported
			• Use RPV with caution when co-administered with a drug having a known risk of torsades de pointes.

Table 6. Advantages and Disadvantages of Antiretroviral Components Recommended as Initial Antiretroviral Therapy (page 2 of 4)

ARV Class	ARV Agent(s)	Advantages	Disadvantages
PIs (in alphabetical order)		**PI Class Advantages:** • Higher genetic barrier to resistance than NNRTIs and RAL • PI resistance at the time of treatment failure uncommon with RTV-boosted PIs	**PI Class Disadvantages:** • Metabolic complications such as dyslipidemia, insulin resistance, and hepatotoxicity • GI adverse effects • CYP3A4 inhibitors and substrates: potential for drug interactions—more pronounced with RTV-based regimens (see Tables 14 and 15a)
	ATV (unboosted)	• Fewer adverse effects on lipids than other PIs • Once-daily dosing • Low pill burden • Good GI tolerability • Signature mutation (I50L) not associated with broad PI cross resistance	• Indirect hyperbilirubinemia sometimes leading to jaundice or scleral icterus • PR interval prolongation, which is generally inconsequential unless ATV is combined with another drug that has a similar effect. • Unboosted ATV should not be co-administered with TDF, EFV, or NVP (see ATV/r). • Nephrolithiasis, cholelithiasis • Skin rash • Food requirement • Absorption depends on food and low gastric pH (see Table 15a for detailed information regarding interactions with H2 antagonists, antacids, and PPIs)
	ATV/r	• RTV boosting: higher trough ATV concentration and greater antiviral effect • Once-daily dosing • Low pill burden	• More adverse effects on lipids than unboosted ATV • More hyperbilirubinemia and jaundice than unboosted ATV • Food requirement • Absorption depends on food and low gastric pH (see Table 15a for interactions with H2 antagonists, antacids, and PPIs) • RTV boosting required with TDF and EFV. With EFV, use ATV 400 mg and RTV 100 mg, once daily (PI-naive patients only). • Should not be co-administered with NVP. • Nephrolithiasis, cholelithiasis
	DRV/r	• Once-daily dosing • Potent virologic efficacy	• Skin rash • Food requirement
	FPV/r	• Twice-daily dosing resulted in efficacy comparable to LPV/r • Once-daily dosing possible with RTV 100 mg or 200 mg daily • No food effect	• Skin rash • Hyperlipidemia • Once-daily dosing results in lower APV concentrations than with twice-daily dosing • For FPV/r 1400/200 mg: requires 200 mg of RTV • Fewer data on FPV/r 1400/100 mg dose than on DRV/r and ATV/r
	LPV/r	• Co-formulated • No food requirement • Greater CD4 count increase than with EFV-based regimens	• Requires 200 mg per day of RTV • Lower drug exposure in pregnant women—may need dose increase in third trimester • Once-daily dosing not recommended in pregnant women • Once-daily dosing results in lower trough concentration than twice-daily dosing • Possible higher risk of MI associated with cumulative use of LPV/r • PR and QT interval prolongation have been reported. Use with caution in patients at risk of cardiac conduction abnormalities or receiving other drugs with similar effect.

Guidelines for the Use of Antiretroviral Agents in HIV-1-Infected Adults and Adolescents

F-17

Table 6. Advantages and Disadvantages of Antiretroviral Components Recommended as Initial Antiretroviral Therapy (page 3 of 4)

ARV Class	ARV Agent(s)	Advantages	Disadvantages

PIs (in alphabetical order)	SQV/r	• Similar efficacy but less hyperlipidemia than with LPV/r	• Highest pill burden (6 pills per day) of available PI regimens
			• Requires 200 mg of RTV
			• Food requirement
			• PR and/or QT interval prolongations in a healthy volunteer study
			• Pretreatment ECG recommended
			• SQV/r is not recommended for patients with any of the following conditions:
			  • congenital or acquired QT prolongation
			  • pretreatment ECG >450 msec
			  • on concomitant therapy with other drugs that prolong QT interval
			  • complete AV block without implanted pacemakers
			  • risk of complete AV block

INSTIs (in alphabetical order)	EVG	• Co-formulation with COBI/TDF/FTC • Once daily dosing • Non-inferior to EFV/TDF/FTC and ATV/r + TDF/FTC	• COBI is a potent CYP3A4 inhibitor, which can result in significant interactions with CYP3A substrates • COBI inhibits active tubular secretion of creatinine and can decrease CrCL without affecting renal glomerular function • Has potential for new onset or worsening of renal impairment • Only recommended for patients with baseline CrCl >70 mL/min; therapy should be discontinued if CrCl decreased to <50mL/min • Lower genetic barrier to resistance than with boosted PI-based regimens • Food requirement
	RAL	• Virologic response noninferior to EFV; superior at 4–5 years • Fewer drug-related adverse events and lipid changes than with EFV • No food effect • Fewer drug-drug interactions than with EVG/COBI/TDF/FTC-, PI-, NNRTI-, or MVC-based regimens	• Twice-daily dosing • Lower genetic barrier to resistance than with boosted PI-based regimens • Increase in creatine kinase, myopathy, and rhabdomyolysis have been reported • Rare cases of severe hypersensitivity reactions (including SJS and TEN) have been reported.
CCR5 Antagonist	MVC	• Virologic response noninferior to EFV in post hoc analysis of MERIT study (see text) • Fewer adverse effects than EFV	• Requires viral tropism testing before initiation of therapy, which results in additional cost and possible delay in initiation of therapy • In the MERIT study, more MVC-treated than EFV-treated patients discontinued therapy due to lack of efficacy • Less long-term experience in ART-naive patients than with boosted PI- or NNRTI-based regimens • Limited experience with dual-NRTIs other than ZDV/3TC • Twice-daily dosing • CYP3A4 substrate; dosing depends on presence or absence of concomitant CYP3A4 inducer(s) or inhibitor(s)

Table 6. Advantages and Disadvantages of Antiretroviral Components Recommended as Initial Antiretroviral Therapy (page 4 of 4)

ARV Class	ARV Agent(s)	Advantages	Disadvantages
Dual-NRTI pairs (in alphabetical order)	ABC/3TC	• Virologic response non-inferior to ZDV/3TC • Better CD4 count responses than with ZDV/3TC • Once-daily dosing • Coformulation • No food effect • No cumulative TAM-mediated resistance	• Potential for ABC HSR in patients with HLA-B*5701 • Inferior virologic responses in patients with baseline HIV RNA >100,000 copies/mL when compared with TDF/FTC in ACTG 5202 study; but not in the HEAT study. • Some observational cohort studies show increased potential for cardiovascular events, especially in patients with cardiovascular risk factors
	TDF/FTC	• Better virologic responses than with ABC/3TC in patients with baseline viral load >100,000 copies/mL in ACTG 5202 study; however, this was not seen in the HEAT study. • Active against HBV; recommended dual-NRTI for HIV/HBV co-infection • Once-daily dosing • No food effect • Co-formulated (TDF/FTC, EFV/TDF/FTC, EVG/COBI/TDF/FTC, and RPV/TDF/FTC) • No cumulative TAM-mediated resistance	• Potential for renal impairment, including proximal tubulopathy and acute or chronic renal insufficiency • Early virologic failure of NVP + TDF + (FTC or 3TC) in small clinical trials • Potential for decrease in BMD
	ZDV/3TC	• Co-formulated (ZDV/3TC and ZDV/3TC/ABC) • No food effect (although better tolerated with food) • Preferred dual NRTI in pregnant women	• Bone marrow suppression, especially anemia and neutropenia • GI intolerance, headache • Mitochondrial toxicity, including lipoatrophy, lactic acidosis, hepatic steatosis • Compared with TDF/FTC, inferior in combination with EFV • Less CD4 increase compared with ABC/3TC • Twice-daily dosing

Key to Abbreviations: 3TC = lamivudine, ABC = abacavir, APV = amprenavir, ART = antiretroviral therapy, ARV = antiretroviral, ATV = atazanavir, ATV/r = atazanavir/ritonavir, AV = atrioventricular, BMD = bone mineral density, CNS = central nervous system, COBI = cobicistat, CrCl = creatinine clearance, CYP = cytochrome P, d4T = stavudine, ddI = didanosine, DRV/r = darunavir/ritonavir, ECG = electrocardiogram, EFV = efavirenz, EVG = elvitegravir, FPV = fosamprenavir, FPV/r = fosamprenavir/ ritonavir, FTC = emtricitabine, GI = gastrointestinal, HBV = hepatitis B virus, HSR = hypersensitivity reaction, INSTI = integrase strand transfer inhibitor, LPV/r = lopinavir/ritonavir, MI = myocardial infarction, msec = milliseconds, MVC = maraviroc, NNRTI = non-nucleoside reverse transcriptase inhibitor, NRTI = nucleoside reverse transcriptase inhibitor, NVP = nevirapine, PI = protease inhibitor, PPI = proton pump inhibitor, RAL = raltegravir, RPV = rilpivirine, RTV = ritonavir, SJS = Stevens-Johnson syndrome, SQV/r = saquinavir/ritonavir, TAM = thymidine analogue mutation, TDF = tenofovir disoproxil fumarate, TEN = toxic epidermal necrosis, ZDV = zidovudine

Table 7. Antiretroviral Components or Regimens Not Recommended as Initial Therapy

ARV drugs or components (in alphabetical order)	Reasons for **NOT** recommending as initial therapy
ABC/3TC/ZDV (co-formulated) as triple-NRTI combination regimen **(BI)**	• Inferior virologic efficacy
ABC + 3TC + ZDV + TDF as quadruple-NRTI combination regimen **(BI)**	• Inferior virologic efficacy
DRV (unboosted)	• Use without RTV has not been studied
DLV **(BIII)**	• Inferior virologic efficacy • Inconvenient (three times daily) dosing
ddI + 3TC (or FTC) **(BIII)**	• Inferior virologic efficacy • Limited clinical trial experience in ART-naive patients • ddI toxicity
ddI + TDF **(BII)**	• High rate of early virologic failure • Rapid selection of resistance mutations • Potential for immunologic nonresponse/CD4 T-cell decline • Increased ddI drug exposure and toxicities
EVG/COBI/TDF/FTC + other ARV drugs **(BIII)**	• Potential for drug-drug interactions, especially with NNRTI, PI, and MVC; appropriate dosages of EVG/COBI/TDF/FTC and other ARV drugs have not been established
T20 **(BIII)**	• No clinical trial experience in ART-naive patients • Requires twice-daily subcutaneous injections
ETR **(BIII)**	• Insufficient data in ART-naive patients
FPV (unboosted) **(BIII)**	• Less potent than RTV-boosted FPV • Virologic failure with unboosted FPV-based regimen may result in selection of mutations that confer resistance to DRV
IDV (unboosted) **(BIII)**	• Inconvenient dosing (three times daily with meal restrictions) • Fluid requirement • IDV toxicities
IDV (RTV-boosted) **(BIII)**	• IDV toxicities • Fluid requirement
NFV **(BI)**	• Inferior virologic efficacy • Diarrhea
RTV as sole PI **(BIII)**	• High pill burden • GI intolerance • Metabolic toxicity
SQV (unboosted) **(BI)**	• Inadequate bioavailability • Inferior virologic efficacy
d4T + 3TC **(BI)**	• Significant toxicities including lipoatrophy; peripheral neuropathy; and hyperlactatemia, including symptomatic and life-threatening lactic acidosis, hepatic steatosis, and pancreatitis
TPV (RTV-boosted) **(BI)**	• Inferior virologic efficacy

Key to Abbreviations: 3TC = lamivudine, ABC = abacavir, ART = antiretroviral therapy, ARV = antiretroviral, COBI = cobicistat, d4T = stavudine, ddI = didanosine, DLV = delavirdine, DRV = darunavir, ETR = etravirine, EVG = elvitegravir, FPV = fosamprenavir, FTC = emtricitabine, GI = gastrointestinal, IDV = indinavir, MVC = maraviroc, NFV = nelfinavir, NRTI = nucleoside reverse transcriptase inhibitor, PI = protease inhibitor, RTV = ritonavir, SQV = sacquinavir, T20 = enfuvirtide, TDF = tenofovir disoproxil fumarate, TPV = tipranavir, ZDV = zidovudine

References

1. Gulick RM, Ribaudo HJ, Shikuma CM, et al. Three- vs four-drug antiretroviral regimens for the initial treatment of HIV-1 infection: a randomized controlled trial. *JAMA*. 2006;296(7):769-781. Available at http://www.ncbi.nlm.nih.gov/entrez/query.fcgi?cmd=Retrieve&db=PubMed&dopt=Citation&list_uids=16905783.

2. Gallant JE, Staszewski S, Pozniak AL, et al. Efficacy and safety of tenofovir DF vs stavudine in combination therapy in antiretroviral-naive patients: a 3-year randomized trial. *JAMA*. 2004;292(2):191-201. Available at http://www.ncbi.nlm.nih.gov/entrez/query.fcgi?cmd=Retrieve&db=PubMed&dopt=Citation&list_uids=15249568.

3. Staszewski S, Morales-Ramirez J, Tashima KT, et al. Efavirenz plus zidovudine and lamivudine, efavirenz plus indinavir, and indinavir plus zidovudine and lamivudine in the treatment of HIV-1 infection in adults. Study 006 Team. *N Engl J Med*. 1999;341(25):1865-1873. Available at http://www.ncbi.nlm.nih.gov/entrez/query.fcgi?cmd=Retrieve&db=PubMed&dopt=Citation&list_uids=10601505.

4. Riddler SA, Haubrich R, DiRienzo AG, et al. Class-sparing regimens for initial treatment of HIV-1 infection. *N Engl J Med*. 2008;358(20):2095-2106. Available at http://www.ncbi.nlm.nih.gov/entrez/query.fcgi?cmd=Retrieve&db=PubMed&dopt=Citation&list_uids=18480202.

5. Squires K, Lazzarin A, Gatell JM, et al. Comparison of once-daily atazanavir with efavirenz, each in combination with fixed-dose zidovudine and lamivudine, as initial therapy for patients infected with HIV. *J Acquir Immune Defic Syndr*. 2004;36(5):1011-1019. Available at http://www.ncbi.nlm.nih.gov/entrez/query.fcgi?cmd=Retrieve&db=PubMed&dopt=Citation&list_uids=15247553.

6. Lennox JL, DeJesus E, Lazzarin A, et al. Safety and efficacy of raltegravir-based versus efavirenz-based combination therapy in treatment-naive patients with HIV-1 infection: a multicentre, double-blind randomised controlled trial. *Lancet*. 2009;374(9692):796-806. Available at http://www.ncbi.nlm.nih.gov/entrez/query.fcgi?cmd=Retrieve&db=PubMed&dopt=Citation&list_uids=19647866.

7. Cooper DA, Heera J, Goodrich J, et al. Maraviroc versus efavirenz, both in combination with zidovudine-lamivudine, for the treatment of antiretroviral-naive subjects with CCR5-tropic HIV-1 infection. *J Infect Dis*. 2010;201(6):803-813. Available at http://www.ncbi.nlm.nih.gov/entrez/query.fcgi?cmd=Retrieve&db=PubMed&dopt=Citation&list_uids=20151839.

8. Sax PE, Tierney C, Collier AC, et al. Abacavir-lamivudine versus tenofovir-emtricitabine for initial HIV-1 therapy. *N Engl J Med*. 2009;361(23):2230-2240. Available at http://www.ncbi.nlm.nih.gov/entrez/query.fcgi?cmd=Retrieve&db=PubMed&dopt=Citation&list_uids=19952143.

9. Post FA, Moyle GJ, Stellbrink HJ, et al. Randomized comparison of renal effects, efficacy, and safety with once-daily abacavir/lamivudine versus tenofovir/emtricitabine, administered with efavirenz, in antiretroviral-naive, HIV-1-infected adults: 48-week results from the ASSERT study. *J Acquir Immune Defic Syndr*. 2010;55(1):49-57. Available at http://www.ncbi.nlm.nih.gov/entrez/query.fcgi?cmd=Retrieve&db=PubMed&dopt=Citation&list_uids=20431394.

10. Smith KY, Patel P, Fine D, et al. Randomized, double-blind, placebo-matched, multicenter trial of abacavir/lamivudine or tenofovir/emtricitabine with lopinavir/ritonavir for initial HIV treatment. *AIDS*. 2009;23(12):1547-1556. Available at http://www.ncbi.nlm.nih.gov/entrez/query.fcgi?cmd=Retrieve&db=PubMed&dopt=Citation&list_uids=19542866.

11. McComsey GA, Kitch D, Daar ES, et al. Bone mineral density and fractures in antiretroviral-naive persons randomized to receive abacavir-lamivudine or tenofovir disoproxil fumarate-emtricitabine along with efavirenz or atazanavir-ritonavir: Aids Clinical Trials Group A5224s, a substudy of ACTG A5202. *J Infect Dis*. 2011;203(12):1791-1801. Available at http://www.ncbi.nlm.nih.gov/entrez/query.fcgi?cmd=Retrieve&db=PubMed&dopt=Citation&list_uids=21606537.

12. Gallant JE, DeJesus E, Arribas JR, et al. Tenofovir DF, emtricitabine, and efavirenz vs. zidovudine, lamivudine, and efavirenz for HIV. *N Engl J Med*. 2006;354(3):251-260. Available at http://www.ncbi.nlm.nih.gov/entrez/query.fcgi?cmd=Retrieve&db=PubMed&dopt=Citation&list_uids=16421366.

13. Daar ES, Tierney C, Fischl MA, et al. Atazanavir plus ritonavir or efavirenz as part of a 3-drug regimen for initial treatment of HIV-1. *Ann Intern Med*. 2011;154(7):445-456. Available at http://www.ncbi.nlm.nih.gov/pubmed/21320923.

14. Cohen CJ, Molina JM, Cahn P, et al. Efficacy and safety of rilpivirine (TMC278) versus efavirenz at 48 weeks in treatment-naive HIV-1-infected patients: pooled results from the phase 3 double-blind randomized ECHO and THRIVE Trials. *J Acquir Immune Defic Syndr*. 2012;60(1):33-42. Available at http://www.ncbi.nlm.nih.gov/pubmed/22343174.

15. Sax PE, DeJesus E, Mills A, et al. Co-formulated elvitegravir, cobicistat, emtricitabine, and tenofovir versus co-formulated efavirenz, emtricitabine, and tenofovir for initial treatment of HIV-1 infection: a randomised, double-blind, phase 3 trial, analysis of results after 48 weeks. *Lancet*. 2012;379(9835):2439-2448. Available at http://www.ncbi.nlm.nih.gov/pubmed/22748591.

16. Aberg JA, Tebas P, Overton ET, et al. Metabolic effects of darunavir/ritonavir versus atazanavir/ritonavir in treatment-naive, HIV type 1-infected subjects over 48 weeks. *AIDS Res Hum Retroviruses*. 2012;28(10):1184-1195. Available at http://www.ncbi.nlm.nih.gov/pubmed/22352336.

17. Anderson PL, Glidden DV, Liu A, et al. Emtricitabine-tenofovir concentrations and pre-exposure prophylaxis efficacy in men who have sex with men. *Sci Transl Med*. 2012;4(151):151ra125. Available at http://www.ncbi.nlm.nih.gov/pubmed/22972843.

18. Kim D, Wheeler W, Ziebell R, et al. Prevalence of transmitted antiretroviral drug resistance among newly-diagnosed HIV-1-infected persons, US, 2007. Paper presented at: 17th Conference on Retroviruses and Opportunistic Infections. 2010. San Francisco, CA.

19. Novak RM, Chen L, MacArthur RD, et al. Prevalence of antiretroviral drug resistance mutations in chronically HIV-infected, treatment-naive patients: implications for routine resistance screening before initiation of antiretroviral therapy. *Clin Infect Dis*. 2005;40(3):468-474. Available at http://www.ncbi.nlm.nih.gov/entrez/query.fcgi?cmd=Retrieve&db=PubMed&dopt=Citation&list_uids=15668873.

20. Wensing AM, van de Vijver DA, Angarano G, et al. Prevalence of drug-resistant HIV-1 variants in untreated individuals in Europe: implications for clinical management. *J Infect Dis*. 2005;192(6):958-966. Available at http://www.ncbi.nlm.nih.gov/entrez/query.fcgi?cmd=Retrieve&db=PubMed&dopt=Citation&list_uids=16107947.

21. Weinstock HS, Zaidi I, Heneine W, et al. The epidemiology of antiretroviral drug resistance among drug-naive HIV-1-infected persons in 10 US cities. *J Infect Dis*. 2004;189(12):2174-2180. Available at http://www.ncbi.nlm.nih.gov/entrez/query.fcgi?cmd=Retrieve&db=PubMed&dopt=Citation&list_uids=15181563.

22. Andries K, Azijn H, Thielemans T, et al. TMC125, a novel next-generation nonnucleoside reverse transcriptase inhibitor active against nonnucleoside reverse transcriptase inhibitor-resistant human immunodeficiency virus type 1. *Antimicrob Agents Chemother*. 2004;48(12):4680-4686. Available at http://www.ncbi.nlm.nih.gov/entrez/query.fcgi?cmd=Retrieve&db=PubMed&dopt=Citation&list_uids=15561844.

23. Food and Drug Administration. Edurant (package insert). 2012. Available at http://www.accessdata.fda.gov/drugsatfda_docs/label/2012/202022s002lbl.pdf. Accessed December 28, 2012.

24. Food and Drug Administration. Intelence (package insert). 2011. Available at http://www.accessdata.fda.gov/drugsatfda_docs/label/2011/022187s008lbl.pdf. Accessed January 18, 2013.

25. Gazzard B, Duvivier C, Zagler C, et al. Phase 2 double-blind, randomised trial of etravirine versus efavirenz in treatment-naive patients: 48 week results. *AIDS*. 2011. Available at http://www.ncbi.nlm.nih.gov/entrez/query.fcgi?cmd=Retrieve&db=PubMed&dopt=Citation&list_uids=21881478.

26. Cassetti I, Madruga JV, Etzel A, et al. The safety and efficacy of tenofovir DF (TDF) in combination with lamivudine (3TC) and efavirenz (EFV) in antiretroviral-naive patients through seven years. Paper presented at:17th International AIDS Conference. 2008. Mexico City, Mexico.

27. van Leth F, Phanuphak P, Ruxrungtham K, et al. Comparison of first-line antiretroviral therapy with regimens including nevirapine, efavirenz, or both drugs, plus stavudine and lamivudine: a randomised open-label trial, the 2NN Study. *Lancet*. 2004;363(9417):1253-1263. Available at http://www.ncbi.nlm.nih.gov/entrez/query.fcgi?cmd=Retrieve&db=PubMed&dopt=Citation&list_uids=15094269.

28. Nunez M, Soriano V, Martin-Carbonero L, et al. SENC (Spanish efavirenz vs. nevirapine comparison) trial: a randomized, open-label study in HIV-infected naive individuals. *HIV Clin Trials*. 2002;3(3):186-194. Available at http://www.ncbi.nlm.nih.gov/entrez/query.fcgi?cmd=Retrieve&db=PubMed&dopt=Citation&list_uids=12032877.

29. Food and Drug Administration. Sustiva (package insert). 2009. Available at http://www.accessdata.fda.gov/drugsatfda_docs/label/2009/020972s033,021360s021lbl.pdf. Accessed January 18, 2013.

30. Fundaro C, Genovese O, Rendeli C, Tamburrini E, Salvaggio E. Myelomeningocele in a child with intrauterine exposure to efavirenz. *AIDS*. 2002;16(2):299-300. Available at http://www.ncbi.nlm.nih.gov/entrez/query.fcgi?cmd=Retrieve&db=PubMed&dopt=Citation&list_uids=11807320.

31. Antiretroviral Pregnancy Registry Steering Committee. Antiretroviral Pregnancy Registry international interim report for 1 January 1989 through 31 January 2012. Available at http://www.apregistry.com/forms/interim_report.pdf. Accessed December 28, 2012.

32. World Health Organization. Technical update on treatment optimization: Use of efavirenz during pregnancy: A public health perspective. Available at http://www.who.int/hiv/pub/treatment2/efavirenz/en/. Accessed June 25, 2012.

33. Ford N, Calmy A, Mofenson L. Safety of efavirenz in the first trimester of pregnancy: an updated systematic review and meta-analysis. *AIDS*. 2011;25(18):2301-2304. Available at http://www.ncbi.nlm.nih.gov/pubmed/21918421.

34. Panel on Treatment of HIV-Infected Pregnant Women and Prevention of Perinatal Transmission. Recommendations for Use of Antiretroviral Drugs in Pregnant HIV-1-Infected Women for Maternal Health and Interventions to Reduce Perinatal HIV Transmission in the United States. Available at http://aidsinfo.nih.gov/contentfiles/lvguidelines/PerinatalGL.pdf.

35. Soriano V, Arasteh K, Migrone H, et al. Nevirapine versus atazanavir/ritonavir, each combined with tenofovir disoproxil fumarate/emtricitabine, in antiretroviral-naive HIV-1 patients: the ARTEN Trial. *Antivir Ther*. 2011;16(3):339-348. Available at http://www.ncbi.nlm.nih.gov/entrez/query.fcgi?cmd=Retrieve&db=PubMed&dopt=Citation&list_uids=21555816.

36. Sanne I, Mommeja-Marin H, Hinkle J, et al. Severe hepatotoxicity associated with nevirapine use in HIV-infected subjects. *J Infect Dis*. 2005;191(6):825-829. Available at http://www.ncbi.nlm.nih.gov/entrez/query.fcgi?cmd=Retrieve&db=PubMed&dopt=Citation&list_uids=15717255.

37. Baylor MS, Johann-Liang R. Hepatotoxicity associated with nevirapine use. *J Acquir Immune Defic Syndr*. 2004;35(5):538-539. Available at http://www.ncbi.nlm.nih.gov/entrez/query.fcgi?cmd=Retrieve&db=PubMed&dopt=Citation&list_uids=15021321.

38. Boehringer Ingelheim. Dear Health Care Professional Letter: Clarification of risk factors for severe, life-threatening and fatal hepatotoxicity with VIRAMUNE® (nevirapine). February 2004. Available at http://www.fda.gov/downloads/Safety/MedWatch/SafetyInformation/SafetyAlertsforHumanMedicalProducts/UCM166534.pdf.

39. Peters P, Stringer J, McConnell MS, et al. Nevirapine-associated hepatotoxicity was not predicted by CD4 count ≥250 cells/muL among women in Zambia, Thailand and Kenya. *HIV Med*. 2010. Available at http://www.ncbi.nlm.nih.gov/entrez/query.fcgi?cmd=Retrieve&db=PubMed&dopt=Citation&list_uids=20659176.

40. Coffie PA, Tonwe-Gold B, Tanon AK, et al. Incidence and risk factors of severe adverse events with nevirapine-based antiretroviral therapy in HIV-infected women. MTCT-Plus program, Abidjan, Cote d'Ivoire. *BMC Infect Dis*. 2010;10:188. Available at http://www.ncbi.nlm.nih.gov/entrez/query.fcgi?cmd=Retrieve&db=PubMed&dopt=Citation&list_uids=20576111.

41. Kesselring AM, Wit FW, Sabin CA, et al. Risk factors for treatment-limiting toxicities in patients starting nevirapine-containing antiretroviral therapy. *AIDS*. 2009;23(13):1689-1699. Available at http://www.ncbi.nlm.nih.gov/entrez/query.fcgi?cmd=Retrieve&db=PubMed&dopt=Citation&list_uids=19487907.

42. Lathouwers E, De Meyer S, Dierynck I, et al. Virological characterization of patients failing darunavir/ritonavir or lopinavir/ritonavir treatment in the ARTEMIS study: 96-week analysis. *Antivir Ther*. 2011;16(1):99-108. Available at http://www.ncbi.nlm.nih.gov/entrez/query.fcgi?cmd=Retrieve&db=PubMed&dopt=Citation&list_uids=21311113.

43. Worm SW, Sabin C, Weber R, et al. Risk of myocardial infarction in patients with HIV infection exposed to specific individual antiretroviral drugs from the 3 major drug classes: the data collection on adverse events of anti-HIV drugs (D:A:D) study. *J Infect Dis*. 2010;201(3):318-330. Available at http://www.ncbi.nlm.nih.gov/entrez/query.fcgi?cmd=Retrieve&db=PubMed&dopt=Citation&list_uids=20039804.

44. Lang S, Mary-Krause M, Cotte L, et al. Impact of individual antiretroviral drugs on the risk of myocardial infarction in human immunodeficiency virus-infected patients: a case-control study nested within the French Hospital Database on HIV ANRS cohort CO4. *Arch Intern Med*. 2010;170(14):1228-1238. Available at http://www.ncbi.nlm.nih.gov/entrez/query.fcgi?cmd=Retrieve&db=PubMed&dopt=Citation&list_uids=20660842.

45. Monforte AD, Reiss P, Ryom L, et al. Atazanavir is not associated with an increased risk of cardio or cerebrovascular disease events. *AIDS*. 2013;27(3):407-415. Available at http://www.ncbi.nlm.nih.gov/pubmed/23291539.

46. Food and Drug Administration (FDA). Invirase (package insert). 2010. Available at http://www.accessdata.fda.gov/drugsatfda_docs/label/2010/020628s033,021785s010lbl.pdf. Accessed January 18, 2013.

47. Malan DR, Krantz E, David N, Wirtz V, Hammond J, McGrath D. Efficacy and safety of atazanavir, with or without ritonavir, as part of once-daily highly active antiretroviral therapy regimens in antiretroviral-naive patients. *J Acquir Immune Defic Syndr*. 2008;47(2):161-7. http://www.ncbi.nlm.nih.gov/entrez/query.fcgi?cmd=Retrieve&db=PubMed&dopt=Citation&list_uids=17971713.

48. Molina JM, Andrade-Villanueva J, Echevarria J, et al. Once-daily atazanavir/ritonavir versus twice-daily lopinavir/ritonavir, each in combination with tenofovir and emtricitabine, for management of antiretroviral-naive HIV-1-infected patients: 48 week efficacy and safety results of the CASTLE study. *Lancet*. 2008;372(9639):646-655. Available at http://www.ncbi.nlm.nih.gov/entrez/query.fcgi?cmd=Retrieve&db=PubMed&dopt=Citation&list_uids=18722869.

49. Molina JM, Andrade-Villanueva J, Echevarria J, et al. Once-daily atazanavir/ritonavir compared with twice-daily lopinavir/ritonavir, each in combination with tenofovir and emtricitabine, for management of antiretroviral-naive HIV-1-infected patients: 96-week efficacy and safety results of the CASTLE study. *J Acquir Immune Defic Syndr*. 2010;53(3):323-332. Available at http://www.ncbi.nlm.nih.gov/entrez/query.fcgi?cmd=Retrieve&db=PubMed&dopt=Citation&list_uids=20032785.

50. Chan-Tack KM, Truffa MM, Struble KA, Birnkrant DB. Atazanavir-associated nephrolithiasis: cases from the US Food and Drug Administration's Adverse Event Reporting System. *AIDS*. 2007;21(9):1215-1218. Available at http://www.ncbi.nlm.nih.gov/entrez/query.fcgi?cmd=Retrieve&db=PubMed&dopt=Citation&list_uids=17502736.

51. Rockwood N, Mandalia S, Bower M, Gazzard B, Nelson M. Ritonavir-boosted atazanavir exposure is associated with an increased rate of renal stones compared with efavirenz, ritonavir-boosted lopinavir and ritonavir-boosted darunavir. *AIDS*. 2011;25(13):1671-1673. Available at http://www.ncbi.nlm.nih.gov/pubmed/21716074.

52. Hamada Y, Nishijima T, Watanabe K, et al. High incidence of renal stones among HIV-infected patients on ritonavir-boosted atazanavir than in those receiving other protease inhibitor-containing antiretroviral therapy. *Clin Infect Dis*. 2012;55(9):1262-1269. Available at http://www.ncbi.nlm.nih.gov/pubmed/22820542.

53. Rakotondravelo S, Poinsignon Y, Borsa-Lebas F, et al. Complicated atazanavir-associated cholelithiasis: a report of 14 cases. *Clin Infect Dis*. 2012;55(9):1270-1272. Available at http://www.ncbi.nlm.nih.gov/pubmed/22820540.

54. Ortiz R, Dejesus E, Khanlou H, et al. Efficacy and safety of once-daily darunavir/ritonavir versus lopinavir/ritonavir in treatment-naive HIV-1-infected patients at week 48. *AIDS*. 2008;22(12):1389-1397. Available at http://www.ncbi.nlm.nih.gov/entrez/query.fcgi?cmd=Retrieve&db=PubMed&dopt=Citation&list_uids=18614861.

55. Orkin C, Dejesus E, Khanlou H, et al. Final 192-week efficacy and safety of once-daily darunavir/ritonavir compared with lopinavir/ritonavir in HIV-1-infected treatment-naive patients in the ARTEMIS trial. *HIV Med*. 2013;14(1):49-59. Available at http://www.ncbi.nlm.nih.gov/pubmed/23088336.

56. Trottier B, Machouf N, Thomas R, et al. Abacavir/lamivudine fixed-dose combination with ritonavir-boosted darunavir: a safe and efficacious regimen for HIV therapy. *HIV Clin Trials*. 2012;13(6):335-342. Available at http://www.ncbi.nlm.nih.gov/pubmed/23195671.

57. Eron J, Jr., Yeni P, Gathe J, Jr., et al. The KLEAN study of fosamprenavir-ritonavir versus lopinavir-ritonavir, each in combination with abacavir-lamivudine, for initial treatment of HIV infection over 48 weeks: a randomised non-inferiority trial. *Lancet*. 2006;368(9534):476-482. Available at http://www.ncbi.nlm.nih.gov/entrez/query.fcgi?cmd=Retrieve&db=PubMed&dopt=Citation&list_uids=16890834.

58. Pulido F, Estrada V, Baril JG, et al. Long-term efficacy and safety of fosamprenavir plus ritonavir versus lopinavir/ritonavir in combination with abacavir/lamivudine over 144 weeks. *HIV Clin Trials*. 2009;10(2):76-87. Available at http://www.ncbi.nlm.nih.gov/entrez/query.fcgi?cmd=Retrieve&db=PubMed&dopt=Citation&list_uids=19487177.

59. Smith KY, Weinberg WG, Dejesus E, et al. Fosamprenavir or atazanavir once daily boosted with ritonavir 100 mg, plus tenofovir/emtricitabine, for the initial treatment of HIV infection: 48-week results of ALERT. *AIDS Res Ther*. 2008;5:5. Available at http://www.ncbi.nlm.nih.gov/entrez/query.fcgi?cmd=Retrieve&db=PubMed&dopt=Citation&list_uids=18373851.

60. Murphy RL, da Silva BA, Hicks CB, et al. Seven-year efficacy of a lopinavir/ritonavir-based regimen in antiretroviral-naive HIV-1-infected patients. *HIV Clin Trials*. 2008;9(1):1-10. Available at http://www.ncbi.nlm.nih.gov/entrez/query.fcgi?cmd=Retrieve&db=PubMed&dopt=Citation&list_uids=18215977.

61. Murphy RL, Sanne I, Cahn P, et al. Dose-ranging, randomized, clinical trial of atazanavir with lamivudine and stavudine in antiretroviral-naive subjects: 48-week results. *AIDS*. 2003;17(18):2603-2614. Available at http://www.ncbi.nlm.nih.gov/entrez/query.fcgi?cmd=Retrieve&db=PubMed&dopt=Citation&list_uids=14685054.

62. Sanne I, Piliero P, Squires K, Thiry A, Schnittman S. Results of a phase 2 clinical trial at 48 weeks (AI424-007): a dose-ranging, safety, and efficacy comparative trial of atazanavir at three doses in combination with didanosine and stavudine in antiretroviral-naive subjects. *J Acquir Immune Defic Syndr*. 2003;32(1):18-29. Available at http://www.ncbi.nlm.nih.gov/entrez/query.fcgi?cmd=Retrieve&db=PubMed&dopt=Citation&list_uids=12514410.

63. Campbell TB, Smeaton LM, Kumarasamy N, et al. Efficacy and safety of three antiretroviral regimens for initial treatment of HIV-1: a randomized clinical trial in diverse multinational settings. *PLoS Med*. 2012;9(8):e1001290. Available at http://www.ncbi.nlm.nih.gov/pubmed/22936892.

64. Walmsley S, Avihingsanon A, Slim J, et al. Gemini: a noninferiority study of saquinavir/ritonavir versus lopinavir/ritonavir as initial HIV-1 therapy in adults. *J Acquir Immune Defic Syndr*. 2009;50(4):367-374. Available at http://www.ncbi.nlm.nih.gov/entrez/query.fcgi?cmd=Retrieve&db=PubMed&dopt=Citation&list_uids=19214123.

65. Rockstroh JK, Lennox JL, Dejesus E, et al. Long-term Treatment With Raltegravir or Efavirenz Combined With Tenofovir/Emtricitabine for Treatment-Naive Human Immunodeficiency Virus-1-Infected Patients: 156-Week Results From STARTMRK. *Clin Infect Dis*. 2011;53(8):807-816. Available at http://www.ncbi.nlm.nih.gov/entrez/query.fcgi?cmd=Retrieve&db=PubMed&dopt=Citation&list_uids=21921224.

66. Young B, Vanig T, Dejesus E, et al. A pilot study of abacavir/lamivudine and raltegravir in antiretroviral-naive HIV-1-infected patients: 48-week results of the SHIELD trial. *HIV Clin Trials*. 2010;11(5):260-269. Available at http://www.ncbi.nlm.nih.gov/entrez/query.fcgi?cmd=Retrieve&db=PubMed&dopt=Citation&list_uids=21126956.

67. Food and Drug Administration. Isentress (package insert). 2011. Available at http://www.accessdata.fda.gov/drugsatfda_docs/label/2011/022145s018lbl.pdf. Accessed February 19, 2012.

68. Mathias AA, West S, Hui J, Kearney BP. Dose-response of ritonavir on hepatic CYP3A activity and elvitegravir oral exposure. *Clin Pharmacol Ther*. 2009;85(1):64-70. Available at http://www.ncbi.nlm.nih.gov/pubmed/18815591.

69. Food and Drug Administration. Stribild (package insert). 2012. Available at http://www.accessdata.fda.gov/drugsatfda_docs/label/2012/203100s000lbl.pdf. Accessed December 28, 2012.

70. DeJesus E, Rockstroh JK, Henry K, et al. Co-formulated elvitegravir, cobicistat, emtricitabine, and tenofovir disoproxil fumarate versus ritonavir-boosted atazanavir plus co-formulated emtricitabine and tenofovir disoproxil fumarate for initial treatment of HIV-1 infection: a randomised, double-blind, phase 3, non-inferiority trial. *Lancet*. 2012;379(9835):2429-2438. Available at http://www.ncbi.nlm.nih.gov/pubmed/22748590.

71. Rockstroh JK, Dejesus E, Henry K, et al. A randomized, double-blind comparison of co-formulated

elvitegravir/cobicistat/emtricitabine/tenofovir versus ritonavir-boosted atazanavir plus co-formulated emtricitabine and tenofovir DF for initial treatment of HIV-1 infection: analysis of week 96 results. *J Acquir Immune Defic Syndr*. 2013. Available at http://www.ncbi.nlm.nih.gov/pubmed/23337366.

72. Zolopa A, Gallant J, Cohen C, et al. Elvitegravir/cobicistat/emtricitabine/tenofovir DF (Quad) has durable efficacy and differentiated safety compared to efavirenz/emtricitabine/tenofovir DF at week 96 in treatment-naive HIV-1-infected patients. *Journal of the International AIDS Society*. 2012;15(6):18219. Available at http://www.ncbi.nlm.nih.gov/pubmed/23234891.

73. German P, Liu HC, Szwarcberg J, et al. Effect of cobicistat on glomerular filtration rate in subjects with normal and impaired renal function. *J Acquir Immune Defic Syndr*. 2012;61(1):32-40. Available at http://www.ncbi.nlm.nih.gov/pubmed/22732469.

74. Sierra-Madero J, Di Perri G, Wood R, et al. Efficacy and safety of maraviroc versus efavirenz, both with zidovudine/lamivudine: 96-week results from the MERIT study. *HIV Clin Trials*. 2010;11(3):125-132. Available at http://www.ncbi.nlm.nih.gov/pubmed/20736149.

75. Ait-Khaled M, Stone C, Amphlett G, et al. M184V is associated with a low incidence of thymidine analogue mutations and low phenotypic resistance to zidovudine and stavudine. *AIDS*. 2002;16(12):1686-1689. Available at http://www.ncbi.nlm.nih.gov/entrez/query.fcgi?cmd=Retrieve&db=PubMed&dopt=Citation&list_uids=12172093.

76. Arribas JR, Pozniak AL, Gallant JE, et al. Tenofovir disoproxil fumarate, emtricitabine, and efavirenz compared with zidovudine/lamivudine and efavirenz in treatment-naive patients: 144-week analysis. *J Acquir Immune Defic Syndr*. 2008;47(1):74-78. Available at http://www.ncbi.nlm.nih.gov/entrez/query.fcgi?cmd=Retrieve&db=PubMed&dopt=Citation&list_uids=17971715.

77. Molina JM, Podsadecki TJ, Johnson MA, et al. A lopinavir/ritonavir-based once-daily regimen results in better compliance and is non-inferior to a twice-daily regimen through 96 weeks. *AIDS Res Hum Retroviruses*. 2007;23(12):1505-1514. Available at http://www.ncbi.nlm.nih.gov/entrez/query.fcgi?cmd=Retrieve&db=PubMed&dopt=Citation&list_uids=18160008.

78. Zimmermann AE, Pizzoferrato T, Bedford J, Morris A, Hoffman R, Braden G. Tenofovir-associated acute and chronic kidney disease: a case of multiple drug interactions. *Clin Infect Dis*. 2006;42(2):283-290. Available at http://www.ncbi.nlm.nih.gov/entrez/query.fcgi?cmd=Retrieve&db=PubMed&dopt=Citation&list_uids=16355343.

79. Karras A, Lafaurie M, Furco A, et al. Tenofovir-related nephrotoxicity in human immunodeficiency virus-infected patients: three cases of renal failure, Fanconi syndrome, and nephrogenic diabetes insipidus. *Clin Infect Dis*. 2003;36(8):1070-1073. Available at http://www.ncbi.nlm.nih.gov/entrez/query.fcgi?cmd=Retrieve&db=PubMed&dopt=Citation&list_uids=12684922.

80. Moore R, Keruly J, Gallant J. Tenofovir and renal dysfunction in clinical practice. Paper presented at: 14th Conference on Retrovirus and Opportunistic Infections. 2007. Los Angeles, CA.

81. Kearney BP, Mathias A, Mittan A, Sayre J, Ebrahimi R, Cheng AK. Pharmacokinetics and safety of tenofovir disoproxil fumarate on co-administration with lopinavir/ritonavir. *J Acquir Immune Defic Syndr*. 2006;43(3):278-283. Available at http://www.ncbi.nlm.nih.gov/entrez/query.fcgi?cmd=Retrieve&db=PubMed&dopt=Citation&list_uids=17079992.

82. Kiser JJ, Carten ML, Aquilante CL, et al. The effect of lopinavir/ritonavir on the renal clearance of tenofovir in HIV-infected patients. *Clin Pharmacol Ther*. 2008;83(2):265-272. Available at http://www.ncbi.nlm.nih.gov/entrez/query.fcgi?cmd=Retrieve&db=PubMed&dopt=Citation&list_uids=17597712.

83. Gallant JE, Moore RD. Renal function with use of a tenofovir-containing initial antiretroviral regimen. *AIDS*. 2009;23(15):1971-1975. Available at http://www.ncbi.nlm.nih.gov/entrez/query.fcgi?cmd=Retrieve&db=PubMed&dopt=Citation&list_uids=19696652.

84. Goicoechea M, Liu S, Best B, et al. Greater tenofovir-associated renal function decline with protease inhibitor-based versus nonnucleoside reverse-transcriptase inhibitor-based therapy. *J Infect Dis*. 2008;197(1):102-108. Available at http://www.ncbi.nlm.nih.gov/entrez/query.fcgi?cmd=Retrieve&db=PubMed&dopt=Citation&list_uids=18171292.

85. Mills AM, Nelson M, Jayaweera D, et al. Once-daily darunavir/ritonavir vs. lopinavir/ritonavir in treatment-naive, HIV-1-

infected patients: 96-week analysis. *AIDS*. 2009;23(13):1679-1688. Available at
http://www.ncbi.nlm.nih.gov/entrez/query.fcgi?cmd=Retrieve&db=PubMed&dopt=Citation&list_uids=19487905.

86. Stellbrink HJ, Orkin C, Arribas JR, et al. Comparison of changes in bone density and turnover with abacavir-lamivudine versus tenofovir-emtricitabine in HIV-infected adults: 48-week results from the ASSERT study. *Clin Infect Dis*. 2010;51(8):963-972. Available at
http://www.ncbi.nlm.nih.gov/entrez/query.fcgi?cmd=Retrieve&db=PubMed&dopt=Citation&list_uids=20828304.

87. DeJesus E, Herrera G, Teofilo E, et al. Abacavir versus zidovudine combined with lamivudine and efavirenz, for the treatment of antiretroviral-naive HIV-infected adults. *Clin Infect Dis*. 2004;39(7):1038-1046. Available at
http://www.ncbi.nlm.nih.gov/entrez/query.fcgi?cmd=Retrieve&db=PubMed&dopt=Citation&list_uids=15472858.

88. Sax PE, Tierney C, Collier AC, et al. Abacavir/Lamivudine Versus Tenofovir DF/Emtricitabine as Part of Combination Regimens for Initial Treatment of HIV: Final Results. *J Infect Dis*. 2011;204(8):1191-1201. Available at
http://www.ncbi.nlm.nih.gov/entrez/query.fcgi?cmd=Retrieve&db=PubMed&dopt=Citation&list_uids=21917892.

89. Mallal S, Phillips E, Carosi G, et al. HLA-B*5701 screening for hypersensitivity to abacavir. *N Engl J Med*. 2008;358(6):568-579. Available at
http://www.ncbi.nlm.nih.gov/entrez/query.fcgi?cmd=Retrieve&db=PubMed&dopt=Citation&list_uids=18256392.

90. Saag M, Balu R, Phillips E, et al. High sensitivity of human leukocyte antigen-b*5701 as a marker for immunologically confirmed abacavir hypersensitivity in white and black patients. *Clin Infect Dis*. 2008;46(7):1111-1118. Available at
http://www.ncbi.nlm.nih.gov/entrez/query.fcgi?cmd=Retrieve&db=PubMed&dopt=Citation&list_uids=18444831.

91. Sabin CA, Worm SW, Weber R, et al. Use of nucleoside reverse transcriptase inhibitors and risk of myocardial infarction in HIV-infected patients enrolled in the D:A:D study: a multi-cohort collaboration. *Lancet*. 2008;371(9622):1417-1426. Available at http://www.ncbi.nlm.nih.gov/entrez/query.fcgi?cmd=Retrieve&db=PubMed&dopt=Citation&list_uids=18387667.

92. Choi AI, Vittinghoff E, Deeks SG, Weekley CC, Li Y, Shlipak MG. Cardiovascular risks associated with abacavir and tenofovir exposure in HIV-infected persons. *AIDS*. 2011;25(10):1289-1298. Available at
http://www.ncbi.nlm.nih.gov/entrez/query.fcgi?cmd=Retrieve&db=PubMed&dopt=Citation&list_uids=21516027.

93. Durand M, Sheehy O, Baril JG, Lelorier J, Tremblay CL. Association between HIV infection, antiretroviral therapy, and risk of acute myocardial infarction: a cohort and nested case-control study using Quebec's public health insurance database. *J Acquir Immune Defic Syndr*. 2011;57(3):245-253. Available at
http://www.ncbi.nlm.nih.gov/entrez/query.fcgi?cmd=Retrieve&db=PubMed&dopt=Citation&list_uids=21499115.

94. Obel N, Farkas DK, Kronborg G, et al. Abacavir and risk of myocardial infarction in HIV-infected patients on highly active antiretroviral therapy: a population-based nationwide cohort study. *HIV Med*. 2010;11(2):130-136. Available at
http://www.ncbi.nlm.nih.gov/entrez/query.fcgi?cmd=Retrieve&db=PubMed&dopt=Citation&list_uids=19682101.

95. The SMART/INSIGHT and the D:A:D Study Groups TSIatDADSG. Use of nucleoside reverse transcriptase inhibitors and risk of myocardial infarction in HIV-infected patients. *AIDS*. 2008;22(14):F17-24. Available at
http://www.ncbi.nlm.nih.gov/entrez/query.fcgi?cmd=Retrieve&db=PubMed&dopt=Citation&list_uids=18753925.

96. Ribaudo HJ, Benson CA, Zheng Y, et al. No risk of myocardial infarction associated with initial antiretroviral treatment containing abacavir: short and long-term results from ACTG A5001/ALLRT. *Clin Infect Dis*. 2011;52(7):929-940. Available at
http://www.ncbi.nlm.nih.gov/entrez/query.fcgi?cmd=Retrieve&db=PubMed&dopt=Citation&list_uids=21427402.

97. Bedimo RJ, Westfall AO, Drechsler H, Vidiella G, Tebas P. Abacavir use and risk of acute myocardial infarction and cerebrovascular events in the highly active antiretroviral therapy era. *Clin Infect Dis*. 2011;53(1):84-91. Available at
http://www.ncbi.nlm.nih.gov/entrez/query.fcgi?cmd=Retrieve&db=PubMed&dopt=Citation&list_uids=21653308.

98. Brothers CH, Hernandez JE, Cutrell AG, et al. Risk of myocardial infarction and abacavir therapy: no increased risk across 52 GlaxoSmithKline-sponsored clinical trials in adult subjects. *J Acquir Immune Defic Syndr*. 2009;51(1):20-28. Available at
http://www.ncbi.nlm.nih.gov/entrez/query.fcgi?cmd=Retrieve&db=PubMed&dopt=Citation&list_uids=19282778.

99. Ding X, Andraca-Carrera E, Cooper C, et al. No association of abacavir use with myocardial infarction: findings of an FDA meta-analysis. *J Acquir Immune Defic Syndr.* 2012;61(4):441-447. Available at http://www.ncbi.nlm.nih.gov/pubmed/22932321.

100. Hsue PY, Hunt PW, Wu Y, et al. Association of abacavir and impaired endothelial function in treated and suppressed HIV-infected patients. *AIDS.* 2009;23(15):2021-2027. Available at http://www.ncbi.nlm.nih.gov/entrez/query.fcgi?cmd=Retrieve&db=PubMed&dopt=Citation&list_uids=19542863.

101. Satchell CS, O'Halloran JA, Cotter AG, et al. Increased Platelet Reactivity in HIV-1-Infected Patients Receiving Abacavir-Containing Antiretroviral Therapy. *J Infect Dis.* 2011;204(8):1202-1210. Available at http://www.ncbi.nlm.nih.gov/entrez/query.fcgi?cmd=Retrieve&db=PubMed&dopt=Citation&list_uids=21917893.

102. Kristoffersen US, Kofoed K, Kronborg G, Benfield T, Kjaer A, Lebech AM. Changes in biomarkers of cardiovascular risk after a switch to abacavir in HIV-1-infected individuals receiving combination antiretroviral therapy. *HIV Med.* 2009;10(10):627-633. Available at http://www.ncbi.nlm.nih.gov/entrez/query.fcgi?cmd=Retrieve&db=PubMed&dopt=Citation&list_uids=19891054.

103. De Pablo C, Orden S, Apostolova N, Blanquer A, Esplugues JV, Alvarez A. Abacavir and didanosine induce the interaction between human leukocytes and endothelial cells through Mac-1 upregulation. *AIDS.* 2010;24(9):1259-1266. Available at http://www.ncbi.nlm.nih.gov/entrez/query.fcgi?cmd=Retrieve&db=PubMed&dopt=Citation&list_uids=20453628.

104. Martinez E, Larrousse M, Podzamczer D, et al. Abacavir-based therapy does not affect biological mechanisms associated with cardiovascular dysfunction. *AIDS.* 2010;24(3):F1-9. Available at http://www.ncbi.nlm.nih.gov/entrez/query.fcgi?cmd=Retrieve&db=PubMed&dopt=Citation&list_uids=20009917.

105. Palella FJ, Jr., Gange SJ, Benning L, et al. Inflammatory biomarkers and abacavir use in the Women's Interagency HIV Study and the Multicenter AIDS Cohort Study. *AIDS.* 2010;24(11):1657-1665. Available at http://www.ncbi.nlm.nih.gov/entrez/query.fcgi?cmd=Retrieve&db=PubMed&dopt=Citation&list_uids=20588104.

106. Martin A, Amin J, Cooper DA, et al. Abacavir does not affect circulating levels of inflammatory or coagulopathic biomarkers in suppressed HIV: a randomized clinical trial. *AIDS.* 2010;24(17):2657-2663. Available at http://www.ncbi.nlm.nih.gov/entrez/query.fcgi?cmd=Retrieve&db=PubMed&dopt=Citation&list_uids=20827168.

107. Jong E, Meijers JC, van Gorp EC, Spek CA, Mulder JW. Markers of inflammation and coagulation indicate a prothrombotic state in HIV-infected patients with long-term use of antiretroviral therapy with or without abacavir. *AIDS Res Ther.* 2010;7:9. Available at http://www.ncbi.nlm.nih.gov/entrez/query.fcgi?cmd=Retrieve&db=PubMed&dopt=Citation&list_uids=20398387.

108. Podzamczer D, Ferrer E, Consiglio E, et al. A randomized clinical trial comparing nelfinavir or nevirapine associated to zidovudine/lamivudine in HIV-infected naive patients (the Combine Study). *Antivir Ther.* 2002;7(2):81-90. Available at http://www.ncbi.nlm.nih.gov/entrez/query.fcgi?cmd=Retrieve&db=PubMed&dopt=Citation&list_uids=12212928.

109. Vibhagool A, Cahn P, Schechter M, et al. Triple nucleoside treatment with abacavir plus the lamivudine/zidovudine combination tablet (COM) compared to indinavir/COM in antiretroviral therapy-naive adults: results of a 48-week open-label, equivalence trial (CNA3014). *Curr Med Res Opin.* 2004;20(7):1103-1114. Available at http://www.ncbi.nlm.nih.gov/entrez/query.fcgi?cmd=Retrieve&db=PubMed&dopt=Citation&list_uids=15265255.

110. Staszewski S, Keiser P, Montaner J, et al. Abacavir-lamivudine-zidovudine vs indinavir-lamivudine-zidovudine in antiretroviral-naive HIV-infected adults: A randomized equivalence trial. *JAMA.* 2001;285(9):1155-1163. Available at http://www.ncbi.nlm.nih.gov/entrez/query.fcgi?cmd=Retrieve&db=PubMed&dopt=Citation&list_uids=11231744.

111. Gulick RM, Ribaudo HJ, Shikuma CM, et al. Triple-nucleoside regimens versus efavirenz-containing regimens for the initial treatment of HIV-1 infection. *N Engl J Med.* 2004;350(18):1850-1861. Available at http://www.ncbi.nlm.nih.gov/entrez/query.fcgi?cmd=Retrieve&db=PubMed&dopt=Citation&list_uids=15115831.

112. Robbins GK, De Gruttola V, Shafer RW, et al. Comparison of sequential three-drug regimens as initial therapy for HIV-1 infection. *N Engl J Med.* 2003;349(24):2293-2303. Available at

http://www.ncbi.nlm.nih.gov/entrez/query.fcgi?cmd=Retrieve&db=PubMed&dopt=Citation&list_uids=14668455.

113. Drake A, Mijch A, Sasadeusz J. Immune reconstitution hepatitis in HIV and hepatitis B coinfection, despite lamivudine therapy as part of HAART. *Clin Infect Dis*. 2004;39(1):129-132. Available at http://www.ncbi.nlm.nih.gov/entrez/query.fcgi?cmd=Retrieve&db=PubMed&dopt=Citation&list_uids=15206064.

114. Bessesen M, Ives D, Condreay L, Lawrence S, Sherman KE. Chronic active hepatitis B exacerbations in human immunodeficiency virus-infected patients following development of resistance to or withdrawal of lamivudine. *Clin Infect Dis*.1999;28(5):1032-1035. Available at http://www.ncbi.nlm.nih.gov/entrez/query.fcgi?cmd=Retrieve&db=PubMed&dopt=Citation&list_uids=10452630.

115. Sellier P, Clevenbergh P, Mazeron MC, et al. Fatal interruption of a 3TC-containing regimen in a HIV-infected patient due to re-activation of chronic hepatitis B virus infection. *Scand J Infect Dis*. 2004;36(6-7):533-535. Available at http://www.ncbi.nlm.nih.gov/entrez/query.fcgi?cmd=Retrieve&db=PubMed&dopt=Citation&list_uids=15307596.

Some antiretroviral (ARV) regimens or components are not generally recommended because of suboptimal antiviral potency, unacceptable toxicities, or pharmacologic concerns. These are summarized below.

Antiretroviral Regimens Not Recommended

Monotherapy with nucleoside reverse transcriptase inhibitor (NRTI). Single-NRTI therapy does not demonstrate potent and sustained antiviral activity and **should not be used (AII)**. For prevention of mother-to-child transmission (PMTCT), zidovudine (ZDV) monotherapy is not recommended but might be considered in certain unusual circumstances in women with HIV RNA <1,000 copies/mL, although the use of a potent combination regimen is preferred. (See Perinatal Guidelines,[1] available at http://aidsinfo.nih.gov.)

Single-drug treatment regimens with a ritonavir (RTV)-boosted protease inhibitor (PI), either lopinavir (LPV),[2] atazanavir (ATV),[3] or darunavir (DRV)[4-5] are under investigation with mixed results, and **cannot be recommended** outside of a clinical trial at this time.

Dual-NRTI regimens. These regimens **are not recommended** because they have not demonstrated potent and sustained antiviral activity compared with triple-drug combination regimens **(AI)**.[6]

Triple-NRTI regimens. In general, triple-NRTI regimens other than abacavir/lamivudine/zidovudine (ABC/3TC/ZDV) **(BI)** and possibly lamivudine/zidovudine + tenofovir (3TC/ZDV + TDF) **(BII) should not be used** because of suboptimal virologic activity[7-9] or lack of data **(AI)**.

Antiretroviral Components Not Recommended

Atazanavir (ATV) + indinavir (IDV). Both of these PIs can cause Grade 3 to 4 hyperbilirubinemia and jaundice. Additive adverse effects may be possible when these agents are used concomitantly. Therefore, these two PIs **are not recommended** for combined use **(AIII)**.

Didanosine (ddI) + stavudine (d4T). The combined use of ddI and d4T as a dual-NRTI backbone can result in a high incidence of toxicities, particularly peripheral neuropathy, pancreatitis, and lactic acidosis.[10-13] This combination has been implicated in the deaths of several HIV-infected pregnant women secondary to severe lactic acidosis with or without hepatic steatosis and pancreatitis.[14] Therefore, the combined use of ddI and d4T **is not recommended (AII)**.

Didanosine (ddI) + tenofovir (TDF). Use of ddI + TDF may increase ddI concentrations[15] and serious ddI-associated toxicities including pancreatitis and lactic acidosis.[16-17] These toxicities may be lessened by ddI dose reduction. The use of this combination has also been associated with immunologic nonresponse or CD4 cell decline despite viral suppression,[18-19] high rates of early virologic failure,[20-21] and rapid selection of resistance mutations.[20-22] Because of these adverse outcomes, this dual-NRTI combination **is not generally recommended (AII)**. Clinicians caring for patients who are clinically stable on regimens containing ddI + TDF should consider altering the NRTIs to avoid this combination.

Two-non-nucleoside reverse transcriptase inhibitor (2-NNRTI) combinations. In the 2NN trial, ARV-naive participants were randomized to receive once- or twice-daily nevirapine (NVP) versus efavirenz (EFV) versus EFV plus NVP, all combined with d4T and 3TC.[23] A higher frequency of clinical adverse events that led to treatment discontinuation was reported in participants randomized to the two-NNRTI arm. Both EFV and NVP may induce metabolism of etravirine (ETR), which leads to reduction in ETR drug exposure.[24] Based on these findings, the Panel **does not recommend using two NNRTIs in combination in any regimen (AI)**.

Efavirenz (EFV) in first trimester of pregnancy and in women with significant childbearing potential. EFV use was associated with significant teratogenic effects in nonhuman primates at drug exposures similar to those representing human exposure. Several cases of congenital anomalies have been reported after early human gestational exposure to EFV.[25-26] EFV **should be avoided** in pregnancy, particularly during the first trimester, and in women of childbearing potential who are trying to conceive or who are not using effective and consistent contraception **(AIII)**. If no other ARV options are available for the woman who is pregnant or at risk of becoming pregnant, the provider should consult with a clinician who has expertise in both HIV infection and pregnancy. (See Perinatal Guidelines,[1] available at http://aidsinfo.nih.gov.)

Emtricitabine (FTC) + lamivudine (3TC). Both of these drugs have similar resistance profiles and have minimal additive antiviral activity. Inhibition of intracellular phosphorylation may occur *in vivo*, as seen with other dual-cytidine analog combinations.[27] These two agents **should not be used** as a dual-NRTI combination **(AIII)**.

Etravirine (ETR) + unboosted PI. ETR may induce the metabolism and significantly reduce the drug exposure of unboosted PIs. Appropriate doses of the PIs have not been established[24] **(AII)**.

Etravirine (ETR) + ritonavir (RTV)-boosted atazanavir (ATV) or fosamprenavir (FPV). ETR may alter the concentrations of these PIs. Appropriate doses of the PIs have not been established[24] **(AII)**.

Etravirine (ETR) + ritonavir (RTV)-boosted tipranavir (TPV). RTV-boosted TPV significantly reduces ETR concentrations. These drugs **should not be co-administered**[24] **(AII)**.

Nevirapine (NVP) initiated in ARV-naive women with CD4 counts >250 cells/mm³ or in ARV-naive men with CD4 counts >400 cells/mm³. Greater risk of symptomatic hepatic events, including serious and life-threatening events, has been observed in these patient groups. NVP **should not be initiated** in these patients **(BI)** unless the benefit clearly outweighs the risk.[28-30] Patients who experience CD4 count increases to levels above these thresholds as a result of antiretroviral therapy (ART) can be safely switched to NVP.[31]

Unboosted darunavir (DRV), saquinavir (SQV), or tipranavir (TPV). The virologic benefit of these PIs has been demonstrated only when they were used with concomitant RTV. Therefore, use of these agents as part of a combination regimen **without RTV is not recommended (AII)**.

Stavudine (d4T) + zidovudine (ZDV). These two NRTIs **should not be used** in combination because of antagonism demonstrated *in vitro*[32] and *in vivo*[33] **(AII)**.

	Rationale	Exception
Antiretroviral Regimens Not Recommended		
Monotherapy with NRTI (AII)	• Rapid development of resistance • Inferior ARV activity when compared with combination of three or more ARV agents	• No exception
Dual-NRTI regimens (AI)	• Rapid development of resistance • Inferior ARV activity when compared with combination of three or more ARV agents	• No exception
Triple-NRTI regimens (AI) except for ABC/ZDV/3TC (BI) or possibly TDF + ZDV/3TC (BII)	• High rate of early virologic nonresponse seen when triple-NRTI combinations, including ABC/TDF/3TC and TDF/ddI/3TC, were used as initial regimen in ART-naive patients. • Other triple-NRTI regimens have not been evaluated.	• ABC/ZDV/3TC (BI) and possibly TDF + ZDV/3TC (BII) in patients in whom other combinations are not desirable
Antiretroviral Components Not Recommended as Part of an Antiretroviral Regimen		
ATV + IDV (AIII)	• Potential additive hyperbilirubinemia	• No exception
ddI + d4T (AII)	• High incidence of toxicities: peripheral neuropathy, pancreatitis, and hyperlactatemia • Reports of serious, even fatal, cases of lactic acidosis with hepatic steatosis with or without pancreatitis in pregnant women	• No exception
ddI + TDF (AII)	• Increased ddI concentrations and serious ddI-associated toxicities • Potential for immunologic nonresponse and/or CD4 cell count decline • High rate of early virologic failure • Rapid selection of resistance mutations at failure	• Clinicians caring for patients who are clinically stable on regimens containing TDF + ddI should consider altering the NRTIs to avoid this combination.
2-NNRTI combination (AI)	• When EFV combined with NVP, higher incidence of clinical adverse events seen when compared with either EFV- or NVP-based regimen. • Both EFV and NVP may induce metabolism and may lead to reductions in ETR exposure; thus, they should not be used in combination with ETR.	• No exception
EFV in first trimester of pregnancy or in women with significant childbearing potential (AIII)	• Teratogenic in nonhuman primates	• When no other ARV options are available and potential benefits outweigh the risks (BIII)
FTC + 3TC (AIII)	• Similar resistance profiles • No potential benefit	• No exception
ETR + unboosted PI (AII)	• ETR may induce metabolism of these PIs; appropriate doses not yet established	• No exception
ETR + RTV-boosted ATV or FPV (AII)	• ETR may alter the concentrations of these PIs; appropriate doses not yet established	• No exception
ETR + RTV-boosted TPV (AII)	• ETR concentration may be significantly reduced by RTV-boosted TPV	• No exception

Table 8. Antiretroviral Regimens or Components That Should Not Be Offered At Any Time (page 2 of 2)

	Rationale	Exception
NVP in ARV-naive women with CD4 count >250 cells/mm³ or men with CD4 count >400 cells/mm³ (BI)	• High incidence of symptomatic hepatotoxicity	• If no other ARV option available; if used, patient should be closely monitored
d4T + ZDV (AII)	• Antagonistic effect on HIV-1	• No exception
Unboosted DRV, SQV, or TPV (AII)	• Inadequate bioavailability	• No exception

Acronyms: 3TC = lamivudine, ABC = abacavir, ATV = atazanavir, d4T = stavudine, ddI = didanosine, DRV = darunavir, EFV = efavirenz, ETR = etravirine, FPV = fosamprenavir, FTC = emitricitabine, IDV = indinavir, NVP = nevirapine, RTV = ritonavir, SQV = saquinavir, TDF = tenofovir, TPV = tipranavir, ZDV = zidovudine

References

1. Panel on Treatment of HIV-Infected Pregnant Women and Prevention of Perinatal Transmission. Recommendations for use of antiretroviral drugs in pregnant HIV-1-infected women for maternal health and interventions to reduce perinatal HIV transmission in the United States. May 24, 2010:1-117. http://aidsinfo.nih.gov/contentfiles/PerinatalGL.pdf.

2. Delfraissy JF, Flandre P, Delaugerre C, et al. Lopinavir/ritonavir monotherapy or plus zidovudine and lamivudine in antiretroviral-naive HIV-infected patients. *AIDS*. 2008;22(3):385-393.

3. Swindells S, DiRienzo AG, Wilkin T, et al. Regimen simplification to atazanavir-ritonavir alone as maintenance antiretroviral therapy after sustained virologic suppression. *JAMA*. 2006;296(7):806-814.

4. Arribas JR, Horban A, Gerstoft J, et al. The MONET trial: darunavir/ritonavir with or without nucleoside analogues, for patients with HIV RNA below 50 copies/ml. *AIDS*. 2010;24(2):223-230.

5. Katlama C, Valantin MA, Algarte-Genin M, et al. Efficacy of darunavir/ritonavir maintenance monotherapy in patients with HIV-1 viral suppression: a randomized open-label, noninferiority trial, MONOI-ANRS 136. *AIDS*. 2010;24(15):2365-2374.

6. Hirsch M, Steigbigel R, Staszewski S, et al. A randomized, controlled trial of indinavir, zidovudine, and lamivudine in adults with advanced human immunodeficiency virus type 1 infection and prior antiretroviral therapy. *J Infect Dis*. 1999;180(3):659-665.

7. Gallant JE, Rodriguez AE, Weinberg WG, et al. Early virologic nonresponse to tenofovir, abacavir, and lamivudine in HIV-infected antiretroviral-naive subjects. *J Infect Dis*. 2005;192(11):1921-1930.

8. Bartlett JA, Johnson J, Herrera G, et al. Long-term results of initial therapy with abacavir and lamivudine combined with efavirenz, amprenavir/ritonavir, or stavudine. *J Acquir Immune Defic Syndr*. 2006;43(3):284-292.

9. Barnas D, Koontz D, Bazmi H, et al. Clonal resistance analyses of HIV type-1 after failure of therapy with didanosine, lamivudine and tenofovir. *Antivir Ther*. 2010;15(3):437-441.

10. Moore RD, Wong WM, Keruly JC, et al. Incidence of neuropathy in HIV-infected patients on monotherapy versus those on combination therapy with didanosine, stavudine and hydroxyurea. *AIDS*. 2000;14(3):273-278.

11. Robbins GK, De Gruttola V, Shafer RW, et al. Comparison of sequential three-drug regimens as initial therapy for HIV-1 infection. *N Engl J Med*. 2003;349(24):2293-2303.

12. Boubaker K, Flepp M, Sudre P, et al. Hyperlactatemia and antiretroviral therapy: the Swiss HIV Cohort Study. *Clin Infect Dis*. 2001;33(11):1931-1937.

13. Coghlan ME, Sommadossi JP, Jhala NC, et al. Symptomatic lactic acidosis in hospitalized antiretroviral-treated patients with human immunodeficiency virus infection: a report of 12 cases. *Clin Infect Dis*. 2001;33(11):1914-1921.

14. FDA FaDA. Caution issued for HIV combination therapy with Zerit and Videx in pregnant women. *HIV Clin.* 2001;13(2):6.

15. Kearney BP, Sayre JR, Flaherty JF, et al. Drug-drug and drug-food interactions between tenofovir disoproxil fumarate and didanosine. *J Clin Pharmacol.* 2005;45(12):1360-1367.

16. Murphy MD, O'Hearn M, Chou S. Fatal lactic acidosis and acute renal failure after addition of tenofovir to an antiretroviral regimen containing didanosine. *Clin Infect Dis.* 2003;36(8):1082-1085.

17. Martinez E, Milinkovic A, de Lazzari E, et al. Pancreatic toxic effects associated with co-administration of didanosine and tenofovir in HIV-infected adults. *Lancet.* 2004;364(9428):65-67.

18. Barrios A, Rendon A, Negredo E, et al. Paradoxical CD4+ T-cell decline in HIV-infected patients with complete virus suppression taking tenofovir and didanosine. *AIDS.* 2005;19(6):569-575.

19. Negredo E, Bonjoch A, Paredes R, et al. Compromised immunologic recovery in treatment-experienced patients with HIV infection receiving both tenofovir disoproxil fumarate and didanosine in the TORO studies. *Clin Infect Dis.* 2005;41(6):901-905.

20. Leon A, Martinez E, Mallolas J, et al. Early virological failure in treatment-naive HIV-infected adults receiving didanosine and tenofovir plus efavirenz or nevirapine. *AIDS.* 2005;19(2):213-215.

21. Maitland D, Moyle G, Hand J, et al. Early virologic failure in HIV-1 infected subjects on didanosine/tenofovir/efavirenz: 12-week results from a randomized trial. *AIDS.* 2005;19(11):1183-1188.

22. Podzamczer D, Ferrer E, Gatell JM, et al. Early virological failure with a combination of tenofovir, didanosine and efavirenz. *Antivir Ther.* 2005;10(1):171-177.

23. van Leth F, Phanuphak P, Ruxrungtham K, et al. Comparison of first-line antiretroviral therapy with regimens including nevirapine, efavirenz, or both drugs, plus stavudine and lamivudine: a randomised open-label trial, the 2NN Study. *Lancet.* 2004;363(9417):1253-1263.

24. Tibotec, Inc. Intelence (package insert) 2009.

25. Fundaro C, Genovese O, Rendeli C, et al. Myelomeningocele in a child with intrauterine exposure to efavirenz. *AIDS.* 2002;16(2):299-300.

26. Antiretroviral Pregnancy Registry Steering Committee. Antiretroviral Pregnancy Registry international interim report for 1 Jan 1989 - 31 January 2007. 2007; http://www.APRegistry.com.

27. Bethell R, Adams J, DeMuys J, et al. Pharmacological evaluation of a dual deoxycytidine analogue combination: 3TC and SPD754. Paper presented at: 11th Conference on Retroviruses and Opportunistic Infections; February 8-11, 2004; San Francisco, California. Abstract 138.

28. Baylor MS, Johann-Liang R. Hepatotoxicity associated with nevirapine use. *J Acquir Immune Defic Syndr.* 2004;35(5):538-539.

29. Sanne I, Mommeja-Marin H, Hinkle J, et al. Severe hepatotoxicity associated with nevirapine use in HIV-infected subjects. *J Infect Dis.* 2005;191(6):825-829.

30. Boehringer Ingelheim. Dear Health Care Professional Letter. *Clarification of risk factors for severe, life-threatening and fatal hepatotoxicity with VIRAMUNE® (nevirapine)* 2004.

31. Kesselring AM, Wit FW, Sabin CA, et al. Risk factors for treatment-limiting toxicities in patients starting nevirapine-containing antiretroviral therapy. *AIDS.* 2009;23(13):1689-1699.

32. Hoggard PG, Kewn S, Barry MG, et al. Effects of drugs on 2',3'-dideoxy-2',3'-didehydrothymidine phosphorylation *in vitro. Antimicrob Agents Chemother.* 1997;41(6):1231-1236.

33. Havlir DV, Tierney C, Friedland GH, et al. *In vivo* antagonism with zidovudine plus stavudine combination therapy. *J Infect Dis.* 2000;182(1):321-325.

Management of the Treatment-Experienced Patient

Virologic and Immunologic Failure (Last updated January 10, 2011; last reviewed January 10, 2011)

Panel's Recommendations

- Assessing and managing an antiretroviral (ARV)-experienced patient experiencing failure of antiretroviral therapy (ART) is complex. Expert advice is critical and should be sought.

- Evaluation of virologic failure should include an assessment of the severity of the patient's HIV disease, ART history, use of concomitant medications with consideration of adverse drug interactions with ARV agents, HIV RNA and CD4 T-cell count trends over time, and prior drug-resistance testing results.

- Drug-resistance testing should be obtained while the patient is taking the failing ARV regimen or within 4 weeks of treatment discontinuation **(AII)**.

- The goal of treatment for ARV-experienced patients with drug resistance who are experiencing virologic failure is to re-establish virologic suppression (e.g., HIV RNA <48 copies/mL) **(AI)**.

- To design a new regimen, the patient's treatment history and past and current resistance test results should be used to identify at least two (preferably three) fully active agents to combine with an optimized background ARV regimen **(AI)**. A fully active agent is one that is likely to have ARV activity on the basis of the patient's treatment history, drug-resistance testing, and/or a novel mechanism of action.

- In general, adding a single, fully active ARV in a new regimen is *not* recommended because of the risk of rapid development of resistance **(BII)**.

- In patients with a high likelihood of clinical progression (e.g., CD4 count <100 cells/mm^3) and limited drug options, adding a single drug may reduce the risk of immediate clinical progression, because even transient decreases in HIV RNA and/or transient increases in CD4 cell counts have been associated with clinical benefits **(CI)**.

- For some highly ART-experienced patients, maximal virologic suppression is not possible. In this case, ART should be continued **(AI)** with regimens designed to minimize toxicity, preserve CD4 cell counts, and avoid clinical progression.

- Discontinuing or briefly interrupting therapy in a patient with viremia may lead to a rapid increase in HIV RNA and a decrease in CD4 cell count and increases the risk of clinical progression. Therefore, this strategy is *not* recommended **(AI)**.

- In the setting of virologic suppression, there is no consensus on how to define or treat immunologic failure.

Rating of Recommendations: A = Strong; B = Moderate; C = Optional

Rating of Evidence: I = Data from randomized controlled trials; II = Data from well-designed nonrandomized trials or observational cohort studies with long-term clinical outcomes; III = Expert opinion

Virologic Definitions

Virologic suppression: A confirmed HIV RNA level below the limit of assay detection (e.g., <48 copies/mL).

Virologic failure: The inability to achieve or maintain suppression of viral replication (to an HIV RNA level <200 copies/mL).

Incomplete virologic response: Two consecutive plasma HIV RNA levels >200 copies/mL after 24 weeks on an ARV regimen. Baseline HIV RNA may affect the time course of response, and some regimens will take longer than others to suppress HIV RNA levels.

Virologic rebound: Confirmed detectable HIV RNA (to >200 copies/mL) after virologic suppression.

Persistent low-level viremia: Confirmed detectable HIV RNA levels that are <1,000 copies/mL.

Virologic blip: After virologic suppression, an isolated detectable HIV RNA level that is followed by a return to virologic suppression.

Causes of Virologic Failure

Virologic failure in a patient can occur for multiple reasons. Data from older patient cohorts suggested that suboptimal adherence and drug intolerance/toxicity accounted for 28% 40% of virologic failure and regimen discontinuations.[1-2] More recent data suggest that most virologic failure on first-line regimens occurred due to either pre-existing (transmitted) drug resistance or suboptimal adherence.[3] Factors associated with virologic failure include:

- Patient characteristics
    - higher pretreatment or baseline HIV RNA level (depending on the specific regimen used)
    - lower pretreatment or nadir CD4 T-cell count
    - prior AIDS diagnosis
    - comorbidities (e.g., active substance abuse, depression)
    - presence of drug-resistant virus, either transmitted or acquired
    - prior treatment failure
    - incomplete medication adherence and missed clinic appointments
- ARV regimen characteristics
    - drug side effects and toxicities
    - suboptimal pharmacokinetics (variable absorption, metabolism, or, theoretically, penetration into reservoirs)
    - food/fasting requirements
    - adverse drug-drug interactions with concomitant medications
    - suboptimal virologic potency
    - prescription errors
- Provider characteristics, such as experience in treating HIV disease
- Other or unknown reasons

Management of Patients with Virologic Failure

Assessment of Virologic Failure

If virologic failure is suspected or confirmed, a thorough work-up is indicated, addressing the following factors:

- change in HIV RNA and CD4 T-cell counts over time
- occurrence of HIV-related clinical events
- ARV treatment history
- results of prior resistance testing (if any)
- medication-taking behavior (including adherence to recommended drug doses, dosing frequency, and food/fasting requirements)

- tolerability of medications
- concomitant medications and supplements (with consideration for adverse drug-drug interactions)
- comorbidities (including substance abuse)

In many cases, the cause(s) of virologic failure will be identified. In some cases, no obvious cause(s) may be identified. It is important to distinguish among the reasons for virologic failure because the approaches to subsequent therapy differ. The following potential causes of virologic failure should be explored in depth.

- **Adherence.** Assess the patient's adherence to the regimen. For incomplete adherence, identify and address the underlying cause(s) (e.g., difficulties accessing or tolerating medications, depression, active substance abuse) and simplify the regimen if possible (e.g., decrease pill count or dosing frequency). (See Adherence.)

- **Medication Intolerance.** Assess the patient's tolerance of the current regimen and the severity and duration of side effects, keeping in mind that even minor side effects can impact adherence. Management strategies for intolerance in the absence of drug resistance may include:
    - using symptomatic treatment (e.g., antiemetics, antidiarrheals)
    - changing one ARV to another within the same drug class, if needed (e.g., change to tenofovir [TDF] or abacavir [ABC] for zidovudine [ZDV]-related toxicities; change to nevirapine [NVP] or etravirine [ETR] for efavirenz [EFV]-related toxicities)[4-5]
    - changing from one drug class to another (e.g., from a non-nucleoside reverse transcriptase inhibitor [NNRTI] to a protease inhibitor [PI], from enfuvirtide [T-20] to raltegravir [RAL]) if necessary and no prior drug resistance is suspected

- **Pharmacokinetic Issues.** Review food/fasting requirements for each medication. Review recent history of gastrointestinal symptoms (such as vomiting or diarrhea) to assess the likelihood of short-term malabsorption. Review concomitant medications and dietary supplements for possible adverse drug-drug interactions (consult Drug Interactions section and tables for common interactions) and make appropriate substitutions for ARV agents and/or concomitant medications, if possible. Therapeutic drug monitoring (TDM) may be helpful if pharmacokinetic drug-drug interactions or impaired drug absorption leading to decreased ARV exposure is suspected. (See also Exposure-Response Relationship and Therapeutic Drug Monitoring.)

- **Suspected Drug Resistance.** Obtain resistance testing while the patient is taking the failing regimen or within 4 weeks after regimen discontinuation if the plasma HIV RNA level is >500 copies/mL **(AII)**. (See Drug-Resistance Testing.) Evaluate the degree of drug resistance and consider the patient's prior treatment history and prior resistance test results. Drug resistance tends to be cumulative for a given individual; thus, all prior treatment history and resistance test results should be taken into account. Routine genotypic or phenotypic testing gives information relevant for selecting nucleoside reverse transcriptase inhibitors (NRTIs), NNRTIs, and PIs. Additional drug-resistance tests for patients experiencing failure on fusion inhibitors and/or integrase strand transfer inhibitors (INSTIs) and viral tropism tests for patients experiencing failure on a CCR5 antagonist also are available. (See Drug-Resistance Testing.)

Changing ART

There is no consensus on the optimal time to change therapy for virologic failure. The goal of ART is to suppress HIV replication to a level where drug-resistance mutations do not emerge. However, the specific level of viral suppression needed to achieve durable virologic suppression remains unknown. Selection of drug resistance does not appear to occur in patients with persistent HIV RNA levels suppressed to <48 copies/mL,[6] although this remains controversial.[7]

The clinical implications of HIV RNA in the range of >48 to <200 copies/mL in a patient on ART are controversial. Unlike the case with higher levels of HIV RNA, most, if not all, circulating virus from individuals with this level of HIV RNA results from the release of HIV from long-lived latently infected cells and does not signify ongoing viral replication with the emergence of drug-resistant virus.[8] Although some studies have suggested that viremia at this low level predicts subsequent failure[9] and can be associated with the evolution of drug resistance,[10] a large retrospective analysis showed that using an HIV RNA threshold for virologic failure of <200 copies/mL had the same predictive value as using a threshold of <50 copies/mL.[11]

Newer technologies (e.g., Taqman assay) have made it possible to detect HIV RNA in more patients with low level viremia (<200 copies/mL) than was possible with previous assays. Use of these newer assays has resulted in more confirmatory viral load testing than may be necessary.[12-14]

Persistent HIV RNA levels >200 copies/mL often are associated with evidence of viral evolution and drug-resistance mutation accumulation;[15] this is particularly common when HIV RNA levels are >500 copies/mL.[16] Persistent plasma HIV RNA levels in the 200 to 1,000 copies/mL range should therefore be considered as virologic failure.

Viremia "blips" (e.g., viral suppression followed by a detectable HIV RNA level and then subsequent return to undetectable levels) usually are not associated with subsequent virologic failure.[17]

Management of Virologic Failure

Once virologic failure is confirmed, generally the regimen should be changed as soon as possible to avoid progressive accumulation of resistance mutations.[18]

Ideally, a new ARV regimen should contain at least two, and preferably three, fully active drugs on the basis of drug treatment history, resistance testing, or new mechanistic class **(AI)**.[19-27] Some ARV drugs (e.g., NRTIs) may contribute partial ARV activity to a regimen, despite drug resistance,[28] while others (e.g., T-20, NNRTIs, RAL) likely do not provide partial activity.[28-30] Because of the potential for drug-class cross resistance that reduces drug activity, using a "new" drug that a patient has not yet taken may not mean that the drug is fully active. In addition, archived drug-resistance mutations may not be detected by standard drug-resistance tests, emphasizing the importance of considering treatment history and prior drug-resistance tests. Drug potency and viral susceptibility are more important than the number of drugs prescribed.

Early studies of ART-experienced patients identified factors associated with better virologic responses to subsequent regimens.[31-32] These factors included lower HIV RNA level and/or higher CD4 cell count at the time of therapy change, using a new (i.e., not yet taken) class of ARV drugs, and using ritonavir (RTV)-boosted PIs in PI-experienced patients.

More recent clinical trials support the strategy of conducting reverse transcriptase (RT) and protease (PT) resistance testing (both genotype and phenotype) while an ART-experienced patient is taking a failing ARV regimen, designing a new regimen based on the treatment history and resistance testing results, and selecting at least two and preferably three active drugs for the new treatment regimen.[20-21, 23-24, 33] Higher genotypic and/or phenotypic susceptibility scores (quantitative measures of drug activity) are associated with better virologic responses.[23-24] Patients who receive more active drugs have a better and more prolonged virologic response than those with fewer active drugs in the regimen. Active ARV drugs include those with activity against drug-resistant viral strains, including newer members of existing classes (the NNRTI ETR, the PIs darunavir [DRV] and tipranavir [TPV]) and drugs with new mechanisms of action (the fusion inhibitor T-20, the CCR5 antagonist maraviroc [MVC] in patients with R5 but not X4 virus, and the INSTI RAL). Drug-resistance tests for patients experiencing failure on fusion inhibitors (FIs) and/or INSTIs and viral tropism tests for patients experiencing failure on a CCR5 antagonist also are available. (See Drug-Resistance Testing.)

Clinical Scenarios of Virologic Failure

- **Low-level viremia (HIV RNA <1,000 copies/mL).** Assess adherence. Consider variability in HIV RNA assays. Patients with HIV RNA <48 copies/mL or isolated increases in HIV RNA ("blips") do not require a change in treatment[13] **(AII)**. There is no consensus regarding how to manage patients with HIV RNA levels >48 copies/mL and <200 copies/mL; HIV RNA levels should be followed over time to assess the need for changes **(AIII)**. Patients with persistent HIV RNA levels >200 copies/mL often select out drug-resistant viral variants, particularly when HIV RNA levels are >500 copies/mL. Persistent plasma HIV RNA levels in the 200 to 1,000 copies/mL range should be considered as possible virologic failure; resistance testing should be attempted if the HIV RNA level is >500 copies/mL. For individuals with sufficient therapeutic options, consider treatment change **(BIII)**.

- **Repeated detectable viremia (HIV RNA >1,000 copies/mL) and NO drug resistance identified.** Consider the timing of the drug-resistance test (e.g., was the patient off ARV for >4 weeks and/or nonadherent?). Consider resuming the same regimen or starting a new regimen and then repeating genotypic testing early (e.g., in 2–4 weeks) to determine whether a resistant viral strain emerges **(CIII)**.

- **Repeated detectable viremia (HIV RNA >1,000 copies/mL) and drug resistance identified.** The goals in this situation are to resuppress HIV RNA levels maximally (i.e., to <48 copies/mL) and to prevent further selection of resistance mutations. With the availability of multiple new ARVs, including some with new mechanisms of action, this goal is now possible in many patients, including those with extensive treatment experience and drug resistance. With virologic failure, consider changing the treatment regimen sooner, rather than later, to minimize continued selection of resistance mutations. In a patient with ongoing viremia and evidence of resistance, some drugs in a regimen (e.g., NNRTI, T-20, RAL) should be discontinued promptly to decrease the risk of selecting additional drug-resistance mutations in order to preserve the activity of these drug classes in future regimens. A new regimen should include at least two, and preferably three, fully active agents **(AII)**.

- **Highly drug resistant HIV.** There is a subset of patients who have experienced toxicity and/or developed resistance to all or most currently available regimens, and designing a regimen with two or three fully active drugs is not possible. Many of these patients received suboptimal ARV regimens (i.e., did not have access to more than one or two of the drugs at the time they became available) or have been unable to adhere to any regimen. If maximal virologic suppression cannot be achieved, the goals are to preserve immunologic function and to prevent clinical progression (even with ongoing viremia). There is no consensus on how to optimize the management of these patients. It is reasonable to observe a patient on the same regimen, rather than changing the regimen, depending on the stage of HIV disease **(BII)**. Even partial virologic suppression of HIV RNA >0.5 $\log_{10}$ copies/mL from baseline correlates with clinical benefits.[34] There is evidence from cohort studies that continuing therapy, even in the presence of viremia and the absence of CD4 T-cell count increases, reduces the risk of disease progression.[35] Other cohort studies suggest continued immunologic and clinical benefits if the HIV RNA level is maintained <10,000–20,000 copies/mL.[36-37] However, these potential benefits all must be balanced with the ongoing risk of accumulating additional resistance mutations.

In general, adding a single, fully active ARV in a new regimen is *not* recommended because of the risk of rapid development of resistance **(BII)**. However, in patients with a high likelihood of clinical progression (e.g., CD4 cell count <100 cells/mm³) and limited drug options, adding a single drug may reduce the risk of immediate clinical progression, because even transient decreases in HIV RNA and/or transient increases in CD4 cell counts have been associated with clinical benefits **(CI)**. Weighing the risks (e.g., selection of drug resistance) and benefits (e.g., ARV activity) of using a single active drug in the heavily ART-experienced patient is complicated, and consultation with an expert is advised.

Patients with ongoing viremia and with an insufficient number of approved treatment options to construct a fully suppressive regimen may be candidates for research studies or expanded access programs, or single-patient access of investigational new drug(s) (IND), as specified in Food and Drug Administration (FDA) regulations: http://www.fda.gov/AboutFDA/CentersOffices/CDER/ucm163982.htm.

Discontinuing or briefly interrupting therapy in a patient with viremia may lead to a rapid increase in HIV RNA and a decrease in CD4 T-cell count and increases the risk of clinical progression.[38-39] Therefore, this strategy is *not* recommended (AI). See Discontinuation or Interruption of Antiretroviral Therapy.

- **Prior treatment and suspected drug resistance, now presenting to care in need of therapy with limited information (i.e., incomplete or absence of self-reported history, medical records, or previous resistance data).** Every effort should be made to obtain medical records and prior drug-resistance testing results; however, this is not always possible. One strategy is to restart the most recent ARV regimen and assess drug resistance in 2 4 weeks to help guide the choice of the next regimen; another strategy is to start two or three drugs known to be active based on treatment history (e.g., MVC with R5 virus, RAL if no prior INSTI).

Immunologic Failure: Definition, Causes, and Management

Immunologic failure can be defined as the failure to achieve and maintain an adequate CD4 response despite virologic suppression. Increases in CD4 counts in ARV-naive patients with initial ARV regimens are approximately 150 cells/mm³ over the first year.[40] A CD4 count plateau may occur after 4 6 years of treatment with suppressed viremia.[41-45]

No accepted specific definition for immunologic failure exists, although some studies have focused on patients who fail to increase CD4 counts above a specific threshold (e.g., >350 or 500 cells/mm³) over a specific period of time (e.g., 4 7 years). Others have focused on an inability to increase CD4 counts above pretherapy levels by a certain threshold (e.g., >50 or 100 cells/mm³) over a given time period. The former criterion may be preferable because of data linking these thresholds with the risk of non-AIDS clinical events.[46]

The proportion of patients experiencing immunologic failure depends on how failure is defined, the observation period, and the CD4 count when treatment was started. In the longest study conducted to date, the percentage of patients with suppressed viremia who reached a CD4 count >500 cells/mm³ through 6 years of treatment was 42% in those starting treatment with a CD4 count <200 cells/mm³, 66% in those starting with a CD4 count 200 350 cells/mm³, and 85% in those starting with a CD4 count >350 cells/mm³.[41]

A persistently low CD4 count while on suppressive ART is associated with a small, but appreciable, risk of AIDS- and non-AIDS-related morbidity and mortality.[47-48] For example, in the FIRST study,[49] a low CD4 count on therapy was associated with an increased risk of AIDS-related complications (adjusted hazard ratio of 0.56 per 100 cells/mm³ higher CD4 count). Similarly, a low CD4 count was associated with an increased risk of non-AIDS events, including cardiovascular, hepatic, and renal disease and cancer. Other studies support these associations.[50-53]

Factors associated with poor CD4 T-cell response:

- CD4 count <200/mm³ when starting ART
- Older age
- Coinfection (e.g., hepatitis C virus [HCV], HIV-2, human T-cell leukemia virus type 1 [HTLV-1], HTLV-2)
- Medications, both ARVs (e.g., ZDV,[54] TDF + didanosine [ddI][55-57]) and other medications.
- Persistent immune activation
- Loss of regenerative potential of the immune system
- Other medical conditions

Assessment of Immunologic Failure. CD4 count should be confirmed by repeat testing. Concomitant medications should be reviewed carefully, with a focus on those known to decrease white blood cells or, specifically, CD4 T-cells (e.g., cancer chemotherapy, interferon, prednisone, ZDV; combination of TDF and ddI), and consideration should be given to substituting or discontinuing these drugs, if possible. Untreated coinfections (e.g., HIV-2, HTLV-1, HTLV-2) and serious medical conditions (e.g., malignancy) also should be considered. In many cases, no obvious cause for immunologic failure can be identified.

Management of Immunologic Failure. No consensus exists on when or how to treat immunologic failure. Given the risk of clinical events, it is reasonable to focus on patients with CD4 counts <200 cells/mm^3 because patients with higher CD4 counts have a lower risk of clinical events. It is not clear that immunologic failure in the setting of virologic suppression should prompt a change in the ARV regimen. Because ongoing immune activation occurs in some patients with suppressed HIV RNA levels, some have suggested adding a drug to an existing regimen. However, this strategy does not result in clear virologic or immunologic benefit.[58] Others suggest changing the regimen to another regimen (e.g., from NNRTI-based to PI-based, INSTI-based, or CCR5 antagonist-based regimens), but this strategy has not shown clear benefit.

An immune-based therapy, interleukin-2, demonstrated CD4 count increases but no clinical benefit in two large randomized studies[59] and therefore is not recommended (**AI**). Other immune-based therapies (e.g., gene therapies, growth hormone, cyclosporine, interleukin-7) are under investigation. Currently, immune-based therapies should not be used unless in the context of a clinical trial (**AIII**).

References

1. d'Arminio Monforte A, Lepri AC, Rezza G, et al. Insights into the reasons for discontinuation of the first highly active antiretroviral therapy (HAART) regimen in a cohort of antiretroviral naive patients. I.CO.N.A. Study Group. Italian Cohort of Antiretroviral-Naive Patients. *AIDS*. 2000;14(5):499-507.

2. Mocroft A, Youle M, Moore A, et al. Reasons for modification and discontinuation of antiretrovirals: results from a single treatment centre. *AIDS*. 2001;15(2):185-194.

3. Paredes R, Lalama CM, Ribaudo HJ, et al. Pre-existing minority drug-resistant HIV-1 variants, adherence, and risk of antiretroviral treatment failure. *J Infect Dis*. 2010;201(5):662-671.

4. Schouten JT, Krambrink A, Ribaudo HJ, et al. Substitution of nevirapine because of efavirenz toxicity in AIDS clinical trials group A5095. *Clin Infect Dis*. 2010;50(5):787-791.

5. Waters L, Fisher M, Winston A, et al. A phase IV, double-blind, multicentre, randomized, placebo-controlled, pilot study to assess the feasibility of switching individuals receiving efavirenz with continuing central nervous system adverse events to etravirine. *AIDS*. 2011;25(1):65-71.

6. Kieffer TL, Finucane MM, Nettles RE, et al. Genotypic analysis of HIV-1 drug resistance at the limit of detection: virus production without evolution in treated adults with undetectable HIV loads. *J Infect Dis*. 2004;189(8):1452-1465.

7. Shiu C, Cunningham CK, Greenough T, et al. Identification of ongoing human immunodeficiency virus type 1 (HIV-1) replication in residual viremia during recombinant HIV-1 poxvirus immunizations in patients with clinically undetectable viral loads on durable suppressive highly active antiretroviral therapy. *J Virol*. 2009;83(19):9731-9742.

8. Siliciano JD, Kajdas J, Finzi D, et al. Long-term follow-up studies confirm the stability of the latent reservoir for HIV-1 in resting CD4+ T cells. *Nat Med*. 2003;9(6):727-728.

9. Eron JJ, Cooper DA, Steigbigel RT, et al. Sustained antiretroviral effect of raltegravir at week 156 in the BENCHMRK studies, and exploratory analysis of late outcomes based on early virologic responses. Paper presented at: 17th Conference on Retroviruses and Opportunistic Infections; February 16-19, 2010; San Francisco, CA. Abstract 515.

10. Taiwo B, Gallien S, Aga S, et al. HIV drug resistance evolution during persistent near-target viral suppression. *Antiviral Therapy* 2010;15:A38.

11. Ribaudo H, Lennox J, Currier J, et al. Virologic failure endpoint definition in clinical trials: Is using HIV-1 RNA threshold <200 copies/mL better than <50 copies/mL? An analysis of ACTG studies. Paper presented at: 16th Conference on Retroviruses and Opportunistic Infections; February 8-11, 2009; Montreal, Canada. Abstract 580.

12. Lima V, Harrigan R, Montaner JS. Increased reporting of detectable plasma HIV-1 RNA levels at the critical threshold of 50 copies per milliliter with the Taqman assay in comparison to the Amplicor assay. *J Acquir Immune Defic Syndr*. 2009;51(1):3-6.

13. Gatanaga H, Tsukada K, Honda H, et al. Detection of HIV type 1 load by the Roche Cobas TaqMan assay in patients with viral loads previously undetectable by the Roche Cobas Amplicor Monitor. *Clin Infect Dis*. 2009;48(2):260-262.

14. Willig JH, Nevin CR, Raper JL, et al. Cost ramifications of increased reporting of detectable plasma HIV-1 RNA levels by the Roche COBAS AmpliPrep/COBAS TaqMan HIV-1 version 1.0 viral load test. *J Acquir Immune Defic Syndr*. 2010;54(4):442-444.

15. Aleman S, Soderbarg K, Visco-Comandini U, et al. Drug resistance at low viraemia in HIV-1-infected patients with antiretroviral combination therapy. *AIDS*. 2002;16(7):1039-1044.

16. Karlsson AC, Younger SR, Martin JN, et al. Immunologic and virologic evolution during periods of intermittent and persistent low-level viremia. *AIDS*. 2004;18(7):981-989.

17. Nettles RE, Kieffer TL, Kwon P, et al. Intermittent HIV-1 viremia (Blips) and drug resistance in patients receiving HAART. *JAMA*. 2005;293(7):817-829.

18. Hosseinipour MC, van Oosterhout JJ, Weigel R, et al. The public health approach to identify antiretroviral therapy failure: high-level nucleoside reverse transcriptase inhibitor resistance among Malawians failing first-line antiretroviral therapy. *AIDS*. 2009;23(9):1127-1134.

19. Cooper DA, Steigbigel RT, Gatell JM, et al. Subgroup and resistance analyses of raltegravir for resistant HIV-1 infection. *N Engl J Med*. 2008;359(4):355-365.

20. Lazzarin A, Clotet B, Cooper D, et al. Efficacy of enfuvirtide in patients infected with drug-resistant HIV-1 in Europe and Australia. *N Engl J Med*. 2003;348(22):2186-2195.

21. Lalezari JP, Henry K, O'Hearn M, et al. Enfuvirtide, an HIV-1 fusion inhibitor, for drug-resistant HIV infection in North and South America. *N Engl J Med*. 2003;348(22):2175-2185.

22. Reynes J, Arasteh K, Clotet B, et al. TORO: ninety-six-week virologic and immunologic response and safety evaluation of enfuvirtide with an optimized background of antiretrovirals. *AIDS Patient Care STDS*. 2007;21(8):533-543.

23. Clotet B, Bellos N, Molina JM, et al. Efficacy and safety of darunavir-ritonavir at week 48 in treatment-experienced patients with HIV-1 infection in POWER 1 and 2: a pooled subgroup analysis of data from two randomised trials. *Lancet*. 2007;369(9568):1169-1178.

24. Steigbigel RT, Cooper DA, Kumar PN, et al. Raltegravir with optimized background therapy for resistant HIV-1 infection. *N Engl J Med*. 2008;359(4):339-354.

25. Katlama C, Haubrich R, Lalezari J, et al. Efficacy and safety of etravirine in treatment-experienced, HIV-1 patients: pooled 48 week analysis of two randomized, controlled trials. *AIDS*. 2009;23(17):2289-2300.

26. Gulick RM, Lalezari J, Goodrich J, et al. Maraviroc for previously treated patients with R5 HIV-1 infection. *N Engl J Med*. 2008;359(14):1429-1441.

27. Fatkenheuer G, Nelson M, Lazzarin A, et al. Subgroup analyses of maraviroc in previously treated R5 HIV-1 infection. *N Engl J Med*. 2008;359(14):1442-1455.

28. Deeks SG, Hoh R, Neilands TB, et al. Interruption of treatment with individual therapeutic drug classes in adults with multidrug-resistant HIV-1 infection. *J Infect Dis*. 2005;192(9):1537-1544.

29. Deeks SG, Lu J, Hoh R, et al. Interruption of enfuvirtide in HIV-1 infected adults with incomplete viral suppression on an enfuvirtide-based regimen. *J Infect Dis*. 2007;195(3):387-391.

30. Wirden M, Simon A, Schneider L, et al. Raltegravir has no residual antiviral activity in vivo against HIV-1 with

resistance-associated mutations to this drug. *J Antimicrob Chemother*. 2009;64(5):1087-1090.

31. Gulick RM, Hu XJ, Fiscus SA, et al. Randomized study of saquinavir with ritonavir or nelfinavir together with delavirdine, adefovir, or both in human immunodeficiency virus-infected adults with virologic failure on indinavir: AIDS Clinical Trials Group Study 359. *J Infect Dis*. 2000;182(5):1375-1384.

32. Hammer SM, Vaida F, Bennett KK, et al. Dual vs single protease inhibitor therapy following antiretroviral treatment failure: a randomized trial. *JAMA*. 2002;288(2):169-180.

33. Hicks CB, Cahn P, Cooper DA, et al. Durable efficacy of tipranavir-ritonavir in combination with an optimised background regimen of antiretroviral drugs for treatment-experienced HIV-1-infected patients at 48 weeks in the Randomized Evaluation of Strategic Intervention in multi-drug reSistant patients with Tipranavir (RESIST) studies: an analysis of combined data from two randomised open-label trials. *Lancet*. 2006;368(9534):466-475.

34. Murray JS, Elashoff MR, Iacono-Connors LC, et al. The use of plasma HIV RNA as a study endpoint in efficacy trials of antiretroviral drugs. *AIDS*. 1999;13(7):797-804.

35. Miller V, Sabin C, Hertogs K, et al. Virological and immunological effects of treatment interruptions in HIV-1 infected patients with treatment failure. *AIDS*. 2000;14(18):2857-2867.

36. Ledergerber B, Lundgren JD, Walker AS, et al. Predictors of trend in CD4-positive T-cell count and mortality among HIV-1-infected individuals with virological failure to all three antiretroviral-drug classes. *Lancet*. 2004;364(9428):51-62.

37. Raffanti SP, Fusco JS, Sherrill BH, et al. Effect of persistent moderate viremia on disease progression during HIV therapy. *J Acquir Immune Defic Syndr*. 2004;37(1):1147-1154.

38. Deeks SG, Wrin T, Liegler T, et al. Virologic and immunologic consequences of discontinuing combination antiretroviral-drug therapy in HIV-infected patients with detectable viremia. *N Engl J Med*. 2001;344(7):472-480.

39. Lawrence J, Mayers DL, Hullsiek KH, et al. Structured treatment interruption in patients with multidrug-resistant human immunodeficiency virus. *N Engl J Med*. 2003;349(9):837-846.

40. Bartlett JA, DeMasi R, Quinn J, et al. Overview of the effectiveness of triple combination therapy in antiretroviral-naive HIV-1 infected adults. *AIDS*. 2001;15(11):1369-1377.

41. Moore RD, Keruly JC. CD4+ cell count 6 years after commencement of highly active antiretroviral therapy in persons with sustained virologic suppression. *Clin Infect Dis*. 2007;44(3):441-446.

42. Kaufmann GR, Perrin L, Pantaleo G, et al. CD4 T-lymphocyte recovery in individuals with advanced HIV-1 infection receiving potent antiretroviral therapy for 4 years: the Swiss HIV Cohort Study. *Arch Intern Med*. 2003;163(18):2187-2195.

43. Garcia F, de Lazzari E, Plana M, et al. Long-term CD4+ T-cell response to highly active antiretroviral therapy according to baseline CD4+ T-cell count. *J Acquir Immune Defic Syndr*. 2004;36(2):702-713.

44. Tarwater PM, Margolick JB, Jin J, et al. Increase and plateau of CD4 T-cell counts in the 3(1/2) years after initiation of potent antiretroviral therapy. *J Acquir Immune Defic Syndr*. 2001;27(2):168-175.

45. Mocroft A, Phillips AN, Ledergerber B, et al. Relationship between antiretrovirals used as part of a cART regimen and CD4 cell count increases in patients with suppressed viremia. *AIDS*. 2006;20(8):1141-1150.

46. Lau B, Gange SJ, Moore RD. Risk of non-AIDS-related mortality may exceed risk of AIDS-related mortality among individuals enrolling into care with CD4+ counts greater than 200 cells/mm^3. *J Acquir Immune Defic Syndr*. 2007;44(2):179-187.

47. Loutfy MR, Walmsley SL, Mullin CM, et al. CD4(+) cell count increase predicts clinical benefits in patients with advanced HIV disease and persistent viremia after 1 year of combination antiretroviral therapy. *J Infect Dis*. 2005;192(8):1407-1411.

48. Moore DM, Hogg RS, Chan K, et al. Disease progression in patients with virological suppression in response to HAART is associated with the degree of immunological response. *AIDS*. 2006;20(3):371-377.

49. Baker JV, Peng G, Rapkin J, et al. CD4+ count and risk of non-AIDS diseases following initial treatment for HIV infection. *AIDS*. 2008;22(7):841-848.

50. Monforte A, Abrams D, Pradier C, et al. HIV-induced immunodeficiency and mortality from AIDS-defining and non-AIDS-defining malignancies. *AIDS*. 2008;22(16):2143-2153.

51. Weber R, Sabin CA, Friis-Moller N, et al. Liver-related deaths in persons infected with the human immunodeficiency virus: the D:A:D study. *Arch Intern Med*. 2006;166(15):1632-1641.

52. El-Sadr WM, Lundgren JD, Neaton JD, et al. CD4+ count-guided interruption of antiretroviral treatment. *N Engl J Med*. 2006;355(22):2283-2296.

53. Lichtenstein KA, Armon C, Buchacz K, et al. Low CD4+ T cell count is a risk factor for cardiovascular disease events in the HIV outpatient study. *Clin Infect Dis*. 2010;51(4):435-447.

54. Huttner AC, Kaufmann GR, Battegay M, et al. Treatment initiation with zidovudine-containing potent antiretroviral therapy impairs CD4 cell count recovery but not clinical efficacy. *AIDS*. 2007;21(8):939-946.

55. Barrios A, Rendon A, Negredo E, et al. Paradoxical CD4+ T-cell decline in HIV-infected patients with complete virus suppression taking tenofovir and didanosine. *AIDS*. 2005;19(6):569-575.

56. Lacombe K, Pacanowski J, Meynard JL, et al. Risk factors for CD4 lymphopenia in patients treated with a tenofovir/didanosine high dose-containing highly active antiretroviral therapy regimen. *AIDS*. 2005;19(10):1107-1108.

57. Negredo E, Bonjoch A, Paredes R, et al. Compromised immunologic recovery in treatment-experienced patients with HIV infection receiving both tenofovir disoproxil fumarate and didanosine in the TORO studies. *Clin Infect Dis*. 2005;41(6):901-905.

58. Hammer S, Bassett R, Fischl MA, et al. Randomized, placebo-controlled trial of abacavir intensification in HIV-1-infect adults with plasma HIV RNA < 500 copies/mL. Paper presented at: 11th Conference on Retroviruses and Opportunistic Infections; February 8-11, 2004; San Francisco, CA. Abstract 56.

59. Abrams D, Levy Y, Losso MH, et al. Interleukin-2 therapy in patients with HIV infection. *N Engl J Med*. 2009;361(16):1548-1559.

Regimen simplification can be defined broadly as a change in established effective therapy to reduce pill burden and dosing frequency, to enhance tolerability, or to decrease specific food and fluid requirements. Many patients on suppressive antiretroviral therapy (ART) may be considered candidates for regimen simplification, especially if (1) they are receiving treatments that are no longer recommended as preferred or alternative choices for initial therapy; (2) they were prescribed a regimen in the setting of treatment failure at a time when there was an incomplete understanding of resistance or drug-drug interaction data; or (3) they were prescribed a regimen prior to the availability of newer options or formulations that might be easier to administer and/or more tolerable.

This section will review situations in which clinicians might consider simplifying treatment in a patient with virologic suppression. Importantly, this section will not review consideration of changes in treatment for reducing ongoing adverse effects. Regimens used in simplification strategies generally should be those that have proven high efficacy in antiretroviral (ARV)-naive patients (see What to Start) or that would be predicted to be highly active for a given patient based on the individual's past treatment history and resistance profile.

Rationale

The major rationales behind regimen simplification are to improve the patient's quality of life, maintain long-term adherence, avoid toxicities that may develop with prolonged ARV use, and reduce the risk of virologic failure. Systematic reviews in the non-HIV literature have shown that adherence is inversely related to the number of daily doses.[1] Some prospective studies in HIV-infected individuals have shown that those on regimens with reduced dosing frequency have higher levels of adherence.[2-3] Patient satisfaction with regimens that contain fewer pills and reduced dosing frequency is also higher.[4]

Candidates for Regimen Simplification

Unlike ARV agents developed earlier in the HIV epidemic, many ARV medications approved in recent years have sufficiently long half-lives to allow for once-daily dosing, and most also do not have dietary restrictions. Patients on regimens initiated earlier in the era of potent combination ART with drugs that pose a high pill burden and/or frequent dosing requirements are often good candidates for regimen simplification.

Patients without suspected drug-resistant virus. Patients on first (or modified) treatment regimens without a history of treatment failure are ideal candidates for regimen simplification. These patients are less likely to harbor drug-resistant virus, especially if a pretreatment genotype did not detect drug resistance. Prospective clinical studies have demonstrated that the likelihood of treatment failure is relatively low in patients after simplification and, indeed, may be lower than in patients who do not simplify treatment.[5] However, some patients may have unrecognized drug-resistant HIV, either acquired at the time of infection or as a consequence of prior treatment, such as patients who were treated with presumably nonsuppressive mono- or dual-nucleoside reverse transcriptase inhibitor (NRTI) regimens before the widespread availability of HIV RNA monitoring and resistance testing.

Patients with documented or suspected drug resistance. Treatment simplification may also be appropriate for selected individuals who achieve viral suppression after having had documented or suspected drug resistance. Often, these patients are on regimens selected when management of drug resistance, understanding of potentially adverse drug-drug interactions, and understanding of treatment options were relatively limited. Regimen simplification may also be considered for patients on two ritonavir (RTV)-boosted protease inhibitors (PIs). Although successful in suppressing viral replication, this treatment may cause patients to be on regimens that are cumbersome, costly, and associated with potential long-term adverse events. The ability to simplify regimens in this setting often reflects the availability of recently approved agents that have activity against drug-resistant virus and are easier to take without sacrificing ARV activity. Specific situations in which drug simplification could be considered in ART-experienced patients with viral drug resistance are outlined below. Simplifying regimens in patients who have extensive prior treatment histories is complicated. In such a case, a patient's treatment history, treatment responses and tolerance, and resistance test results should be thoroughly reviewed before designing a new regimen. Expert consultation should be considered whenever possible.

Types of Treatment Simplification

Within-Class Simplifications. Within-class substitutions offer the advantage of not exposing patients to still-unused drug classes, which potentially preserves other classes for future regimens. In general, within-class substitutions use a newer agent; coformulated drugs; or a formulation that has a lower pill burden, a lower dosing frequency, or would be less likely to cause toxicity.

- ***NRTI Substitutions*** *(e.g., changing from zidovudine [ZDV] or stavudine [d4T] to tenofovir [TDF] or abacavir [ABC]):* This may be considered for a patient who has no history of viral resistance on an NRTI-containing regimen. Other NRTIs may be substituted to create a regimen with lower dosing frequency (e.g., once daily) that takes advantage of coformulated agents and potentially avoids some long-term toxicities (e.g., pancreatitis, peripheral neuropathy, lipoatrophy).

- ***Switching of Non-Nucleoside Reverse Transcriptase Inhibitors (NNRTIs)*** *(e.g., from nevirapine [NVP] to efavirenz [EFV]):* This may be considered to reduce dosing frequency or to take advantage of coformulated agents.

- ***Switching of PIs:*** This switch can be from one PI to another PI, to the same PI at a lower dosing frequency (such as from twice-daily to once-daily RTV-boosted lopinavir [LPV/r] or RTV-boosted darunavir [DRV/r]) or, in the case of atazanavir (ATV), to administration without RTV boosting.[6] (Unboosted ATV is presently not a preferred PI component and not recommended if the patient is taking TDF or if the patient has HIV with reduced susceptibility to ATV.) Such changes can reduce dosing frequency, pill count, drug-drug or drug-food interactions, or dyslipidemia or can take advantage of coformulation. These switches can be done with relative ease in patients without PI-resistant virus. However, these switches are not recommended in patients who have a history of documented or suspected PI resistance because convincing data in this setting are lacking.

Out-of-Class Substitutions. One common out-of-class substitution for regimen simplification involves a change from a PI-based to an NNRTI-based regimen. An important study in this regard was the NEFA trial, which evaluated substitution of a PI-based regimen in virologically suppressed patients with NVP, EFV, or ABC.[7] Although the baseline regimens in the study are no longer in widespread use, the NEFA findings are still relevant and provide information about the risks and benefits of switching treatment in patients with virologic suppression. In this study, 460 patients on stable, PI-based regimens with virologic suppression (<200 copies/mL for the previous 6 months) were switched to their randomized treatment arms. After 36 months of follow-up, virologic failure occurred more frequently in patients switched to ABC than in patients switched to EFV or NVP. The increased risk of treatment failure was particularly high in patients who had previous suboptimal treatment with mono- and dual-NRTI therapy. This emphasizes the need to consider the potential for drug-resistant virus prior to attempting simplification.[8]

Newer agents that target different sites in the HIV life cycle, such as the integrase strand transfer inhibitor (INSTI) raltegravir (RAL) and the CCR5 antagonist maraviroc (MVC), also offer opportunities for out-of-class substitutions, particularly in patients who have a history of virus resistant to older HIV drugs. Three randomized studies have evaluated replacing a boosted PI with RAL in virologically suppressed patients. In two of these studies,[9-10] the switch to RAL was associated with an increased risk of virologic failure in patients with documented or suspected pre-existing NRTI resistance; a third study did not find this higher risk, possibly due to a longer period of virologic suppression before the change.[11] Overall, these results suggest that in ART-experienced patients, RAL should be used with caution as a substitute for a boosted PI.

This strategy should be avoided in patients with documented NRTI resistance unless there are other fully active drugs in the regimen.

Because enfuvirtide (T-20) requires twice-daily injections, causes injection-site reactions, and is more expensive than other available ARV agents, patients who are virologically suppressed on T-20-containing regimens may wish to substitute T-20 with an active oral agent. Because the majority of patients on T-20 have highly drug-resistant virus, substitution must be with another fully active agent. Data from one randomized trial and one observational study suggest that RAL can safely substitute for T-20 in patients not previously treated with INSTI.[12-13] Although this strategy generally maintains virologic suppression and is well tolerated, clinicians should be aware that any drug substitution may introduce unanticipated adverse effects or drug-drug interactions.[14]

Other newer agents that might be considered as substitutes for T-20 are etravirine (ETR) or MVC. Use of ETR in this setting would optimally be considered only when viral susceptibility to ETR can be assured from resistance testing performed prior to virologic suppression and after carefully assessing for possible deleterious drug-drug interactions (e.g., ETR cannot be administered with several PIs [see Table 16b]). In the ETR early access program, switching from T-20 to ETR showed promise in maintaining viral suppression at 24 weeks, but only 37 subjects were included in this report.[15] MVC is only active in those with documented R5-only virus, a determination that cannot routinely be made in those with undetectable HIV RNA on a stable regimen. Although there is a commercially available proviral DNA assay to assess viral tropism in virologically suppressed patients, there are no clinical data on whether results of this test predict the successful use of MVC as a substitute for another active drug.

Reducing the number of active drugs in a regimen. This approach to treatment simplification involves switching a patient from a suppressive regimen to fewer active drugs. In early studies, this approach was associated with a higher risk of treatment failure than continuation of standard treatment with two NRTIs plus a PI.[16] More recently, studies have evaluated the use of an RTV-boosted PI as monotherapy after virologic suppression with a two-NRTI + boosted-PI regimen.[17-18] The major motivations for this approach are a reduction in NRTI-related toxicity and lower cost. In a randomized clinical trial,[18] low-level viremia was more common in those on maintenance LPV/r alone than on a three-drug combination regimen. Viral suppression was achieved by resuming the NRTIs. Studies of DRV/r monotherapy, both as once- or twice-daily dosing, have reported mixed results.[19-20] In aggregate, boosted-PI monotherapy as initial[21] or as simplification treatment has been somewhat less effective in achieving complete virologic suppression and avoiding resistance. Therefore, this strategy cannot be recommended outside of a clinical trial.

Monitoring After Treatment Simplification

Patients should be evaluated 2 6 weeks after treatment simplification to assess tolerance and to undergo laboratory monitoring, including HIV RNA, CD4 cell count, and markers of renal and liver function. Assessment of fasting cholesterol subsets and triglycerides should be performed within 3 months after the change in therapy. In the absence of any specific complaints, laboratory abnormalities, or viral rebound at that visit, patients may resume regularly scheduled clinical and laboratory monitoring.

References

1. Claxton AJ, Cramer J, Pierce C. A systematic review of the associations between dose regimens and medication compliance. *Clin Ther.* 2001;23(8):1296-1310.

2. Gallant JE, DeJesus E, Arribas JR, et al. Tenofovir DF, emtricitabine, and efavirenz vs. zidovudine, lamivudine, and efavirenz for HIV. *N Engl J Med.* 2006;354(3):251-260.

3. Molina JM, Podsadecki TJ, Johnson MA, et al. A lopinavir/ritonavir-based once-daily regimen results in better compliance and is non-inferior to a twice-daily regimen through 96 weeks. *AIDS Res Hum Retroviruses.*

2007;23(12):1505-1514.

4. Stone VE, Jordan J, Tolson J, et al. Perspectives on adherence and simplicity for HIV-infected patients on antiretroviral therapy: self-report of the relative importance of multiple attributes of highly active antiretroviral therapy (HAART) regimens in predicting adherence. *J Acquir Immune Defic Syndr*. 2004;36(3):808-816.

5. Gatell J, Salmon-Ceron D, Lazzarin A, et al. Efficacy and safety of atazanavir-based highly active antiretroviral therapy in patients with virologic suppression switched from a stable, boosted or unboosted protease inhibitor treatment regimen: the SWAN Study (AI424-097) 48-week results. *Clin Infect Dis*. 2007;44(11):1484-1492.

6. Squires KE, Young B, Dejesus E, et al. Similar efficacy and tolerability of atazanavir compared with atazanavir/ritonavir, each with abacavir/lamivudine after initial suppression with abacavir/lamivudine plus ritonavir-boosted atazanavir in HIV-infected patients. *AIDS*. 2010;24(13):2019-2027.

7. Martinez E. The NEFA study: results at three years. *AIDS Rev*. 2007;9(1):62.

8. Ochoa de Echaguen A, Arnedo M, Xercavins M, et al. Genotypic and phenotypic resistance patterns at virological failure in a simplification trial with nevirapine, efavirenz or abacavir. *AIDS*. 2005;19(13):1385-1391.

9. Eron JJ, Young B, Cooper DA, et al. Switch to a raltegravir-based regimen versus continuation of a lopinavir-ritonavir-based regimen in stable HIV-infected patients with suppressed viraemia (SWITCHMRK 1 and 2): two multicentre, double-blind, randomised controlled trials. *Lancet*. 2010;375(9712):396-407.

10. Vispo E, Barreiro P, Maida I, et al. Simplification From Protease Inhibitors to Once- or Twice-Daily Raltegravir: The ODIS Trial. *HIV Clin Trials*. 2010;11(4):197-204.

11. Martinez E, Larrousse M, Llibre JM, et al. Substitution of raltegravir for ritonavir-boosted protease inhibitors in HIV-infected patients: the SPIRAL study. *AIDS*. 2010;24(11):1697-1707.

12. Harris M, Larsen G, Montaner JS. Outcomes of multidrug-resistant patients switched from enfuvirtide to raltegravir within a virologically suppressive regimen. *AIDS*. 2008;22(10):1224-1226.

13. De Castro N, Braun J, Charreau I, et al. Switch from enfuvirtide to raltegravir in virologically suppressed multidrug-resistant HIV-1-infected patients: a randomized open-label trial. *Clin Infect Dis*. 2009;49(8):1259-1267.

14. Harris M, Larsen G, Montaner JS. Exacerbation of depression associated with starting raltegravir: a report of four cases. *AIDS*. 2008;22(14):1890-1892.

15. Loutfy M, Ribera E, Florence E, et al. Sustained HIV RNA suppression after switching from enfuvirtide to etravirine in the early access programme. *J Antimicrob Chemother*. 2009;64(6):1341-1344.

16. Havlir DV, Marschner IC, Hirsch MS, et al. Maintenance antiretroviral therapies in HIV infected patients with undetectable plasma HIV RNA after triple-drug therapy. AIDS Clinical Trials Group Study 343 Team. *N Engl J Med*. 1998;339(18):1261-1268.

17. Swindells S, DiRienzo AG, Wilkin T, et al. Regimen simplification to atazanavir-ritonavir alone as maintenance antiretroviral therapy after sustained virologic suppression. *JAMA*. 2006;296(7):806-814.

18. Pulido F, Arribas JR, Delgado R, et al. Lopinavir-ritonavir monotherapy versus lopinavir-ritonavir and two nucleosides for maintenance therapy of HIV. *AIDS*. 2008;22(2):F1-9.

19. Arribas JR, Horban A, Gerstoft J, et al. The MONET trial: darunavir/ritonavir with or without nucleoside analogues, for patients with HIV RNA below 50 copies/ml. *AIDS*. 2010;24(2):223-230.

20. Katlama C, Valantin MA, Algarte-Genin M, et al. Efficacy of darunavir/ritonavir maintenance monotherapy in patients with HIV-1 viral suppression: a randomized open-label, noninferiority trial, MONOI-ANRS 136. *AIDS*. 2010;24(15):2365-2374.

21. Delfraissy JF, Flandre P, Delaugerre C, et al. Lopinavir/ritonavir monotherapy or plus zidovudine and lamivudine in antiretroviral-naive HIV-infected patients. *AIDS*. 2008;22(3):385-393.

Exposure-Response Relationship and Therapeutic Drug Monitoring (TDM) for Antiretroviral Agents (Last updated January 10, 2011; last reviewed January 10, 2011)

Panel's Recommendations
• Therapeutic drug monitoring (TDM) for antiretroviral (ARV) agents is not recommended for routine use in the management of the HIV-infected adult **(CIII)**.
• TDM may be considered in selected clinical scenarios, as discussed in the text below.

Rating of Recommendations: A = Strong; B = Moderate; C = Optional

Rating of Evidence: I = Data from randomized controlled trials; II = Data from well-designed nonrandomized trials or observational cohort studies with long-term clinical outcomes; III = Expert opinion

Knowledge of the relationship between systemic exposure (or concentration) and drug responses (beneficial and/or adverse) is key in selecting the dose of a drug, in understanding the variability in the response of patients to a drug, and in designing strategies to optimize response and tolerability.

TDM is a strategy applied to certain antiarrhythmics, anticonvulsants, antineoplastics, and antibiotics that utilizes measured drug concentrations to design dosing regimens to improve the likelihood of the desired therapeutic and safety outcomes. The key characteristic of a drug that is a candidate for TDM is knowledge of the exposure-response relationship and a therapeutic range of concentrations. The therapeutic range is a range of concentrations established through clinical investigations that are associated with a greater likelihood of achieving the desired therapeutic response and/or reducing the frequency of drug-associated adverse reactions.

Several ARV agents meet most of the characteristics of agents that can be considered candidates for a TDM strategy.[1] The rationale for TDM in managing antiretroviral therapy (ART) derives from the following:

- data showing that considerable interpatient variability in drug concentrations exists among patients who take the same dose;
- data indicating that relationships exist between the concentration of drug in the body and anti-HIV effect and, in some cases, toxicities; and
- data from small prospective studies demonstrating that TDM improved virologic response and/or decreased the incidence of concentration-related drug toxicities.[2-3]

TDM for ARV agents, however, is not recommended for routine use in the management of the HIV-infected adult (CIII).

Multiple factors limit the routine use of TDM in HIV-infected adults.[4-5] These factors include:

- lack of large prospective studies demonstrating that TDM improves clinical and virologic outcomes. (This is the most important limiting factor for the implementation of TDM at present.);
- lack of established therapeutic range of concentrations for all ARV drugs that is associated with achieving the desired therapeutic response and/or reducing the frequency of drug-associated adverse reactions;
- intrapatient variability in ARV drug concentrations;
- lack of widespread availability of clinical laboratories that perform quantitation of ARV concentrations under rigorous quality assurance/quality control standards; and
- shortage of experts to assist with interpretation of ARV concentration data and application of such data to revise patients' dosing regimens.

Exposure-Response Relationships and TDM with Different ARV Classes

Protease Inhibitors (PIs), Non-Nucleoside Reverse Transcriptase Inhibitors (NNRTIs), and Integrase Inhibitors. Relationships between the systemic exposure to PIs and NNRTIs and treatment response have been reviewed in various publications.[4-7] Although there are limitations and unanswered questions, the consensus among clinical pharmacologists from the United States and Europe is that the data provide a framework for the potential implementation of TDM for PIs and NNRTIs. However, information on relationships between concentrations and drug-associated toxicities are sparse. Clinicians who use TDM as a strategy to manage either ARV response or toxicities should consult the most current data on the proposed therapeutic concentration range. Exposure-response data for darunavir (DRV), etravirine (ETR), and raltegravir (RAL) are accumulating but are not sufficient to recommend minimum trough concentrations. The median trough concentrations for these agents in HIV-infected persons receiving the recommended dose are included in Table 9b.

CCR5 Antagonists. Trough maraviroc (MVC) concentrations have been shown to be an important predictor of virologic success in studies conducted in ART-experienced persons.[8-9] Clinical experience in the use of TDM for MVC, however, is very limited. Nonetheless, as with PIs and NNRTIs, the exposure-response data provide a framework for TDM, and that information is presented in these guidelines (Table 9b).

Nucleoside Reverse Transcriptase Inhibitors (NRTIs). Relationships between plasma concentrations of NRTIs and their intracellular pharmacologically active moieties have not yet been established. Therefore, monitoring of plasma or intracellular NRTI concentrations for an individual patient largely remains a research tool. Measurement of plasma concentrations, however, is routinely used for studies of drug-drug interactions.

Scenarios for Use of TDM. Multiple scenarios exist in which both ARV concentration data and expert opinion may be useful in patient management. Consultation with a clinical pharmacologist or a clinical pharmacist with HIV expertise may be advisable in these cases. These scenarios include the following:

- Suspect clinically significant drug-drug or drug-food interactions that may result in reduced efficacy or increased dose-related toxicities;
- Changes in pathophysiologic states that may impair gastrointestinal, hepatic, or renal function, thereby potentially altering drug absorption, distribution, metabolism, or elimination;
- Pregnant women who may be at risk of virologic failure as a result of changes in their pharmacokinetic parameters during the later stage of pregnancy, which may result in plasma concentrations lower than those achieved in the earlier stages of pregnancy and in the nonpregnant patient;
- Heavily pretreated patients experiencing virologic failure and who may have viral isolates with reduced susceptibility to ARVs;
- Use of alternative dosing regimens and ARV combinations for which safety and efficacy have not been established in clinical trials;
- Concentration-dependent, drug-associated toxicities; and
- Lack of expected virologic response in medication-adherent persons.

TDM

- **For patients who have drug-susceptible virus.** Table 9a includes a synthesis of recommendations[2-7] for minimum target trough PI and NNRTI concentrations in persons with drug-susceptible virus.
- **For ART-experienced patients with virologic failure** (see Table 9b). Fewer data are available to formulate suggestions for minimum target trough concentrations in ART-experienced patients who have viral isolates with reduced susceptibility to ARV agents. Concentration recommendations for tipranavir

(TPV) and MVC were derived only from studies in ART-experienced persons. It is likely that use of PIs and NNRTIs in the setting of reduced viral susceptibility may require higher trough concentrations than those needed for wild-type virus. The inhibitory quotient (IQ), which is the ratio of ARV drug concentration to a measure of susceptibility (genotype or phenotype) of the patient's strain of HIV to that drug, may additionally improve prediction of virologic response as has been shown, for example, with DRV in ART-experienced persons.[10-11] Exposure-response data for DRV, ETR, and RAL are accumulating but are not sufficient to recommend minimum trough concentrations. The median trough concentrations for these agents in HIV-infected persons receiving the recommended dose are included in Table 9b.

Using Drug Concentrations to Guide Therapy. There are several challenges and considerations for implementation of TDM in the clinical setting. Use of TDM to monitor ARV concentrations in a patient requires multiple steps:

- quantification of the concentration of the drug, usually in plasma or serum;
- determination of the patient's pharmacokinetic characteristics;
- integration of information on patient adherence;
- interpretation of the concentrations; and
- adjustment of the drug dose to achieve concentrations within the therapeutic range, if necessary.

Guidelines for the collection of blood samples and other practical suggestions can be found in a position paper by the Adult AIDS Clinical Trials Group Pharmacology Committee.[4]

A final caveat to the use of measured drug concentrations in patient management is a general one drug concentration information cannot be used alone; it must be integrated with other clinical information. In addition, as knowledge of associations between ARV concentrations and virologic response continues to accumulate, clinicians who employ a TDM strategy for patient management should consult the most current literature.

Table 9a. Trough Concentrations of Antiretroviral Drugs for Patients Who Have Drug-Susceptible Virus

Drug	Concentration (ng/mL)
Suggested minimum target trough concentrations in patients with HIV-1 susceptible to the ARV drugs[2-9]	
Fosamprenavir (FPV)	400 (measured as amprenavir concentration)
Atazanavir (ATV)	150
Indinavir (IDV)	100
Lopinavir (LPV)	1000
Nelfinavir[a] (NFV)	800
Saquinavir (SQV)	100–250
Efavirenz (EFV)	1000
Nevirapine (NVP)	3000

[a] Measurable active (M8) metabolite

Table 9b. Trough Concentrations of Antiretroviral Drugs for Treatment-Experienced Patients with Virologic Failure

Drug	Concentration (ng/mL)
Suggested minimum target trough concentrations for ART-experienced patients who have resistant HIV-1 strains	
Maraviroc (MVC)	>50
Tipranavir (TPV)	20,500
Median (Range) Trough Concentrations from Clinical Trials[12-1]	
Darunavir (DRV) (600 mg twice daily)	3300 (1255–7368)
Etravirine (ETR)	275 (81–2980)
Raltegravir (RAL)	72 (29–118)

References

1. Spector R, Park GD, Johnson GF, et al. Therapeutic drug monitoring. *Clin Pharmacol Ther*. 1988;43(4):345-353.

2. Fletcher CV, Anderson PL, Kakuda TN, et al. Concentration-controlled compared with conventional antiretroviral therapy for HIV infection. *AIDS*. 2002;16(4):551-560.

3. Fabbiani M, Di Giambenedetto S, Bracciale L, et al. Pharmacokinetic variability of antiretroviral drugs and correlation with virological outcome: 2 years of experience in routine clinical practice. *J Antimicrob Chemother*. 2009;64(1):109-117.

4. Acosta EP, Gerber JG. Position paper on therapeutic drug monitoring of antiretroviral agents. *AIDS Res Hum Retroviruses*. 2002;18(12):825-834.

5. van Luin M, Kuks PF, Burger DM. Use of therapeutic drug monitoring in HIV disease. *Curr Opin HIV AIDS*. 2008;3(3):266-271.

6. Boffito M, Acosta E, Burger D, et al. Current status and future prospects of therapeutic drug monitoring and applied clinical pharmacology in antiretroviral therapy. *Antivir Ther*. 2005;10(3):375-392.

7. LaPorte CJL, Back BJ, Blaschke T, et al. Updated guidelines to perform therapeutic drug monitoring for antiretroviral agents. *Rev Antivir Ther*. 2006;3:4-14.

8. Pfizer Inc. Selzentry (maraviroc) tablets prescribing information NY. 2007.

9. McFayden L, Jacqmin P, Wade J, et al. Maraviroc exposure response analysis: phase 3 antiviral efficacy in treatment-experienced HIV+ patients. Paper presented at: 16th Population Approach Group in Europe Meeting; June 2007, 2007; Kobenhavn, Denmark. Abstract P4-13.

10. Molto J, Santos JR, Perez-Alvarez N, et al. Darunavir inhibitory quotient predicts the 48-week virological response to darunavir-based salvage therapy in human immunodeficiency virus-infected protease inhibitor-experienced patients. *Antimicrob Agents Chemother*. 2008;52(11):3928-3932.

11. Sekar V, DeMeyer S, Vangeneugden T, et al. Pharmacokinetic/pharmacodynamic (PK/PD) analysis of TMC114 in the POWER 1 and POWER 2 trials in treatment-experienced HIV-infected patients. Paper presented at: 13th Conference on Retroviruses and Opportunistic Infections; February 5, 2006, 2006; Denver, CO. Abstract J-121.

12. Markowitz M, Morales-Ramirez JO, Nguyen BY, et al. Antiretroviral activity, pharmacokinetics, and tolerability of MK-0518, a novel inhibitor of HIV-1 integrase, dosed as monotherapy for 10 days in treatment-naive HIV-1-infected individuals. *J Acquir Immune Defic Syndr*. 2006;43(5):509-515.

13. Kakuda TN, Wade JR, Snoeck E, et al. Pharmacokinetics and pharmacodynamics of the non-nucleoside reverse-transcriptase inhibitor etravirine in treatment-experienced HIV-1-infected patients. *Clin Pharmacol Ther*. 2010;88(5):695-703.

14. Food and Drug Administration (FDA). Prezista (package insert). 2010. http://www.accessdata.fda.gov/drugsatfda_docs/label/2010/021976s016lbl.pdf.

Discontinuation or Interruption of Antiretroviral Therapy (Last updated January 10, 2011; last reviewed January 10, 2011)

Discontinuation of antiretroviral therapy (ART) may result in viral rebound, immune decompensation, and clinical progression. Unplanned interruption of ART may become necessary because of severe drug toxicity, intervening illness, surgery that precludes oral therapy, or unavailability of antiretroviral (ARV) medication. Some investigators have studied planned treatment discontinuation strategies in situations or for reasons that include: in patients who achieve viral suppression and wish to enhance adherence; to reduce inconvenience, long-term toxicities, and costs for patients; or in extensively treated patients who experience treatment failure due to resistant HIV, to allow reversion to wild-type virus. Potential risks and benefits of interruption vary according to a number of factors, including the clinical and immunologic status of the patient, the reason for the interruption, the type and duration of the interruption, and the presence or absence of resistant HIV at the time of interruption. Below are brief discussions on what is currently known about the risks and benefits of treatment interruption in some of these circumstances.

Short-Term Therapy Interruptions

Reasons for short-term interruption (days to weeks) of ART vary and may include drug toxicity; intercurrent illnesses that preclude oral intake, such as gastroenteritis or pancreatitis; surgical procedures; or unavailability of drugs. Stopping ARV drugs for a short time (i.e., <1 to 2 days) due to medical/surgical procedures can usually be done by holding all drugs in the regimen. Recommendations for some other scenarios are listed below:

Unanticipated Need for Short-Term Interruption

- **When a patient experiences a severe or life-threatening toxicity or unexpected inability to take oral medications** all components of the drug regimen should be stopped simultaneously, regardless of drug half-life.

Planned Short Term Interruption (>2 3 days)

- **When all regimen components have similar half-lives and do not require food for proper absorption** all drugs may be given with a sip of water, if allowed; otherwise, all drugs should be stopped simultaneously. All discontinued regimen components should be restarted simultaneously.

- **When all regimen components have similar half-lives and require food for adequate absorption, and the patient cannot take anything by mouth for a sustained period of time** temporary discontinuation of all drug components is indicated. The regimen should be restarted as soon as the patient can resume oral intake.

- **When the ARV regimen contains drugs with differing half-lives** stopping all drugs simultaneously may result in functional monotherapy with the drug with the longest half-life (typically a non-nucleoside reverse transcriptase inhibitor [NNRTI]). Options in this circumstance are discussed below. (See Discontinuation of efavirenz, etravirine, or nevirapine.)

Interruption of Therapy after Pregnancy

ARV drugs for prevention of perinatal transmission of HIV are recommended for all pregnant women, regardless of whether they have indications for ART for their own health. Following delivery, considerations regarding continuation of the ARV regimen for maternal therapeutic indications are the same as for other nonpregnant individuals. The decision of whether to continue therapy after delivery should take into account current recommendations for initiation of ART, current and nadir CD4 T-cell counts and trajectory, HIV RNA levels, adherence issues, and patient preference.

Planned Long-Term Therapy Interruptions

Planned therapy interruptions have been contemplated in various scenarios, listed below. Research is ongoing in several of the scenarios. Therapy interruptions *cannot be recommended* at this time outside of controlled clinical trials **(AI)**.

- **In patients who initiated therapy during acute HIV infection and achieved virologic suppression** the optimal duration of treatment and the consequences of treatment interruption are not known at this time. (See Acute HIV Infection.)

- **In patients who have had exposure to multiple ARV agents, have experienced ARV treatment failure, and have few treatment options available because of extensive resistance mutations** interruption is *not recommended* unless done in a clinical trial setting **(AI)**. Several clinical trials, largely yielding negative results, but some with conflicting results, have been conducted to better understand the role of treatment interruption in these patients.[1-4] The largest of these studies showed negative clinical impact of treatment interruption in these patients.[1] The Panel notes that partial virologic suppression from combination therapy has been associated with clinical benefit;[5] therefore, interruption of therapy is not recommended.

- **In patients on ART who have maintained a CD4 count above the level currently recommended for treatment initiation and irrespective of whether their baseline CD4 counts were either above or below that recommended threshold** interruption is also *not recommended* unless done in a clinical trial setting **(BI)**. (See discussion below highlighting potential adverse outcomes seen in some treatment interruption trials.)

Temporary treatment interruption to reduce inconvenience, potential long-term toxicity, and/or overall treatment cost has been considered as a strategy for patients on ART who have maintained CD4 counts above those currently recommended for initiating therapy. Several clinical trials have been designed to determine the safety of such interruptions, in which reinitiation is triggered by predetermined CD4 count thresholds. In these trials, various CD4 count levels have been set to guide both treatment interruption and reinitiation. In the SMART study, the largest of such trials with more than 5,000 subjects, interrupting treatment with CD4 counts >350 cells/mm^3 and reinitiating when <250 cells/mm^3 was associated with an increased risk of disease progression and all cause mortality compared with the trial arm of continuous ART.[6] In the TRIVACAN study, the same CD4 count thresholds were used for stopping and restarting treatment.[7] This study also showed that interruption was an inferior strategy; the interventions in both trials were stopped early because of these findings. Data from the DART trial reported a twofold increase in rates of World Health Organization (WHO) Stage 4 events/deaths in the 12-week ART cycling group among African patients achieving a CD4 count >300/mm^3 compared with the continuous ART group.[8] Observational data from the EuroSIDA cohort noted a twofold increase in risk of death after a treatment interruption of >3 months. Factors linked to increased risk of death or progression included lower CD4 counts, higher viral loads, and a prior history of AIDS.[9] Other studies have reported no major safety concerns,[10-12] but these studies had smaller sample sizes. Results have been reported from several small observational studies evaluating treatment interruption in patients doing well with nadir CD4 counts >350/mm^3, but further studies are needed to determine the safety of treatment interruption in this population.[13-14] There is concern that CD4 counts <500 cells/mm^3 are associated with a range of non-AIDS clinical events (e.g., cancer and heart, liver, and kidney disease).[6, 15-16]

Planned long-term therapy interruption strategies *cannot be recommended* at this time outside of controlled clinical trials **(BI)** based on available data and a range of ongoing concerns.

If therapy has to be discontinued, patients should be counseled about the need for close clinical and laboratory monitoring. They should also be aware of the risks of viral rebound, acute retroviral syndrome, increased risk of HIV transmission, decline of CD4 count, HIV disease progression or death, development of minor HIV-associated manifestations such as oral thrush, development of serious non-AIDS complications, development of drug resistance, and the need for chemoprophylaxis against opportunistic infections depending on the CD4 count. Treatment interruptions often result in rapid reductions in CD4 counts.

Prior to any planned treatment interruption, a number of ARV-specific issues should be taken into consideration. These include:

- **Discontinuation of efavirenz (EFV), etravirine (ETR), or nevirapine (NVP).** The optimal interval between stopping EFV, ETR, or NVP and other ARV drugs is not known. The duration of detectable levels of EFV or NVP after discontinuation ranges from less than 1 week to more than 3 weeks.[17-18] Simultaneously stopping all drugs in a regimen containing these agents may result in functional monotherapy with the NNRTIs because NNRTIs have much longer half-lives than other agents. This may increase the risk of selection of NNRTI-resistant mutations. It is further complicated by evidence that certain host genetic polymorphisms may result in slower rates of clearance. Such polymorphisms may be more common among specific ethnic groups, such as African Americans and Hispanics.[18-19] Some experts recommend stopping the NNRTI but continuing the other ARV drugs for a period of time. The optimal time sequence for staggered component discontinuation has not been determined. A study in South Africa demonstrated that giving 4 or 7 days of zidovudine (ZDV) + lamivudine (3TC) after a single dose of NVP reduced the risk of postnatal NVP resistance from 60% to 10% 12%.[20] Use of nucleoside reverse transcriptase inhibitors (NRTIs) with a longer half-life such as tenofovir (TDF) plus emtricitabine (FTC) has also been shown to decrease NVP resistance after single-dose treatment.[21] The findings may, however, differ in patients on chronic NVP treatment. An alternative strategy is to substitute a protease inhibitor (PI) for the NNRTI and to continue the PI with dual NRTIs for a period of time. In a post-study analysis of the patients who interrupted therapy in the SMART trial, patients who were switched from an NNRTI- to a PI-based regimen prior to interruption had a lower rate of NNRTI-resistant mutation after interruption and a greater chance of resuppression of HIV RNA after restarting therapy than those who stopped all the drugs simultaneously or stopped the NNRTI before the 2-NRTI.[22] The optimal duration needed to continue the PI-based regimen after stopping the NNRTI is not known. Given the potential of prolonged detectable NNRTI concentrations for more than 3 weeks, some suggest that the PI-based regimen may need to be continued for up to 4 weeks. Further research to determine the best approach to discontinuing NNRTIs is needed. Clinical data on ETR and treatment interruption is lacking but its long half-life of approximately 40 hours suggests that stopping ETR needs to be done carefully using the same suggestions for NVP and EFV for the time being.

- **Discontinuation and reintroduction of NVP.** Because NVP is an inducer of the drug-metabolizing hepatic enzymes, administration of full therapeutic doses of NVP without a 2-week, low-dose escalation phase will result in excess plasma drug levels and potentially increase the risk of toxicity. Therefore, in a patient who has interrupted treatment with NVP for more than 2 weeks, NVP should be reintroduced with a dose escalation period of 200 mg once daily for 14 days and then a 200 mg twice-daily regimen **(AII)**.

- **Discontinuation of FTC, 3TC, or TDF in patients with hepatitis B virus (HBV) coinfection.** Patients with HBV coinfection (hepatitis B surface antigen [HbsAg] or hepatitis B e antigen [HBeAg] positive) and receiving one or a combination of these NRTIs may experience an exacerbation of hepatitis upon drug discontinuation.[23-24] (See Hepatitis B (HBV)/HIV Coinfection.)

References

1. Lawrence J, Mayers DL, Hullsiek KH, et al. Structured treatment interruption in patients with multidrug-resistant human immunodeficiency virus. *N Engl J Med.* 2003;349(9):837-846.

2. Ruiz L, Ribera E, Bonjoch A, et al. Role of structured treatment interruption before a 5-drug salvage antiretroviral

regimen: the Retrogene Study. *J Infect Dis*. 2003;188(7):977-985.

3. Ghosn J, Wirden M, Ktorza N, et al. No benefit of a structured treatment interruption based on genotypic resistance in heavily pretreated HIV-infected patients. *AIDS*. 2005;19(15):1643-1647.

4. Jaafar A, Massip P, Sandres-Saune K, et al. HIV therapy after treatment interruption in patients with multiple failure and more than 200 CD4+ T lymphocyte count. *J Med Virol*. 2004;74(1):8-15.

5. Kousignian I, Abgrall S, Grabar S, et al. Maintaining antiretroviral therapy reduces the risk of AIDS-defining events in patients with uncontrolled viral replication and profound immunodeficiency. *Clin Infect Dis*. 2008;46(2):296-304.

6. El-Sadr WM, Lundgren JD, Neaton JD, et al. CD4+ count-guided interruption of antiretroviral treatment. *N Engl J Med*. 2006;355(22):2283-2296.

7. Danel C, Moh R, Minga A, et al. CD4-guided structured antiretroviral treatment interruption strategy in HIV-infected adults in west Africa (Trivacan ANRS 1269 trial): a randomised trial. *Lancet*. 2006;367(9527):1981-1989.

8. DART Trial Team DTT. Fixed duration interruptions are inferior to continuous treatment in African adults starting therapy with CD4 cell counts < 200 cells/microl. *AIDS*. 2008;22(2):237-247.

9. Holkmann Olsen C, Mocroft A, Kirk O, et al. Interruption of combination antiretroviral therapy and risk of clinical disease progression to AIDS or death. *HIV Med*. 2007;8(2):96-104.

10. Maggiolo F, Ripamonti D, Gregis G, et al. Effect of prolonged discontinuation of successful antiretroviral therapy on CD4 T cells: a controlled, prospective trial. *AIDS*. 2004;18(3):439-446.

11. Cardiello PG, Hassink E, Ananworanich J, et al. A prospective, randomized trial of structured treatment interruption for patients with chronic HIV type 1 infection. *Clin Infect Dis*. 2005;40(4):594-600.

12. Ananworanich J, Siangphoe U, Hill A, et al. Highly active antiretroviral therapy (HAART) retreatment in patients on CD4-guided therapy achieved similar virologic suppression compared with patients on continuous HAART: the HIV Netherlands Australia Thailand Research Collaboration 001.4 study. *J Acquir Immune Defic Syndr*. 2005;39(5):523-529.

13. Pogany K, van Valkengoed IG, Prins JM, et al. Effects of active treatment discontinuation in patients with a CD4+ T-cell nadir greater than 350 cells/mm^3: 48-week Treatment Interruption in Early Starters Netherlands Study (TRIESTAN). *J Acquir Immune Defic Syndr*. 2007;44(4):395-400.

14. Skiest DJ, Su Z, Havlir DV, et al. Interruption of antiretroviral treatment in HIV-infected patients with preserved immune function is associated with a low rate of clinical progression: a prospective study by AIDS Clinical Trials Group 5170. *J Infect Dis*. 2007;195(10):1426-1436.

15. Monforte A, Abrams D, Pradier C, et al. HIV-induced immunodeficiency and mortality from AIDS-defining and non-AIDS-defining malignancies. *AIDS*. 2008;22(16):2143-2153.

16. Phillips AN, Neaton J, Lundgren JD. The role of HIV in serious diseases other than AIDS. *AIDS*. 2008;22(18):2409-2418.

17. Cressey TR, Jourdain G, Lallemant MJ, et al. Persistence of nevirapine exposure during the postpartum period after intrapartum single-dose nevirapine in addition to zidovudine prophylaxis for the prevention of mother-to-child transmission of HIV-1. *J Acquir Immune Defic Syndr*. 2005;38(3):283-288.

18. Ribaudo HJ, Haas DW, Tierney C, et al. Pharmacogenetics of plasma efavirenz exposure after treatment discontinuation: an Adult AIDS Clinical Trials Group Study. *Clin Infect Dis*. 2006;42(3):401-407.

19. Haas DW, Ribaudo HJ, Kim RB, et al. Pharmacogenetics of efavirenz and central nervous system side effects: an Adult AIDS Clinical Trials Group study. *AIDS*. 2004;18(18):2391-2400.

20. McIntyre JA, Hopley M, Moodley D, et al. Efficacy of short-course AZT plus 3TC to reduce nevirapine resistance in the prevention of mother-to-child HIV transmission: a randomized clinical trial. *PLoS Med*. 2009;6(10):e1000172.

21. Chi BH, Sinkala M, Mbewe F, et al. Single-dose tenofovir and emtricitabine for reduction of viral resistance to non-nucleoside reverse transcriptase inhibitor drugs in women given intrapartum nevirapine for perinatal HIV prevention: an open-label randomised trial. *Lancet*. 2007;370(9600):1698-1705.

22. Fox Z, Phillips A, Cohen C, et al. Viral resuppression and detection of drug resistance following interruption of a suppressive non-nucleoside reverse transcriptase inhibitor-based regimen. *AIDS*. 2008;22(17):2279-2289.

23. Bessesen M, Ives D, Condreay L, et al. Chronic active hepatitis B exacerbations in human immunodeficiency virus-infected patients following development of resistance to or withdrawal of lamivudine. *Clin Infect Dis*. 1999;28(5):1032-1035.

24. Sellier P, Clevenbergh P, Mazeron MC, et al. Fatal interruption of a 3TC-containing regimen in a HIV-infected patient due to re-activation of chronic hepatitis B virus infection. *Scand J Infect Dis*. 2004;36(6-7):533-535.

Considerations for Antiretroviral Use in Special Patient Populations

Acute and Recent (Early*) HIV Infection (Last updated February 12, 2013; last reviewed February 12, 2013)

Panel's Recommendations
• Antiretroviral therapy (ART) is recommended for all persons with HIV infection and should be offered to those with early* HIV infection **(BII)**, although definitive data are lacking as to whether this approach will result in long-term virologic, immunologic, or clinical benefits.
• All pregnant women with early HIV infection should start ART as soon as possible to prevent perinatal transmission of HIV **(AI)**.
• If treatment is initiated in a patient with early HIV infection, the goal is to suppress plasma HIV RNA to below detectable levels **(AIII)**.
• For patients with early HIV infection in whom therapy is initiated, testing for plasma HIV RNA levels, CD4 count, and toxicity monitoring should be performed as described for patients with chronic HIV infection **(AII)**.
• Genotypic drug-resistance testing should be performed before initiation of ART to guide the selection of the regimen **(AII)**. If therapy is deferred, genotypic resistance testing should still be performed because the results will be useful in selecting a regimen with the greatest potential for achieving optimal virologic response when therapy is ultimately initiated **(AII)**.
• For patients without transmitted drug resistant virus, therapy should be initiated with a regimen that is recommended for patients with chronic HIV infection (see What to Start) **(AIII)**.
• ART can be initiated before drug resistance test results are available. Since resistance to ritonavir (RTV)-boosted protease inhibitors (PIs) emerges slowly and since clinically significant transmitted resistance to PIs is uncommon, these drugs combined with nucleoside reverse transcriptase inhibitors (NRTIs) should be used in this setting **(AIII)**.
• Patients starting ART should be willing and able to commit to treatment and should understand the possible benefits and risks of therapy and the importance of adherence **(AIII)**. Patients may choose to postpone therapy, and providers, on a case-by-case basis, may elect to defer therapy because of clinical and/or psychosocial factors.
* Early infection represents either acute or recent infection as defined in the first paragraph below.
Rating of Recommendations: A = Strong; B = Moderate; C = Optional   *Rating of Evidence: I = Data from randomized controlled trials; II = Data from well-designed nonrandomized trials or observational cohort studies with long-term clinical outcomes; III = Expert opinion*

Definitions: Acute HIV infection is the phase of HIV disease immediately after infection during which the initial burst of viremia in newly infected patients occurs; anti-HIV antibodies are undetectable at this time while HIV RNA or p24 antigen are present. Recent infection generally is considered the phase up to 6 months after infection during which anti-HIV antibodies are detectable. Throughout this section, the term "early HIV infection" is used to refer to either acute or recent HIV infection.

An estimated 40% to 90% of patients with acute HIV infection will experience symptoms of acute retroviral syndrome, characterized by fever, lymphadenopathy, pharyngitis, skin rash, myalgias/arthralgias, and other symptoms.[1-6] Primary care clinicians, however, often do not recognize acute HIV infection because the self-limiting symptoms are similar to those of many other viral infections, such as influenza and infectious mononucleosis. Acute infection can also be asymptomatic. Table 10 provides practitioners with guidance to recognize, diagnose, and manage acute HIV infection.

Diagnosis of Acute HIV Infection

Health care providers should maintain a high level of suspicion of acute HIV infection in patients who have a compatible clinical syndrome—especially in those who report recent high-risk behavior (Table 10).[7] Patients may not always disclose or admit to high-risk behaviors or they may not perceive that their behaviors put them at risk for HIV acquisition. Thus, signs and symptoms consistent with acute retroviral syndrome should motivate consideration of a diagnosis of acute HIV infection even in the absence of reported high-risk behaviors.

Acute HIV infection is usually defined as detectable HIV RNA or p24 antigen, the latter often used in currently available HIV antigen/antibody (Ag/Ab) combination assays, in serum or plasma in the setting of a negative or indeterminate HIV antibody test.[7, 8] When the acute retroviral syndrome is suspected in a patient with a negative or indeterminate HIV antibody test result, a test for HIV RNA should be performed to diagnose acute infection **(AII)**. A low-positive HIV RNA level (<10,000 copies/mL) may represent a false-positive test result because values in acute infection are generally very high (>100,000 copies/mL).[5, 6] A presumptive diagnosis of acute HIV infection can be made on the basis of a negative or indeterminate HIV antibody test result and a positive HIV RNA test result. However, if the results of an HIV RNA test are low-positive, the test should be repeated using a different specimen from the same patient. It is highly unlikely that a second test will reproduce a false-positive result.[6] Interest in routine screening for acute infection has led select centers to use the HIV Ag/Ab test as the primary HIV screening assay or to test all HIV antibody negative samples for HIV RNA.[9] Combination HIV Ag/Ab tests (ARCHITECT HIV Ag/Ab Combo and GS HIV Combo Ag/Ab) now are approved by the Food and Drug Administration; however, the currently available tests do not differentiate between a positive antibody test result and a positive antigen result. Thus HIV Ag/Ab-reactive specimens should be tested with an antibody assay, and if the test results are negative or indeterminate and if acute HIV infection is suspected, be further tested for HIV RNA.[10, 11] Because HIV RNA or Ag/Ab combination assays are not yet used routinely for HIV screening in all settings, clinicians should not assume that a laboratory report of a negative HIV test result indicates that screening for acute HIV infection has been conducted. Patients also should know that home HIV testing only detects HIV antibodies and therefore will not detect very early acute HIV infection. Persons diagnosed presumptively with acute HIV infection should have serologic testing repeated over the next 3 to 6 months to document seroconversion **(AI)** (see Table 10).

Treatment for Early HIV Infection

Clinical trial data regarding the treatment of early HIV infection is limited. Many patients who enrolled in studies to assess the role of antiretroviral therapy (ART) in early HIV infection, as outlined below, were identified as trial participants because they presented with signs or symptoms of acute infection. With the introduction of HIV screening tests that include assays for HIV RNA or p24 antigen and wider HIV screening in healthcare systems, the number of asymptomatic patients identified with early infection may be increasing. The natural history of HIV disease in these patients may differ from that in persons with symptomatic infections, thus further studies on the impact of ART on the natural history of asymptomatic acute HIV infection are needed. The initial burst of high level viremia in infected adults usually declines shortly after acute infection (e.g., within 2 months); however, a rationale for treatment during recent infection (e.g., 2–6 months after infection) remains because the immune system may not yet have maximally contained viral replication in the lymphoid tissue during this time.[12] Several trials have addressed the question of the long-term benefit of potent treatment regimens initiated during early HIV infection. The potential benefits and risks of treating HIV during this stage of disease are discussed below:

- **Potential Benefits of Treatment During Early HIV Infection.** Preliminary data indicate that treatment of early HIV infection with combination ART improves laboratory markers of disease progression.[13-17] The data, though limited, indicate that treatment of early HIV infection may also decrease the severity of acute disease; lower the viral set point,[18-20] which can affect disease progression rates in the event therapy is stopped; reduce the size of the viral reservoir;[21] and decrease the rate of viral mutation by suppressing viral replication and preserving immune function.[22] Because early HIV infection often is associated with high viral loads and increased infectiousness,[23] and ART use by HIV-infected individuals reduces transmission to serodiscordant sexual partners,[24] treatment during this stage of infection is expected to substantially reduce the risk of HIV transmission. In addition, although data are limited and the clinical relevance unclear, the profound loss of gastrointestinal lymphoid tissue that occurs during the first weeks of infection may be mitigated by initiating ART during early HIV infection.[25, 26] Many of the potential benefits described above may be more likely to occur with treatment of acute infection, but they also may occur if treatment is initiated during recent HIV infection.

- **Potential Risks of Treatment During Early HIV Infection.** The potential disadvantages of initiating therapy during early HIV infection include more prolonged exposure to ART without a known long-term clinical benefit. This could result in drug toxicities, development of drug resistance, and adverse effects on an individual's quality of life due to earlier initiation of lifelong therapy that requires strict adherence.

Several randomized controlled trials have studied the effect of ART during acute and recent infection to assess whether initiating early therapy would allow patients to stop treatment and maintain lower viral loads and higher CD4 counts while off ART for prolonged periods of time. This objective was of interest when these studies were initiated but is less relevant in an era in which treatment is recommended for virtually all HIV-infected patients and treatment interruptions are not recommended (see Initiating Antiretroviral Therapy in Treatment-Naive Patients).

The Setpoint Study (ACTG A5217 Study) randomized patients with recent but not acute HIV infection to either defer therapy or immediately initiate ART for 36 weeks and then stop.[18] The primary study end point was a composite of meeting criteria for ART or re-initiation of ART and viral load results at week 72 in both groups and at week 36 in the deferred treatment group. The study was stopped prematurely by the Data and Safety Monitoring Board because of an apparent benefit associated with early therapy that was driven mostly by greater proportion of participants meeting criteria for ART initiation in the deferred treatment group (50%) than in the immediate treatment group (10%). Nearly half of the patients in the deferred treatment group needed to start therapy during the first year of study enrollment.

The Randomized Primo-SHM Trial randomized patients with acute (~70%) or recent (~30%) infection to either defer ART or to undergo treatment for 24 or 60 weeks and then stop.[19] Significantly lower viral loads were observed 36 weeks after treatment interruption in the patients who had been treated early. These patients also experienced a longer time before the need to initiate therapy, primarily on the basis of reaching a CD4 count of <350 cells/mm³. The median time to starting treatment was 0.7 years for the deferred therapy group and 3.0 and 1.8 years for the 24- and 60-week treatment arms, respectively. The time to reaching a CD4 count of <500 cells/mm³ was only 0.5 years in the deferred group.

Finally, the SPARTAC Trial included patients with acute and recent infection randomized to either defer therapy or to undergo treatment for 12 or 48 weeks and then stop.[20] In this case, the time to CD4 <350 cells/mm³ or initiation of therapy was significantly longer in the group treated for 48 weeks than in the deferred treatment group or the group treated for 12 weeks. However, no difference was observed comparing persons who received 12 weeks of ART with those who deferred treatment during early infection.

The strategies tested in these studies are of limited relevance in the current treatment era in which treatment interruption is not recommended. The study results may not fully reflect the natural history of HIV disease in persons with asymptomatic acute infection because most patients in these trials were enrolled on the basis of identified early symptomatic HIV infections. Nevertheless, the results do demonstrate that some immunologic and virologic benefits may be associated with the treatment of early HIV infection. Moreover, all the findings suggest, at least in the population recruited for these studies, that the time to initiating ART after identification of early infection is quite short when the threshold for ART initiation is 350 CD4 cells/mm^3, and nonexistent when therapy is advised for all individuals regardless of CD4 cell count as currently recommended in these guidelines. These observations must be balanced with the risks of early treatment, risks that are largely the same as those of therapy initiated in chronically infected asymptomatic patients with high CD4 counts. Consequently, the health care provider and the patient should be fully aware that the rationale for initiating therapy during early HIV infection is based on theoretical benefits and the extrapolation of data from the strategy trials outlined above. These potential benefits must be weighed against the risks. For these reasons, and because ART is currently recommended for all HIV-infected patients (see Initiating Antiretroviral Therapy in Treatment-Naive Patients), ART should be offered to all patients with early HIV infection **(BII)**. However, patients must be willing and able to commit to treatment and providers, on a case-by-case basis, may elect to defer therapy for clinical and/or psychosocial reasons. Providers also should consider enrolling patients with early HIV infection in clinical studies to further evaluate the natural history of this stage of HIV infection and to further define the role of ART in this setting. Providers can obtain information regarding such trials at www.clinicaltrials.gov or from local HIV treatment experts.

Treatment for Early HIV Infection During Pregnancy

Because early HIV infection is associated with a high risk of perinatal transmission, all HIV-infected pregnant women should start combination ART as soon as possible to prevent perinatal transmission of HIV **(AI)**.[27]

Treatment Regimen for Early HIV Infection

Data from the United States and Europe demonstrate that transmitted virus may be resistant to at least 1 antiretroviral in 6% to 16% of patients.[28-30] Up to 21% of isolates from contemporary patients with acute HIV infection demonstrated resistance to at least 1 drug.[31] Therefore, before initiation of ART in a person with early HIV infection, genotypic antiretroviral drug-resistance testing should be performed to guide the selection of a regimen **(AII)**. If the decision to initiate therapy during early infection is made, especially in the setting of acute infection, treatment initiation should not be delayed pending resistance testing results. Once results are available, the treatment regimen can be modified if warranted. If therapy is deferred, resistance testing still should be performed because the results will help guide selection of a regimen to optimize virologic response once therapy is initiated **(AII)**.

The goal of therapy during early HIV infection is to suppress plasma HIV RNA to undetectable levels **(AIII)**. Because data to draw firm conclusions regarding specific drug combinations to use in this stage of HIV infection are insufficient, ART should be initiated with one of the combination regimens recommended for patients with chronic infection **(AIII)** (see What to Start). If therapy is started before the results of drug-resistance testing are available, because resistance to RTV-boosted protease inhibitors (PIs) emerge slowly and clinically significant transmitted resistance to PIs is uncommon **(AIII)**. If available, the results of ARV drug-resistance testing or the ARV resistance pattern of the source person's virus should be used to guide the selection of the ARV regimen. Given the recent approval of daily tenofovir DF/emtricitabine (TDF/FTC) for pre-exposure prophylaxis (PrEP),[32-34] early infection may be diagnosed in some patients while they are taking TDF/FTC as PrEP. In this setting, resistance testing should be performed; however, because PI resistance is unlikely, use of a RTV-boosted PI with TDF/FTC remains a reasonable option pending resistance testing results (see What to Start).

Patient Follow-up

Testing for plasma HIV RNA levels, CD4 cell counts, and toxicity monitoring should be performed as described in Laboratory Testing for Initial Assessment and Monitoring While on Antiretroviral Therapy (i.e., HIV RNA at initiation of therapy, after 2 to 8 weeks, then every 4 to 8 weeks until viral suppression, and thereafter, every 3 to 4 months) **(AII)**.

Duration of Therapy for Early HIV Infection

The optimal duration of therapy for patients with early HIV infection is unknown. Recent studies of early HIV infection have evaluated the potential for starting and then stopping treatment.[18-20] Although these studies showed some benefits associated with this strategy, a large randomized controlled trial of patients with chronic HIV infection found that treatment interruption was harmful in terms of increased risk of AIDS and non-AIDS events,[35] and that the strategy was associated with increased markers of inflammation, immune activation and coagulation.[36] For these reasons and because of the potential benefit of ART in reducing the risk of HIV transmission, the Panel recommends against discontinuation of ART in patients treated for early HIV infection **(AIII)**.

Table 10. Identifying, Diagnosing, and Managing Acute and Recent HIV-1 Infection

- **Suspecting acute HIV infection:** Signs or symptoms of acute HIV infection with recent (within 2 to 6 weeks) high risk of exposure to HIV[a]
    - Signs/symptoms/laboratory findings may include but are not limited to one or more of the following: fever, lymphadenopathy, skin rash, myalgia/arthralgia, headache, diarrhea, oral ulcers, leucopenia, thrombocytopenia, transaminase elevation.
    - High-risk exposures include sexual contact with an HIV-infected person or a person at risk of HIV infection, sharing injection drug use paraphernalia, or contact of mucous membranes or breaks in skin with potentially infectious fluids.

- **Differential diagnosis:** Includes but is not limited to viral illnesses such as Epstein-Barr virus (EBV)- and non-EBV (e.g., cytomegalovirus) infectious mononucleosis syndromes, influenza, viral hepatitis, streptococcal infection, or syphilis.

- **Evaluation/diagnosis of acute HIV infection:**
    - Acute infection is defined as detectable HIV RNA or p24 antigen (the antigen used in currently available HIV antigen/antibody [Ag/Ab] combination assays), in serum or plasma in the setting of a negative or indeterminate HIV antibody test result
        - A reactive HIV antibody test or Ag/Ab test must be followed by supplemental confirmatory testing.
        - A negative or indeterminate HIV antibody test in a person with a positive Ag/Ab test or in whom acute HIV infection is suspected requires assessment of plasma HIV RNA[b] to assess for acute HIV infection.
        - A positive plasma HIV RNA test in the setting of a negative or indeterminate antibody result is consistent with acute HIV infection.
    - Patients presumptively diagnosed with acute HIV infection should have serologic testing repeated over the next 3 to 6 months to document seroconversion.

- **Considerations for antiretroviral therapy (ART) during early HIV infection:**
    - All pregnant women with early HIV infection should begin taking combination ART as soon as possible because of the high risk of perinatal HIV transmission **(AI)**.
    - Treatment for early HIV infection should be offered to all non-pregnant persons **(BII)**.
    - The risks of ART during early HIV infection are largely the same as those for ART initiated in chronically infected asymptomatic patients with high CD4 counts.
    - If therapy is initiated, the goal should be sustained plasma virologic suppression **(AIII)**.
    - Providers should consider enrolling patients with early HIV infection in clinical studies.

[a] In some settings, behaviors conducive to acquisition of HIV infection might not be ascertained or might not be perceived as high risk by the health care provider or the patient or both. Thus, symptoms and signs consistent with acute retroviral syndrome should motivate consideration of this diagnosis even in the absence of reported high-risk behaviors.

[b] Plasma HIV RNA can be measured by a variety of quantitative assays, including branched DNA (bDNA) and reverse transcriptase-polymerase chain reaction (RT-PCR)-based assays as well as by a qualitative transcription-mediated amplification assay (APTIMA, GenProbe).

References

1. Tindall B, Cooper DA. Primary HIV infection: host responses and intervention strategies. *AIDS*. 1991;5(1):1-14. Available at http://www.ncbi.nlm.nih.gov/entrez/query.fcgi?cmd=Retrieve&db=PubMed&dopt=Citation&list_uids=1812848.

2. Niu MT, Stein DS, Schnittman SM. Primary human immunodeficiency virus type 1 infection: review of pathogenesis and early treatment intervention in humans and animal retrovirus infections. *J Infect Dis*. 1993;168(6):1490-1501. Available at http://www.ncbi.nlm.nih.gov/entrez/query.fcgi?cmd=Retrieve&db=PubMed&dopt=Citation&list_uids=8245534.

3. Kinloch-de Loes S, de Saussure P, Saurat JH, Stalder H, Hirschel B, Perrin LH. Symptomatic primary infection due to human immunodeficiency virus type 1: review of 31 cases. *Clin Infect Dis*. 1993;17(1):59-65. Available at http://www.ncbi.nlm.nih.gov/entrez/query.fcgi?cmd=Retrieve&db=PubMed&dopt=Citation&list_uids=8353247.

4. Schacker T, Collier AC, Hughes J, Shea T, Corey L. Clinical and epidemiologic features of primary HIV infection. *Ann Intern Med*. 1996;125(4):257-264. Available at http://www.ncbi.nlm.nih.gov/entrez/query.fcgi?cmd=Retrieve&db=PubMed&dopt=Citation&list_uids=8678387.

5. Daar ES, Little S, Pitt J, et al. Diagnosis of primary HIV-1 infection. Los Angeles County Primary HIV Infection Recruitment Network. *Ann Intern Med*. 2001;134(1):25-29. Available at http://www.ncbi.nlm.nih.gov/entrez/query.fcgi?cmd=Retrieve&db=PubMed&dopt=Citation&list_uids=11187417.

6. Hecht FM, Busch MP, Rawal B, et al. Use of laboratory tests and clinical symptoms for identification of primary HIV infection. *AIDS*. 2002;16(8):1119-1129. Available at http://www.ncbi.nlm.nih.gov/entrez/query.fcgi?cmd=Retrieve&db=PubMed&dopt=Citation&list_uids=12004270.

7. Branson BM, Handsfield HH, Lampe MA, et al. Revised recommendations for HIV testing of adults, adolescents, and pregnant women in health-care settings. *MMWR Recomm Rep*. 2006;55(RR-14):1-17; quiz CE11-14. Available at http://www.ncbi.nlm.nih.gov/pubmed/16988643.

8. Pilcher CD, Christopoulos KA, Golden M. Public health rationale for rapid nucleic acid or p24 antigen tests for HIV. *J Infect Dis*. 2010;201(1):S7-15. Available at http://www.ncbi.nlm.nih.gov/pubmed/20225950.

9. Pilcher CD, Fiscus SA, Nguyen TQ, et al. Detection of acute infections during HIV testing in North Carolina. *N Engl J Med*. 2005;352(18):1873-1883. Available at http://www.ncbi.nlm.nih.gov/entrez/query.fcgi?cmd=Retrieve&db=PubMed&dopt=Citation&list_uids=15872202.

10. Branson BM. The future of HIV testing. *J Acquir Immune Defic Syndr*. Dec 2010;55 Suppl 2:S102-105. Available at http://www.ncbi.nlm.nih.gov/pubmed/21406978.

11. Branson BM, Stekler JD. Detection of acute HIV infection: we can't close the window. *J Infect Dis*. Feb 15 2012;205(4):521-524. Available at http://www.ncbi.nlm.nih.gov/pubmed/22207652.

12. Pantaleo G, Cohen OJ, Schacker T, et al. Evolutionary pattern of human immunodeficiency virus (HIV) replication and distribution in lymph nodes following primary infection: implications for antiviral therapy. *Nat Med*. 1998;4(3):341-345. Available at http://www.ncbi.nlm.nih.gov/entrez/query.fcgi?cmd=Retrieve&db=PubMed&dopt=Citation&list_uids=9500610.

13. Hoen B, Dumon B, Harzic M, et al. Highly active antiretroviral treatment initiated early in the course of symptomatic primary HIV-1 infection: results of the ANRS 053 trial. *J Infect Dis*. 1999;180(4):1342-1346. Available at http://www.ncbi.nlm.nih.gov/entrez/query.fcgi?cmd=Retrieve&db=PubMed&dopt=Citation&list_uids=10479169.

14. Lafeuillade A, Poggi C, Tamalet C, Profizi N, Tourres C, Costes O. Effects of a combination of zidovudine, didanosine, and lamivudine on primary human immunodeficiency virus type 1 infection. *J Infect Dis*. 1997;175(5):1051-1055. Available at http://www.ncbi.nlm.nih.gov/entrez/query.fcgi?cmd=Retrieve&db=PubMed&dopt=Citation&list_uids=9129065.

15. Lillo FB, Ciuffreda D, Veglia F, et al. Viral load and burden modification following early antiretroviral therapy of primary HIV-1 infection. *AIDS*. 1999;13(7):791-796. Available at http://www.ncbi.nlm.nih.gov/entrez/query.fcgi?cmd=Retrieve&db=PubMed&dopt=Citation&list_uids=10357377.

16. Malhotra U, Berrey MM, Huang Y, et al. Effect of combination antiretroviral therapy on T-cell immunity in acute human immunodeficiency virus type 1 infection. *J Infect Dis*. 2000;181(1):121-131. Available at http://www.ncbi.nlm.nih.gov/entrez/query.fcgi?cmd=Retrieve&db=PubMed&dopt=Citation&list_uids=10608758.

17. Smith DE, Walker BD, Cooper DA, Rosenberg ES, Kaldor JM. Is antiretroviral treatment of primary HIV infection clinically justified on the basis of current evidence? *AIDS*. 2004;18(5):709-718. Available at

http://www.ncbi.nlm.nih.gov/entrez/query.fcgi?cmd=Retrieve&db=PubMed&dopt=Citation&list_uids=15075505.

18. Hogan CM, Degruttola V, Sun X, et al. The setpoint study (ACTG A5217): effect of immediate versus deferred antiretroviral therapy on virologic set point in recently HIV-1-infected individuals. *J Infect Dis*. 2012;205(1):87-96. Available at http://www.ncbi.nlm.nih.gov/pubmed/22180621.

19. Grijsen ML, Steingrover R, Wit FW, et al. No treatment versus 24 or 60 weeks of antiretroviral treatment during primary HIV infection: the randomized Primo-SHM trial. *PLoS Med*. 2012;9(3):e1001196. Available at http://www.ncbi.nlm.nih.gov/pubmed/22479156.

20. The SPARTAC Trial Investigators. Short-Course Antiretroviral Therapy in Primary HIV Infection. *N Engl J Med*. 2013;368(3):207-217. Available at http://www.ncbi.nlm.nih.gov/pubmed/23323897.

21. Strain MC, Little SJ, Daar ES, et al. Effect of treatment, during primary infection, on establishment and clearance of cellular reservoirs of HIV-1. *J Infect Dis*. 2005;191(9):1410-1418. Available at http://www.ncbi.nlm.nih.gov/pubmed/15809898.

22. Rosenberg ES, Altfeld M, Poon SH, et al. Immune control of HIV-1 after early treatment of acute infection. *Nature*. S2000;407(6803):523-526. Available at http://www.ncbi.nlm.nih.gov/pubmed/11029005.

23. Wawer MJ, Gray RH, Sewankambo NK, et al. Rates of HIV-1 transmission per coital act, by stage of HIV-1 infection, in Rakai, Uganda. *J Infect Dis*. 2005;191(9):1403-1409. Available at http://www.ncbi.nlm.nih.gov/pubmed/15809897.

24. Cohen MS, Chen YQ, McCauley M, et al. Prevention of HIV-1 infection with early antiretroviral therapy. *N Engl J Med*. 2011;365(6):493-505. Available at http://www.ncbi.nlm.nih.gov/pubmed/21767103.

25. Mehandru S, Poles MA, Tenner-Racz K, et al. Primary HIV-1 infection is associated with preferential depletion of CD4+ T lymphocytes from effector sites in the gastrointestinal tract. *J Exp Med*. 2004;200(6):761-770. Available at http://www.ncbi.nlm.nih.gov/entrez/query.fcgi?cmd=Retrieve&db=PubMed&dopt=Citation&list_uids=15365095.

26. Guadalupe M, Reay E, Sankaran S, et al. Severe CD4+ T-cell depletion in gut lymphoid tissue during primary human immunodeficiency virus type 1 infection and substantial delay in restoration following highly active antiretroviral therapy. *J Virol*. 2003;77(21):11708-11717. Available at http://www.ncbi.nlm.nih.gov/entrez/query.fcgi?cmd=Retrieve&db=PubMed&dopt=Citation&list_uids=14557656.

27. Panel on Treatment of HIV-Infected Pregnant Women and Prevention of Perinatal Transmission. *Recommendations for Use of Antiretroviral Drugs in Pregnant HIV-1-Infected Women for Maternal Health and Interventions to Reduce Perinatal HIV Transmission in the United States*. Available at http://aidsinfo.nih.gov/contentfiles/lvguidelines/PerinatalGL.pdf.

28. Wheeler WH, Ziebell RA, Zabina H, et al. Prevalence of transmitted drug resistance associated mutations and HIV-1 subtypes in new HIV-1 diagnoses, U.S.-2006. *AIDS*. 2010;24(8):1203-1212. Available at http://www.ncbi.nlm.nih.gov/entrez/query.fcgi?cmd=Retrieve&db=PubMed&dopt=Citation&list_uids=20395786.

29. Kim D, Wheeler W, Ziebell R, al e. Prevalence of transmitted antiretroviral drug resistance among newly-diagnosed HIV-1-infected persons, US, 2007. Paper presented at: 17th Conference on Retroviruses and Opportunistic Infections; 2010; San Francisco, CA.

30. Wensing AM, van de Vijver DA, Angarano G, et al. Prevalence of drug-resistant HIV-1 variants in untreated individuals in Europe: implications for clinical management. *J Infect Dis*. 2005;192(6):958-966. Available at http://www.ncbi.nlm.nih.gov/entrez/query.fcgi?cmd=Retrieve&db=PubMed&dopt=Citation&list_uids=16107947.

31. Yanik EL, Napravnik S, Hurt CB, et al. Prevalence of transmitted antiretroviral drug resistance differs between acutely and chronically HIV-infected patients. *J Acquir Immune Defic Syndr*. 2012;61(2):258-262. Available at http://www.ncbi.nlm.nih.gov/pubmed/22692092.

32. Grant RM, Lama JR, Anderson PL, et al. Preexposure chemoprophylaxis for HIV prevention in men who have sex with men. *N Engl J Med*. 2010;363(27):2587-2599. Available at http://www.ncbi.nlm.nih.gov/pubmed/21091279.

33. Baeten JM, Donnell D, Ndase P, et al. Antiretroviral prophylaxis for HIV prevention in heterosexual men and women. *N Engl J Med*. 2012;367(5):399-410. Available at http://www.ncbi.nlm.nih.gov/pubmed/22784037.

34. Thigpen MC, Kebaabetswe PM, Paxton LA, et al. Antiretroviral preexposure prophylaxis for heterosexual HIV transmission in Botswana. *N Engl J Med*. 2012;367(5):423-434. Available at http://www.ncbi.nlm.nih.gov/pubmed/22784038.

35. Strategies for Management of Antiretroviral Therapy Study G, El-Sadr WM, Lundgren J, et al. CD4+ count-guided interruption of antiretroviral treatment. *N Engl J Med*. 2006;355(22):2283-2296. Available at http://www.ncbi.nlm.nih.gov/pubmed/17135583.

36. Kuller LH, Tracy R, Belloso W, et al. Inflammatory and coagulation biomarkers and mortality in patients with HIV infection. *PLoS Med*. 2008;5(10):e203. Available at http://www.ncbi.nlm.nih.gov/pubmed/18942885.

HIV-Infected Adolescents and Young Adults (Last updated January 10, 2011; last reviewed January 10, 2011)

Older children and adolescents now make up the largest percentage of HIV-infected children cared for at pediatric HIV clinics in the United States. The Centers for Disease Control and Prevention (CDC) estimates that 15% of the 35,314 new HIV diagnoses reported among the 33 states that participated in confidential, name-based HIV infection reporting in 2006 were among youth 13 24 years of age.[1] Recent trends in HIV prevalence reveal that the disproportionate burden of HIV/AIDS among racial minorities is even greater among youth 13 19 years of age than among young adults 20 24 years of age.[2] Furthermore, trends for all HIV/AIDS diagnoses in 33 states from 2001 to 2006 decreased for all transmission categories except among men who have sex with men (MSM). Notably, among all black MSM, the largest increase in HIV/AIDS diagnoses occurred among youth 13 24 years of age.[3] HIV-infected adolescents represent a heterogeneous group in terms of sociodemographics, mode of HIV infection, sexual and substance abuse history, clinical and immunologic status, psychosocial development, and readiness to adhere to medications. Many of these factors may influence decisions concerning when to start antiretroviral therapy (ART) and what antiretroviral (ARV) medications should be used.

Most adolescents who acquire HIV are infected through high-risk behaviors. Many of them are recently infected and unaware of their HIV infection status. Thus, many are in an early stage of HIV infection, which makes them ideal candidates for early interventions, such as prevention counseling, linkage, and engagement to care. A recent study among HIV-infected adolescents and young adults presenting for care identified primary genotypic resistance mutations to ARV medications in up to 18% of the evaluable sample of recently infected youth, as determined by the detuned antibody testing assay strategy that defined recent infection as occurring within 180 days of testing.[4] This transmission dynamic reflects that a substantial proportion of youth's sexual partners are likely older and may be more ART experienced; thus, awareness of the importance of baseline resistance testing among recently infected youth naive to ART is imperative.

A limited but increasing number of HIV-infected adolescents are long-term survivors of HIV infection acquired perinatally or in infancy through blood products. Such adolescents are usually heavily ART experienced and may have a unique clinical course that differs from that of adolescents infected later in life.[5] If these heavily ART-experienced adolescents harbor resistant virus, optimal ARV regimens should be based on the same guiding principles as for heavily ART-experienced adults. (See Virologic and Immunogic Failure.)

Adolescents are developmentally at a difficult crossroad. Their needs for autonomy and independence and their evolving decisional capacity intersect and compete with concrete thinking processes, risk-taking behaviors, preoccupation with self-image, and the need to "fit in" with their peers. This makes it challenging to attract and sustain adolescents' focus on maintaining their health, particularly for those with chronic illnesses. These challenges are not specific to any particular transmission mode or stage of disease. Thus, irrespective of disease duration or mode of HIV transmission, every effort must be made to engage them in care so they can improve and maintain their health for the long term.

Antiretroviral Therapy Considerations in Adolescents

Adult guidelines for ART are usually appropriate for postpubertal adolescents, because the clinical course of HIV-infected adolescents who were infected sexually or through injection drug use during adolescence is more similar to that of adults than to that of children. Adult guidelines can also be useful for postpubertal youth who were perinatally infected because these patients often have treatment challenges associated with the use of long-term ART that mirror those of ART-experienced adults, such as extensive resistance, complex regimens, and adverse drug effects.

Dosage of medications for HIV infection and opportunistic infections should be prescribed according to Tanner staging of puberty and not solely on the basis of age.[6-7] Adolescents in early puberty (i.e., Tanner

Stages I and II) should be administered doses on pediatric schedules, whereas those in late puberty (i.e., Tanner Stage V) should follow adult dosing schedules. However, Tanner stage and age are not necessarily directly predictive of drug pharmacokinetics. Because puberty may be delayed in children who were infected with HIV perinatally,[8] continued use of pediatric doses in puberty-delayed adolescents can result in medication doses that are higher than the usual adult doses. Because data are not available to predict optimal medication doses for each ARV medication for this group of children, issues such as toxicity, pill or liquid volume burden, adherence, and virologic and immunologic parameters should be considered in determining when to transition from pediatric to adult doses. Youth who are in their growth spurt period (i.e., Tanner Stage III in females and Tanner Stage IV in males) and following adult or pediatric dosing guidelines and adolescents who have transitioned from pediatric to adult doses should be closely monitored for medication efficacy and toxicity. Therapeutic drug monitoring can be considered in selected circumstances to help guide therapy decisions in this context. Pharmacokinetic studies of drugs in youth are needed to better define appropriate dosing. For a more detailed discussion, see Guidelines for the Use of Antiretroviral Agents in Pediatric HIV Infection.[9]

Adherence Concerns in Adolescents

HIV-infected adolescents are especially vulnerable to specific adherence problems based on their psychosocial and cognitive developmental trajectory. Comprehensive systems of care are required to serve both the medical and psychosocial needs of HIV-infected adolescents, who are frequently inexperienced with health care systems and who lack health insurance. Many HIV-infected adolescents face challenges in adhering to medical regimens for reasons that include:

- denial and fear of their HIV infection;
- misinformation;
- distrust of the medical establishment;
- fear and lack of belief in the effectiveness of medications;
- low self-esteem;
- unstructured and chaotic lifestyles;
- mood disorders and other mental illness;
- lack of familial and social support;
- absence of or inconsistent access to care or health insurance; and
- incumbent risk of inadvertent parental disclosure of the youth's HIV infection status if parental health insurance is used.

In selecting treatment regimens for adolescents, clinicians must balance the goal of prescribing a maximally potent ART regimen with realistic assessment of existing and potential support systems to facilitate adherence. Adolescents benefit from reminder systems (e.g., beepers, timers, and pill boxes) that are stylish and inconspicuous.[10] It is important to make medication adherence as user friendly and as little stigmatizing as possible for the older child or adolescent. The concrete thought processes of adolescents make it difficult for them to take medications when they are asymptomatic, particularly if the medications have side effects. Adherence to complex regimens is particularly challenging at a time of life when adolescents do not want to be different from their peers.[11-13] Directly observed therapy might be considered for selected HIV-infected adolescents such as those with mental illness.[14-18]

Difficult Adherence Problems

Because adolescence is characterized by rapid changes in physical maturation, cognitive processes, and life style, predicting long-term adherence in an adolescent can be very challenging. The ability of youth to adhere to therapy needs to be included as part of therapeutic decision making concerning the risks and benefits of starting treatment. Erratic adherence may result in the loss of future regimens because of the development of resistance mutations. Clinicians who care for HIV-infected adolescents frequently manage youth who, while needing therapy, pose significant concerns regarding their ability to adhere to therapy. In these cases, alternative considerations to initiation of therapy can be the following: (1) a short-term deferral of treatment until adherence is more likely or while adherence-related problems are aggressively addressed; (2) an adherence testing period in which a placebo (e.g., vitamin pill) is administered; and (3) the avoidance of any regimens with low genetic resistance barriers. Such decisions are ideally individualized to each patient and should be made carefully in context with the individual's clinical status. For a more detailed discussion on specific therapy and adherence issues for HIV-infected adolescents, see Guidelines for Use of Antiretroviral Agents in Pediatric HIV Infection.[9]

Special Considerations in Adolescents

Sexually transmitted infections (STIs), in particular human papilloma virus (HPV), should also be addressed in all adolescents. For a more detailed discussion on STIs, see the most recent CDC guidelines[19] and the pediatric opportunistic infection treatment guidelines on HPV among HIV-infected adolescents.[20] Family planning counseling, including a discussion of the risks of perinatal transmission of HIV and methods to reduce risks, should be provided to all youth. Providing gynecologic care for the HIV-infected female adolescent is especially important. Contraception, including the interaction of specific ARV drugs on hormonal contraceptives, and the potential for pregnancy also may alter choices of ART. As an example, efavirenz (EFV) should be used with caution in females of childbearing age and should only be prescribed after intensive counseling and education about the potential effects on the fetus, the need for close monitoring including periodic pregnancy testing and a commitment on the part of the teen to use effective contraception. For a more detailed discussion, see HIV-Infected Women and the Perinatal Guidelines.[21]

Transitioning Care

Given lifelong infection with HIV and the need for treatment through several stages of growth and development, HIV care programs and providers need flexibility to appropriately transition care for HIV-infected children, adolescents, and young adults. A successful transition requires an awareness of some fundamental differences between many adolescent and adult HIV care models. In most adolescent HIV clinics, care is more "teen-centered" and multidisciplinary, with primary care being highly integrated into HIV care. Teen services, such as sexual and reproductive health, substance abuse treatment, mental health, treatment education, and adherence counseling are all found in one clinic setting. In contrast, some adult HIV clinics may rely more on referral of the patient to separate subspecialty care settings, such as gynecology. Transitioning the care of an emerging young adult includes considerations of areas such as medical insurance, independence, autonomy, decisional capacity, confidentiality, and consent. Also, adult clinic settings tend to be larger and can easily intimidate younger, less motivated patients. As an additional complication to this transition, HIV-infected adolescents belong to two epidemiologically distinct subgroups: (1) those perinatally infected who would likely have more disease burden history, complications, and chronicity; less functional autonomy; greater need for ART; and higher mortality risk; and (2) those more recently infected due to high-risk behaviors. Thus, these subgroups have unique biomedical and psychosocial considerations and needs.

To maximize the likelihood of a successful transition, facilitators to successful transitioning are best implemented early on. These include the following: (1) optimizing provider communication between adolescent and adult clinics; (2) addressing patient/family resistance caused by lack of information, stigma or disclosure concerns, and differences in practice styles; (3) preparing youth for life skills development, including counseling them on the appropriate use of a primary care provider and appointment management, the importance of prompt symptom recognition and reporting, and the importance of self-efficacy with medication management, insurance, and entitlements; (4) identifying an optimal clinic model for a given setting (i.e., simultaneous transition of mental health and/or case management versus a gradual phase-in); (5) implementing ongoing evaluation to measure the success of a selected model; (6) engaging in regular multidisciplinary case conferences between adult and adolescent care providers; (7) implementing interventions that may be associated with improved outcomes, such as support groups and mental health consultation; and (8) incorporating a family planning component into clinical care. Attention to these key areas will likely improve adherence to appointments and avert the potential for a youth to "fall through the cracks," as it is commonly referred to in adolescent medicine.

References

1.   Centers for Disease Control and Prevention (CDC). HIV and AIDS in the United States: A picture of today's epidemic. 2008; http://www.cdc.gov/hiv/topics/surveillance/united states.htm

2.   Centers for Disease Control and Prevention (CDC). HIV/AIDS surveillance in adolescents and young adults (through 2007). 2009; http://www.cdc.gov/hiv/topics/surveillance/resources/slides/adolescents/index.htm.

3.   MMWR. Trends in HIV/AIDS diagnoses among men who have sex with men—33 states, 2001-2006. *MMWR Morb Mortal Wkly Rep*. 2008;57(25):681-686.

4.   Viani RM, Peralta L, Aldrovandi G, et al. Prevalence of primary HIV-1 drug resistance among recently infected adolescents: a multicenter adolescent medicine trials network for HIV/AIDS interventions study. *J Infect Dis*. 2006;194(11):1505-1509.

5.   Grubman S, Gross E, Lerner-Weiss N, et al. Older children and adolescents living with perinatally acquired human immunodeficiency virus infection. *Pediatrics*. 1995;95(5):657-663.

6.   Rogers A (ed). Pharmacokinetics and pharmacodynamics in adolescents. *J Adolesc Health*. 1994;15:605-678.

7.   El-Sadar W, Oleske JM, Agins BD, et al. Evaluation and management of early HIV infection. Clinical Practice Guideline No. 7 (AHCPR Publication No. 94-0572). Rockville, MD: Agency for Health Care Policy and Research, Public Health Service, US Department of Health and Human Services, 1994.

8.   Buchacz K, Rogol AD, Lindsey JC, et al. Delayed onset of pubertal development in children and adolescents with perinatally acquired HIV infection. *J Acquir Immune Defic Syndr*. 2003;33(1):56-65.

9.   Working Group on Antiretroviral Therapy and Medical Management of HIV-Infected Children. Guidelines for the use of antiretroviral agents in pediatric HIV infection. August 16, 2010:1-219. http://aidsinfo.nih.gov/contentfiles/PediatricGuidelines.pdf.

10. Lyon ME, Trexler C, Akpan-Townsend C, et al. A family group approach to increasing adherence to therapy in HIV-infected youths: results of a pilot project. *AIDS Patient Care STDS*. 2003;17(6):299-308.

11. Brooks-Gunn J, Graber JA. Puberty as a biological and social event: implications for research on pharmacology. *J Adolesc Health*. 1994;15(8):663-671.

12. Kyngas H, Hentinen M, Barlow JH. Adolescents' perceptions of physicians, nurses, parents and friends: help or hindrance in compliance with diabetes self-care? *J Adv Nurs*. 1998;27(4):760-769.

13. La Greca AM. Peer influences in pediatric chronic illness: an update. J Pediatr Psychol. 1992;17(6):775-784.

14. Murphy DA, Wilson CM, Durako SJ, et al. Antiretroviral medication adherence among the REACH HIV-infected adolescent cohort in the USA. *AIDS Care*. 2001;13(1):27-40.

15. Stenzel MS, McKenzie M, Mitty JA, et al. Enhancing adherence to HAART: a pilot program of modified directly observed therapy. *AIDS Read*. 2001;11(6):317-319, 324-318.

16. Purdy JB, Freeman AF, Martin SC, et al. Virologic response using directly observed therapy in adolescents with HIV: an adherence tool. *J Assoc Nurses AIDS Care*. 2008;19(2):158-165.

17. Garvie PA, Lawford J, Flynn PM, et al. Development of a directly observed therapy adherence intervention for adolescents with human immunodeficiency virus-1: application of focus group methodology to inform design, feasibility, and acceptability. *J Adolesc Health*. 2009;44(2):124-132.

18. Gaur A BM, Britto P, et al. Directly observed therapy for non-adherent HIV-infected adolescents - lessons learned, challenges ahead. Paper presented at: 15th Conference on Retroviruses and Opportunistic Infections. Paper presented at: 15th Conference on Retroviruses and Opportunistic Infections; 2008; Boston, MA.

19. Workowski KA, Berman SM. Sexually transmitted diseases treatment guidelines, 2006. *MMWR Recomm Rep*. 2006;55(RR-11):1-94.

20. Centers for Disease Control and Prevention (CDC). Guidelines for the Prevention and Treatment of Opportunistic Infections among HIV-exposed and HIV-infected children: recommendations from CDC, the National Institutes of Health, the HIV Medicine Association of the Infectious Diseases Society of America, the Pediatric Infectious Diseases Society, and the American Academy of Pediatrics. *MMWR Recomm Rep*. 2009;58(RR-11):1-166.

21. Panel on Treatment of HIV-Infected Pregnant Women and Prevention of Perinatal Transmission. Recommendations for use of antiretroviral drugs in pregnant HIV-1-infected women for maternal health and interventions to reduce perinatal HIV transmission in the United States. May 24, 2010:1-117. http://aidsinfo.nih.gov/contentfiles/PerinatalGL.pdf.

Treatment Challenges of HIV-Infected Illicit Drug Users

Injection drug use is the second most common mode of HIV transmission in the United States. In addition, noninjection illicit drug use may facilitate sexual transmission of HIV. Injection and noninjection illicit drugs include the following: heroin, cocaine, marijuana, and club drugs (i.e., methamphetamine, ketamine, gamma-hydroxybutyrate [GHB], and amyl nitrate [i.e., poppers]). The most commonly used illicit drugs associated with HIV infection are heroin and stimulants (e.g., cocaine and amphetamines); however, the use of club drugs has increased substantially in the past several years and is common among individuals who have HIV infection or who are at risk of HIV infection. The association between club drugs and high-risk sexual behavior in men who have sex with men (MSM) is strongest for methamphetamine and amyl nitrate; this association is less consistent with the other club drugs.[1]

Illicit drug use has been associated with depression and anxiety, either as part of the withdrawal process or as a consequence of repeated use. This is particularly relevant in the treatment of HIV infection because depression is one of the strongest predictors of poor adherence and poor treatment outcomes.[2] Treatment of HIV disease in illicit drug users can be successful but HIV-infected illicit drug users present special treatment challenges. These challenges may include the following: (1) an array of complicating comorbid medical and mental health conditions; (2) limited access to HIV care; (3) inadequate adherence to therapy; (4) medication side effects and toxicities; (5) the need for substance abuse treatment; and (6) drug interactions that can complicate HIV treatment.[3]

Underlying health problems in injection and noninjection drug users result in increased morbidity and mortality, either independent of or accentuated by HIV disease. Many of these problems are the consequence of prior exposures to infectious pathogens from nonsterile needle and syringe use. Such problems can include hepatitis B or C virus infection, tuberculosis (TB), skin and soft tissue infections, recurrent bacterial pneumonia, and endocarditis. Other morbidities such as alteration in levels of consciousness and neurologic and renal disease are not uncommon. Furthermore, these comorbidities are associated with a higher risk of drug overdoses in illicit drug users with HIV disease than in HIV-uninfected illicit drug users, due in part to respiratory, hepatic, and neurological impairments associated with HIV infection.[4] Successful HIV therapy for illicit drug users often depends on clinicians becoming familiar with and managing these comorbid conditions and providing overdose prevention support.

Illicit drug users have less access to HIV care and are less likely to receive antiretroviral therapy (ART) than other populations.[5-6] Factors associated with low rates of ART use among illicit drug users include active drug use, younger age, female gender, suboptimal health care, recent incarceration, lack of access to rehabilitation programs, and health care providers' lack of expertise in HIV treatment.[5-6] The typically unstable, chaotic life patterns of many illicit drug users; the powerful pull of addictive substances; and common misperceptions about the dangers, impact, and benefits of ART all contribute to decreased adherence.[7] The chronic and relapsing nature of substance abuse as a biologic and medical disease, compounded by the high rate of mental illness that antedates and/or is exacerbated by illicit substance use, additionally complicate the relationship between health care workers and illicit drug users.[8-9] The first step in provision of care and treatment for these individuals is to recognize the existence of a substance abuse problem. It is often obvious that the problem exists, but some patients may hide these problem behaviors from clinicians. Assessment of a patient for substance abuse should be part of routine medical history taking and should be done in a professional, straightforward, and nonjudgmental manner.

Treatment Efficacy in HIV-Infected Illicit Drug Use Populations

Although illicit drug users are underrepresented in HIV therapy clinical trials, available data indicate that efficacy of ART in illicit drug users   when they are not actively using drugs   is similar to that seen in other populations.[10] Furthermore, therapeutic failure in this population generally correlates with the degree that drug use disrupts daily activities rather than with drug use per se.[11] Providers need to remain attentive to the possible impact of disruptions caused by drug use on the patient both before and while receiving ART. Although many illicit drug users can sufficiently control their drug use for long enough time to benefit from care, substance abuse treatment is often necessary for successful HIV management.

Close collaboration with substance abuse treatment programs and proper support and attention to this population's special multidisciplinary needs are critical components of successful HIV treatment. Essential to this end are accommodating, flexible, community-based HIV care sites that are characterized by familiarity with and nonjudgmental expertise in management of drug users' wide array of needs and in development of effective strategies to promote medication adherence.[9] These strategies should include, if available, the use of adherence support mechanisms such as modified directly observed therapy (mDOT), which has shown promise in this population.[12]

Antiretroviral Agents and Opioid Substitution Therapy

Compared with noninjection drug users receiving ART, injection drug users (IDUs) receiving ART are more likely to experience an increased frequency of side effects and toxicities of ART. Although not systematically studied, this is likely because underlying hepatic, renal, neurologic, psychiatric, gastrointestinal (GI), and hematologic disorders are highly prevalent among IDUs. These comorbid conditions should be considered when selecting antiretroviral (ARV) agents in this population. Opioid substitution therapies such as methadone and buprenorphine/naloxone and extended-release naltrexone are commonly used for management of opioid dependence in HIV-infected patients.

Methadone and Antiretroviral Therapy. Methadone, an orally administered, long-acting opioid agonist, is the most common pharmacologic treatment for opioid addiction. Its use is associated with decreased heroin use, decreased needle sharing, and improved quality of life. Because of its opioid-induced effects on gastric emptying and the metabolism of cytochrome P (CYP) 450 isoenzymes 2B6, 3A4, and 2D6, pharmacologic effects and interactions with ARV agents may commonly occur.[13] These may diminish the effectiveness of either or both therapies by causing opioid withdrawal or overdose, increased methadone toxicity, and/or decreased ARV efficacy. Efavirenz (EFV), nevirapine (NVP), and lopinavir/ritonavir (LPV/r) have been associated with significant decreases in methadone levels. Patients and substance abuse treatment facilities should be informed of the likelihood of this interaction. The clinical effect is usually seen after 7 days of co-administration and may be managed by increasing the methadone dosage, usually in 5-mg to 10-mg increments daily until the desired effect is achieved.

Buprenorphine and Antiretroviral Therapy. Buprenorphine, a partial μ-opioid agonist, is administrated sublingually and is often coformulated with naloxone. It is increasingly used for opioid dependence treatment. Compared with methadone, buprenorphine has a lower risk of respiratory depression and overdose. This allows physicians in primary care to prescribe buprenorphine for the treatment of opioid dependency. The flexibility of the primary care setting can be of significant value to opioid-addicted HIV-infected patients who require ART because it enables one physician or program to provide both medical and substance abuse services. Limited information is currently available about interactions between buprenorphine and ARV agents.[13-14] Findings from available studies show that the drug interaction profile of buprenorphine is more favorable than that of methadone.

Naltrexone and Antiretroviral Therapy. A once-monthly extended-release intramuscular formulation of naltrexone was recently approved for prevention of relapse in patients who have undergone an opioid detoxification program. Naltrexone is also indicated for treatment of alcohol dependency. Naltrexone is not metabolized via the CYP450 enzyme system and is not expected to interact with protease inhibitors (PIs) or non-nucleoside reverse transcriptase inhibitors (NNRTIs).[15]

Table 11 provides the currently available pharmacokinetic (PK) interaction data that clinicians can use as a guide for managing patients receiving ART and methadone or buprenorphine. Particular attention is needed concerning communication between HIV care providers and drug treatment programs regarding additive drug toxicities and drug interactions resulting in opiate withdrawal or excess.

Methylenedioxymethamphetamine (MDMA), GHB, ketamine, and methamphetamine all have the potential to interact with ARV agents because all are metabolized, at least in part, by the CYP450 system. Overdoses secondary to interactions between the party drugs (i.e., MDMA or GHB) and PI-based ART have been reported.[16]

Summary

It is usually possible over time to support most active drug users such that acceptable adherence levels with ARV agents can be achieved.[17-18] Providers must work to combine all available resources to stabilize an active drug user in preparation for ART. This should include identification of concurrent medical and psychiatric illnesses, drug treatment and needle and syringe exchange programs, strategies to reduce high-risk sexual behavior, and harm-reduction strategies. A history of drug use alone is insufficient reason to withhold ART because individuals with a history of prior drug use have adherence rates similar to those who do not abuse drugs.

Important considerations in the selection of successful regimens and the provision of appropriate patient monitoring in this population include need for supportive clinical sites; linkage to substance abuse treatment; and awareness of the interactions between illicit drugs and ARV agents, including the increased risk of side effects and toxicities. Simple regimens should be considered to enhance medication adherence. Preference should be given to ARV agents that have a lower risk of hepatic and neuropsychiatric side effects, simple dosing schedules, and minimal interaction with methadone.

Table 11. Drug Interactions between Antiretroviral Agents and Drugs Used to Treat Opioid Addiction (page 1 of 2)

Concomitant Drug	Antiretroviral Drug	Pharmacokinetic Interactions Clinical Comments/Recommendations
Buprenorphine	EFV	buprenorphine AUC ↓ 50%; norbuprenorphine[a] AUC ↓ 71% No withdrawal symptoms reported. No dosage adjustment recommended; however, monitor for withdrawal symptoms.
	ETR	buprenorphine AUC ↓ 25% No dosage adjustment necessary.
	ATV	buprenorphine AUC ↑ 93%; norbuprenorphine AUC ↑ 76%; ↓ ATV levels possible Do not co-administer buprenorphine with unboosted ATV.
	ATV/r	buprenorphine AUC ↑ 66%; norbuprenorphine AUC ↑ 105% Monitor for sedation. Buprenorphine dose reduction may be necessary.
	DRV/r	buprenorphine: no significant effect; norbuprenorphine AUC ↑ 46% and C_{min} ↑ 71% No dose adjustment necessary.
	FPV/r	buprenorphine: no significant effect; norbuprenorphine AUC ↓ 15% No dosage adjustment necessary.
	TPV/r	buprenorphine: no significant effect; norbuprenorphine AUC, C_{max}, and C_{min} ↓ 80%; TPV C_{min} ↓ 19%–40% Consider monitoring TPV level.
	3TC, ddl, TDF, ZDV, NVP, LPV/r, NFV	No significant effect No dosage adjustment necessary.
	ABC, d4T, FTC, ETR, IDV +/- RTV, SQV/r, RAL, MVC, T20	No data
Methadone	ABC	methadone clearance ↑ 22% No dosage adjustment necessary.
	d4T	d4T AUC ↓ 23% and C_{max} ↓ 44% No dosage adjustment necessary.
	ZDV	ZDV AUC ↑ 29%–43% Monitor for ZDV-related adverse effects.
	EFV	methadone AUC ↓ 52% Opioid withdrawal common; increased methadone dose often necessary.

Table 11. Drug Interactions between Antiretroviral Agents and Drugs Used to Treat Opioid Addiction (page 2 of 2)

Methadone, cont'd	NVP	methadone AUC ↓ 41% NVP: no significant effect Opioid withdrawal common; increased methadone dose often necessary.
	ATV/r, DRV/r, FPV/r, IDV/r, LPV/r, SQV/r, TPV/r	With ATV/r, DRV/r, FPV/r: R-methadone[b] AUC ↓ 16%–18%; With LPV/r: methadone AUC ↓ 26%–53%; With SQV/r 1000/100 mg BID: R-methadone AUC ↓ 19%; With TPV/r: R-methadone AUC ↓ 48% Opioid withdrawal unlikely but may occur. Adjustment of methadone dose usually not required; however, monitor for opioid withdrawal and increase methadone dose as clinically indicated.
	FPV	No data with FPV (unboosted) With APV: R-methadone C_{min} ↓ 21%, no significant change in AUC Monitor and titrate methadone as clinically indicated. The interaction with FPV is presumed to be similar.
	NFV	methadone AUC ↓ 40% Opioid withdrawal rarely occurs. Monitor and titrate dose as clinically indicated. May require increased methadone dose.
	ddI (EC capsule), 3TC, TDF, ETR, RTV, ATV, IDV, RAL	No significant effect No dosage adjustment necessary.
	FTC, MVC, T20	No data

[a] Norbuprenorphine is an active metabolite of buprenorphine.
[b] R-methadone is the active form of methadone.

Key to Abbreviations: 3TC = lamivudine, ABC = abacavir, APV = amprenavir, ATV = atazanavir, ATV/r = atazanavir/ ritonavair, AUC = area under the curve, BID = twice daily, C_{max} = maximum plasma concentration, C_{min} = minimum plasma concentration, d4T = stavudine, ddI = didanosine, DRV/r = darunavir/ritonavir, EC = enteric coated, EFV = efavirenz, ETR = etravirine, FPV = fosamprenavir, FPV/r = fosamprenavir/ritonavir, FTC = emtricitabine, IDV = indinavir, IDV/r = indinavir/ritonavir, LPV/r = lopinavir/ritonavir, MVC = maraviroc, NFV = nelfinavir, NVP = nevirapine, RAL = raltegravir, RTV = ritonavir, SQV/r = sacquinavir/ritonavir, T20 = enfuvirtide, TDF = tenofovir, TPV = tipranavir, TPV/r = tipranavir/ritonavir, ZDV = zidovudine

References

1. Colfax G, Guzman R. Club drugs and HIV infection: a review. *Clin Infect Dis.* May 15 2006;42(10):1463-1469.

2. Tucker JS, Burnam MA, Sherbourne CD, Kung FY, Gifford AL. Substance use and mental health correlates of nonadherence to antiretroviral medications in a sample of patients with human immunodeficiency virus infection. *Am J Med.* May 2003;114(7):573-580.

3. Bruce RD, Altice FL, Gourevitch MN, Friedland GH. Pharmacokinetic drug interactions between opioid agonist therapy and antiretroviral medications: implications and management for clinical practice. *J Acquir Immune Defic Syndr.* Apr 15 2006;41(5):563-572.

4. Wang C, Vlahov D, Galai N, et al. The effect of HIV infection on overdose mortality. *AIDS.* Jun 10 2005;19(9):935-942.

5. Strathdee SA, Palepu A, Cornelisse PG, et al. Barriers to use of free antiretroviral therapy in injection drug users. *JAMA.* Aug 12 1998;280(6):547-549.

6. Celentano DD, Vlahov D, Cohn S, Shadle VM, Obasanjo O, Moore RD. Self-reported antiretroviral therapy in injection

drug users. *JAMA*. Aug 12 1998;280(6):544-546.

7. Altice FL, Mostashari F, Friedland GH. Trust and the acceptance of and adherence to antiretroviral therapy. *J Acquir Immune Defic Syndr*. Sep 1 2001;28(1):47-58.

8. Altice FL, Kamarulzaman A, Soriano VV, Schechter M, Friedland GH. Treatment of medical, psychiatric, and substance-use comorbidities in people infected with HIV who use drugs. *Lancet*. Jul 31 2010;376(9738):367-387.

9. Bruce RD, Altice FL, Friedland GH, Volberding P. HIV Disease Among Substance Misusers: Treatment Issues. *Global AIDS/HIV Medicine*. San Diego, CA: Elsevier Inc; 2007:513-526.

10. Morris JD, Golub ET, Mehta SH, Jacobson LP, Gange SJ. Injection drug use and patterns of highly active antiretroviral therapy use: an analysis of ALIVE, WIHS, and MACS cohorts. *AIDS Res Ther*. 2007;4:12.

11. Bouhnik AD, Chesney M, Carrieri P, et al. Nonadherence among HIV-infected injecting drug users: the impact of social instability. *J Acquir Immune Defic Syndr*. Dec 15 2002;31(Suppl 3):S149-153.

12. Altice FL, Maru DS, Bruce RD, Springer SA, Friedland GH. Superiority of directly administered antiretroviral therapy over self-administered therapy among HIV-infected drug users: a prospective, randomized, controlled trial. *Clin Infect Dis*. Sep 15 2007;45(6):770-778.

13. Gruber VA, McCance-Katz EF. Methadone, buprenorphine, and street drug interactions with antiretroviral medications. *Curr HIV/AIDS Rep*. Aug 2010;7(3):152-160.

14. Bruce RD, McCance-Katz E, Kharasch ED, Moody DE, Morse GD. Pharmacokinetic interactions between buprenorphine and antiretroviral medications. *Clin Infect Dis*. Dec 15 2006;43(Suppl 4):S216-223.

15. Food and Drug Administration (FDA). Vivitrol (package insert). October 2010. http://www.accessdata.fda.gov/drugsatfda_docs/label/2010/021897s015lbl.pdf.

16. Bruce RD, Altice FL, Gourevitch MN, Friedland GH. A review of pharmacokinetic drug interactions between drugs of abuse and antiretroviral medications: Implications and management for clinical practice. *Exp Rev of Clin Pharmacol*. 2008;1(1):115-127.

17. Hicks PL, Mulvey KP, Chander G, et al. The impact of illicit drug use and substance abuse treatment on adherence to HAART. *AIDS Care*. Oct 2007;19(9):1134-1140.

18. Cofrancesco J, Jr., Scherzer R, Tien PC, et al. Illicit drug use and HIV treatment outcomes in a US cohort. *AIDS*. Jan 30 2008;22(3):357-365.

HIV-Infected Women (Last updated February 12, 2013; last reviewed February 12, 2013)

Panel's Recommendations
• The indications for initiation of antiretroviral therapy (ART) and the goals of treatment are the same for HIV-infected women as for other HIV-infected adults and adolescents **(AI)**.
• Women taking antiretroviral (ARV) drugs that have significant pharmacokinetic interactions with oral contraceptives should use an additional or alternative contraceptive method to prevent unintended pregnancy **(AIII)**.
• In pregnant women, an additional goal of therapy is prevention of perinatal transmission of HIV, with a goal of maximal viral suppression to reduce the risk of transmission of HIV to the fetus and newborn **(AI)**.
• When selecting an ARV combination regimen for a pregnant woman, clinicians should consider the known safety, efficacy, and pharmacokinetic data on use during pregnancy for each agent **(AIII)**.
• Women of childbearing potential should undergo pregnancy testing before initiation of efavirenz (EFV) and receive counseling about the potential risk to the fetus and desirability of avoiding pregnancy while on EFV-based regimens **(AIII)**.
• Alternative regimens that do not include EFV should be strongly considered in women who are planning to become pregnant or sexually active and not using effective contraception, assuming these alternative regimens are acceptable to the provider and are not thought to compromise the woman's health **(BIII)**.
• Because the risk of neural tube defects is restricted to the first 5 to 6 weeks of pregnancy and pregnancy is rarely recognized before 4 to 6 weeks of pregnancy, EFV can be continued in pregnant women receiving an EFV-based regimen who present for antenatal care in the first trimester, provided the regimen produces virologic suppression **(CIII)**.
• When designing a regimen for a pregnant woman, clinicians should consult the most current Health and Human Services (HHS) Perinatal Guidelines **(AIII)**.
Rating of Recommendations: A = Strong; B = Moderate; C = Optional
Rating of Evidence: I = Data from randomized controlled trials; II = Data from well-designed nonrandomized trials or observational cohort studies with long-term clinical outcomes; III = Expert opinion

This section provides discussion of some basic principles and unique considerations to follow when caring for HIV-infected women, including during pregnancy. Clinicians who provide care for pregnant women should consult the current *Perinatal Guidelines*[1] for more in-depth discussion and management assistance. Additional guidance on the management of HIV-infected women can be found at http://hab.hrsa.gov/deliverhivaidscare/clinicalguide11.

Gender Considerations in Antiretroviral Therapy

In general, studies to date have not shown gender differences in virologic responses to antritretroviral therapy (ART),[2-4] but a number of studies have suggested that gender may influence the frequency, presentation, and severity of selected antiretroviral (ARV)-related adverse events.[5] Although data are limited, evidence also exists that pharmacokinetics for some ARV drugs may differ between men and women, possibly because of variations between men and women in factors such as body weight, plasma volume, gastric emptying time, plasma protein levels, cytochrome P (CYP) 450 activity, drug transporter function, and excretion activity.[6-8]

Adverse Effects:

• *Nevirapine (NVP)-associated hepatotoxicity:* NVP has been associated with an increased risk of symptomatic, potentially fatal, and often rash-associated liver toxicity in ARV-naive individuals; women with higher CD4 counts (>250 cells/mm^3) or elevated baseline transaminase levels appear to be at greatest risk.[9-12] It is generally recommended that NVP not be prescribed to ARV-naive women who have CD4 counts >250 cells/mm^3 unless there is no other alternative and the benefit from NVP outweighs the risk of hepatotoxicity (**AI**).

- *Lactic acidosis:* There is a female predominance in the increased incidence of symptomatic and even fatal lactic acidosis associated with prolonged exposure to nucleoside reverse transcriptase inhibitors (NRTIs). Lactic acidosis is most common with stavudine (d4T), didanosine (ddI), and zidovudine (ZDV) but it can occur with other NRTIs.[13]

- *Metabolic complications:* A few studies have compared women and men in terms of metabolic complications associated with ARV use. Compared with HIV-infected men, HIV-infected women are more likely to experience increases in central fat with ART and are less likely to have triglyceride elevations on treatment.[14, 15] Women have an increased risk of osteopenia/osteoporosis, particularly after menopause, and this risk is exacerbated by HIV and ART.[16, 17] At the present time, none of these differences requires women-specific recommendations regarding treatment or monitoring.

Women of Childbearing Potential

All women of childbearing potential should be offered pre-conception counseling and care as a component of routine primary medical care. Counseling should include discussion of special considerations pertaining to ARV use when trying to conceive and during pregnancy (see *Perinatal Guidelines*[1]). Safe sexual practices, reproductive desires and options for conception, HIV status of sexual partner(s), and use of effective contraception to prevent unintended pregnancy should be discussed. An HIV-infected woman who wishes to conceive with an HIV-uninfected male partner should be informed of options to prevent sexual transmission of HIV while attempting conception. Interventions include initiation of maximally suppressive ART, which significantly decreases the risk of sexual transmission (see Preventing Secondary Transmission of HIV), and artificial insemination, including the option to self-inseminate with the partner's sperm during the periovulatory period[18] (for more extensive discussion on this topic, see the Reproductive Options for HIV-Concordant and Serodiscordant Couples section of the *Perinatal Guidelines*.[1]

Efavirenz (EFV) is teratogenic in non-human primates. Women of childbearing potential should undergo pregnancy testing before initiation of EFV and receive counseling about the potential risk to the fetus and desirability of avoiding pregnancy while on EFV-based regimens (**AIII**). Alternative regimens that do not include EFV should be strongly considered in women who are planning to become pregnant or who are sexually active and not using effective contraception, assuming these alternative regimens are acceptable to the provider and are not thought to compromise the woman's health (**BIII**). The most vulnerable period in fetal organogenesis is early in gestation, before pregnancy is recognized.

Hormonal Contraception

Safe and effective reproductive health and family planning services to reduce unintended pregnancy and perinatal transmission of HIV are an essential component of care for HIV-infected women of childbearing age. Counseling about reproductive issues should be provided on an ongoing basis.

Providers should be aware of potential interactions between ARV drugs and hormonal contraceptives that could lower contraceptive efficacy. Several protease inhibitors (PIs) and non-nucleoside reverse transcriptase inhibitors (NNRTIs) have drug interactions with combined oral contraceptives (COCs). Interactions include either a decrease or an increase in blood levels of ethinyl estradiol, norethindrone, or norgestimate (see Tables 15a and 15b), which potentially decreases contraceptive efficacy or increases estrogen- or progestin-related adverse effects (e.g., thromboembolism). Small studies of HIV-infected women receiving injectable depot-medroxyprogesterone acetate (DMPA) while on ART showed no significant interactions between DMPA and EFV, NVP, nelfinavir (NFV), or NRTI drugs.[19-21] Contraceptive failure of the etonogestrel implant in two patients on EFV-based therapy has been reported and a study has shown EFV may decrease plasma progestin concentrations of COCs containing ethinyl estradiol and norgestimate.[22, 23] Several RTV-boosted PIs decrease oral contraceptive estradiol levels.[24, 25] A small study from Malawi showed that NVP use did not significantly affect estradiol or progestin levels in HIV-infected women.[26] Overall, data are relatively limited and the clinical implications of these findings are unclear. The magnitudes of change in drug levels that may reduce contraceptive efficacy or increase adverse effects are unknown. Concerns about pharmacokinetic interactions between oral and implant hormonal contraceptives and ARVs should not prevent clinicians from prescribing hormonal contraceptives for women on ART if that is their preferred contraceptive method. However, when women wish to use hormonal contraceptives and drug interactions with ARVs are known, additional or alternative contraceptive methods may be recommended (see drug interaction Tables 15a, 15b, and 15d and *Perinatal Guidelines*[1]). Consistent use of male or female condoms to prevent transmission of HIV and protect against other sexually transmitted diseases (STDs) is recommended for all HIV-infected women and their partners, regardless of contraceptive use.

The data on the association between hormonal contraception and the risk of acquisition of HIV are conflicting.[27] A retrospective secondary analysis of two studies of serodiscordant couples in Africa in which the HIV-infected partner was not receiving ART found that women using hormonal contraception (the vast majority using injectable DMPA) had a twofold increased risk of acquiring HIV (for HIV-infected male/HIV-uninfected female couples) or transmitting HIV (HIV-infected female/HIV-uninfected male couples). HIV-infected women using hormonal contraception had higher genital HIV RNA concentrations than did women not using hormonal contraceptives.[28] Oral contraceptive use was not significantly associated with transmission of HIV; however, the number of women using oral contraceptives in this study was insufficient to adequately assess risk. It is important to note that not all studies have supported a link between hormonal contraception and transmission or acquisition of HIV and that the individuals in this study were not receiving ART. Further research is needed to definitively determine if hormonal contraceptive use is an independent risk factor for acquisition and transmission of HIV, particularly in the setting of ART.[27, 29]

Intrauterine devices (IUDs) appear to be a safe and effective contraceptive option for HIV-infected women.[30-33] Although studies have focused primarily on non-hormone-containing IUDs (e.g., copper IUD), several small studies have also found levonorgestrel-releasing IUDs to be safe and not associated with increased genital tract shedding of HIV.[31, 34, 35]

Pregnant Women

Clinicians should review the *Perinatal Guidelines*[1] for a detailed discussion of the management of HIV-infected pregnant women. The use of combination ARV regimens is recommended for all HIV-infected pregnant women, regardless of virologic, immunologic, or clinical parameters **(AI)**. Pregnant HIV-infected women should be counseled regarding the known benefits and risks of ARV use during pregnancy to the woman, fetus, and newborn. A woman's decision regarding ARV use should be respected. Coercive and punitive approaches undermine provider-patient trust and could discourage women from seeking prenatal care and adopting health care behaviors that optimize maternal, fetal, and neonatal well-being.

Prevention of Perinatal Transmission of HIV. The use of ARVs and the resultant reduction of HIV RNA levels decrease perinatal transmission of HIV.[36-38] The goal of ARV use is to achieve maximal and sustained suppression of HIV RNA levels during pregnancy.

As in non-pregnant individuals, genotypic resistance testing is recommended for all pregnant women before ARV initiation **(AIII)** and for pregnant women with detectable HIV RNA levels while on therapy **(AI)**. Optimal prevention of perinatal transmission may require initiation of ARV drugs before results of resistance testing are available. If results demonstrate the presence of significant mutation(s) that may confer resistance to the prescribed ARV regimen, the regimen should be modified.

Long-term follow-up is recommended for all infants born to women who have received ARVs during pregnancy, regardless of the infant's HIV status (see the *Perinatal Guidelines*[1]).

Regimen Considerations. Pregnancy should not preclude the use of optimal drug regimens. Because recommendations on ARVs to use for treatment of HIV-infected pregnant women are subject to unique considerations, recommendations specific to the timing of therapy initiation and the choice of ARVs for pregnant women may differ from those for non-pregnant individuals. These considerations include the following:

- Potential changes in pharmacokinetics and, thus, dosing requirements, which result from physiologic changes associated with pregnancy;

- potential ARV-associated adverse effects in pregnant women and the woman's ability to adhere to a particular regimen during pregnancy; and

- potential short- and long-term effects of the ARV on the fetus and newborn, which are unknown for many drugs.

Combination drug regimens are considered the standard of care in pregnancy, both for the treatment of HIV infection and for the prevention of perinatal transmission of HIV. Because the risk of neural tube defects is restricted to the first 5 to 6 weeks of pregnancy and pregnancy is rarely recognized before 4 to 6 weeks of pregnancy, and unnecessary changes in ARV drugs during pregnancy may be associated with loss of viral control and increased risk of perinatal transmission, EFV can be continued in pregnant women receiving an EFV-based regimen who present for antenatal care in the first trimester, provided the regimen produces virologic suppression **(CIII)**. Detailed recommendations on ARV choice in pregnancy are discussed in detail in the Perinatal Guidelines (see *Perinatal Guidelines*[1]).

Intravenous (IV) zidovudine (ZDV) infusion to the mother during labor is recommended if maternal HIV RNA is ≥400 copies/mL (or with unknown HIV RNA levels) near delivery, regardless of antepartum regimen or mode of delivery **(AI)**. Consideration can be given to omitting IV ZDV infusion during labor for HIV-infected women receiving combination ART regimens who have HIV RNA <400 copies/mL near delivery **(BII)**; however, the combination ART should continue to be administered during labor.

Clinicians who are treating HIV-infected pregnant women are strongly encouraged to report cases of prenatal exposure to ARVs (either administered alone or in combinations) to the Antiretroviral Pregnancy Registry (http://www.apregistry.com). The registry collects observational data regarding exposure to Food and Drug Administration-approved ARV drugs during pregnancy for the purpose of assessing potential teratogenicity. For more information regarding selection and use of ART during pregnancy, refer to the *Perinatal Guidelines*.[1]

Postpartum Management

Following delivery, clinical, immunologic, and virologic follow-up should continue as recommended for non-pregnant adults and adolescents. Because maternal ART reduces but does not eliminate the risk of transmission of HIV in breast milk and postnatal transmission can occur despite maternal ART, women should also be counseled to avoid breastfeeding.[1] HIV-infected women should avoid pre-mastication of food fed to their infants because the practice has been associated with transmission of HIV from mother to child.[39] Considerations regarding continuation of ART for maternal therapeutic indications are the same as those for ART use in other non-pregnant individuals. For more information regarding postpartum discontinuation of ART, refer to the *Perinatal Guidelines*.[1]

Several studies have demonstrated that adherence to ART may worsen in the postpartum period.[40-44] Clinicians caring for women postpartum who are receiving ART should specifically address adherence, including an evaluation of specific facilitators and barriers to adherence. Clinicians may consider an intervention to improve adherence (see Adherence to Antiretroviral Therapy).

References

1. Panel on Treatment of HIV-Infected Pregnant Women and Prevention of Perinatal Transmission. Recommendations for Use of Antiretroviral Drugs in Pregnant HIV-1-Infected Women for Maternal Health and Interventions to Reduce Perinatal HIV Transmission in the United States. Available at http://aidsinfo.nih.gov/contentfiles/lvguidelines/PerinatalGL.pdf.

2. Collazos J, Asensi V, Carton JA. Sex differences in the clinical, immunological and virological parameters of HIV-infected patients treated with HAART. *AIDS*. 2007;21(7):835-843. Available at http://www.ncbi.nlm.nih.gov/entrez/query.fcgi?cmd=Retrieve&db=PubMed&dopt=Citation&list_uids=17415038.

3. Fardet L, Mary-Krause M, Heard I, Partisani M, Costagliola D. Influence of gender and HIV transmission group on initial highly active antiretroviral therapy prescription and treatment response. *HIV Med*. 2006;7(8):520-529. Available at http://www.ncbi.nlm.nih.gov/entrez/query.fcgi?cmd=Retrieve&db=PubMed&dopt=Citation&list_uids=17105511.

4. Currier J, Averitt Bridge D, Hagins D, et al. Sex-based outcomes of darunavir-ritonavir therapy: a single-group trial. *Ann Intern Med*. 2010;153(6):349-357. Available at http://www.ncbi.nlm.nih.gov/entrez/query.fcgi?cmd=Retrieve&db=PubMed&dopt=Citation&list_uids=20855799.

5. Clark RA, Squires KE. Gender-specific considerations in the antiretroviral management of HIV-infected women. *Expert Rev Anti Infect Ther*. 2005;3(2):213-227. Available at http://www.ncbi.nlm.nih.gov/entrez/query.fcgi?cmd=Retrieve&db=PubMed&dopt=Citation&list_uids=15918779.

6. Gandhi M, Aweeka F, Greenblatt RM, Blaschke TF. Sex differences in pharmacokinetics and pharmacodynamics. *Annu Rev Pharmacol Toxicol*. 2004;44:499-523. Available at http://www.ncbi.nlm.nih.gov/entrez/query.fcgi?cmd=Retrieve&db=PubMed&dopt=Citation&list_uids=14744256.

7. Floridia M, Giuliano M, Palmisano L, Vella S. Gender differences in the treatment of HIV infection. *Pharmacol Res*. 2008;58(3-4):173-182. Available at http://www.ncbi.nlm.nih.gov/entrez/query.fcgi?cmd=Retrieve&db=PubMed&dopt=Citation&list_uids=18708144.

8. Ofotokun I, Chuck SK, Hitti JE. Antiretroviral pharmacokinetic profile: a review of sex differences. *Gend Med*. 2007;4(2):106-119. Available at http://www.ncbi.nlm.nih.gov/entrez/query.fcgi?cmd=Retrieve&db=PubMed&dopt=Citation&list_uids=17707845.

9. Baylor MS, Johann-Liang R. Hepatotoxicity associated with nevirapine use. *J Acquir Immune Defic Syndr*. 2004;35(5):538-539. Available at http://www.ncbi.nlm.nih.gov/entrez/query.fcgi?cmd=Retrieve&db=PubMed&dopt=Citation&list_uids=15021321.

10. Wit FW, Kesselring AM, Gras L, et al; for the ATHENA cohort study. Discontinuation of nevirapine because of hypersensitivity reactions in patients with prior treatment experience, compared with treatment-naive patients. *Clin Infect Dis*. 2008;46(6):933-940. Available at http://www.ncbi.nlm.nih.gov/entrez/query.fcgi?cmd=Retrieve&db=PubMed&dopt=Citation&list_uids=18271750.

11. Dieterich DT, Robinson PA, Love J, Stern JO. Drug-induced liver injury associated with the use of nonnucleoside reverse-transcriptase inhibitors. *Clin Infect Dis*. 2004;38 Suppl 2:S80-89. Available at http://www.ncbi.nlm.nih.gov/entrez/query.fcgi?cmd=Retrieve&db=PubMed&dopt=Citation&list_uids=14986279.

12. Leith J, Piliero P, Storfer S, Mayers D, Hinzmann R. Appropriate use of nevirapine for long-term therapy. *J Infect Dis*. 2005;192(3):545-546; author reply 546. Available at http://www.ncbi.nlm.nih.gov/entrez/query.fcgi?cmd=Retrieve&db=PubMed&dopt=Citation&list_uids=15995971.

13. Lactic Acidosis International Study Group (LAISG). Risk factors for lactic acidosis and severe hyperlactataemia in HIV-1-infected adults exposed to antiretroviral therapy. *AIDS*. 2007;21(18):2455-2464. Available at http://www.ncbi.nlm.nih.gov/entrez/query.fcgi?cmd=Retrieve&db=PubMed&dopt=Citation&list_uids=18025882.

14. Thiebaut R, Dequae-Merchadou L, Ekouevi DK, et al. Incidence and risk factors of severe hypertriglyceridaemia in the era of highly active antiretroviral therapy: the Aquitaine Cohort, France, 1996-99. *HIV Med*. 2001;2(2):84-88. Available

at http://www.ncbi.nlm.nih.gov/entrez/query.fcgi?cmd=Retrieve&db=PubMed&dopt=Citation&list_uids=11737383.

15. Galli M, Veglia F, Angarano G, et al. Gender differences in antiretroviral drug-related adipose tissue alterations. Women are at higher risk than men and develop particular lipodystrophy patterns. *J Acquir Immune Defic Syndr*. 2003;34(1):58-61. Available at http://www.ncbi.nlm.nih.gov/entrez/query.fcgi?cmd=Retrieve&db=PubMed&dopt=Citation&list_uids=14501794.

16. Yin M, Dobkin J, Brudney K, et al. Bone mass and mineral metabolism in HIV+ postmenopausal women. *Osteoporos Int*. 2005;16(11):1345-1352. Available at http://www.ncbi.nlm.nih.gov/entrez/query.fcgi?cmd=Retrieve&db=PubMed&dopt=Citation&list_uids=15754081.

17. Brown TT, Qaqish RB. Response to Berg et al. "Antiretroviral therapy and the prevalence of osteopenia and osteoporosis: a meta-analytic review." *AIDS*. 20 2007;21(13):1830-1831. Available at http://www.ncbi.nlm.nih.gov/entrez/query.fcgi?cmd=Retrieve&db=PubMed&dopt=Citation&list_uids=17690589.

18. Lampe MA, Smith DK, Anderson GJ, Edwards AE, Nesheim SR. Achieving safe conception in HIV-discordant couples: the potential role of oral preexposure prophylaxis (PrEP) in the United States. *Am J Obstet Gynecol*. 2011;204(6):488 e481-488. Available at http://www.ncbi.nlm.nih.gov/pubmed/21457911.

19. Cohn SE, Park JG, Watts DH, et al. Depo-medroxyprogesterone in women on antiretroviral therapy: effective contraception and lack of clinically significant interactions. *Clin Pharmacol Ther*. 2007;81(2):222-227. Available at http://www.ncbi.nlm.nih.gov/entrez/query.fcgi?cmd=Retrieve&db=PubMed&dopt=Citation&list_uids=17192768.

20. Nanda K, Amaral E, Hays M, Viscola MA, Mehta N, Bahamondes L. Pharmacokinetic interactions between depot medroxyprogesterone acetate and combination antiretroviral therapy. *Fertil Steril*. 2008;90(4):965-971. Available at http://www.ncbi.nlm.nih.gov/entrez/query.fcgi?cmd=Retrieve&db=PubMed&dopt=Citation&list_uids=17880953.

21. Watts DH, Park JG, Cohn SE, et al. Safety and tolerability of depot medroxyprogesterone acetate among HIV-infected women on antiretroviral therapy: ACTG A5093. *Contraception*. 2008;77(2):84-90. Available at http://www.ncbi.nlm.nih.gov/entrez/query.fcgi?cmd=Retrieve&db=PubMed&dopt=Citation&list_uids=18226670.

22. Leticee N, Viard JP, Yamgnane A, Karmochkine M, Benachi A. Contraceptive failure of etonogestrel implant in patients treated with antiretrovirals including efavirenz. *Contraception*. 2011. Available at http://www.ncbi.nlm.nih.gov/pubmed/22036046.

23. Sevinsky H, Eley T, Persson A, et al. The effect of efavirenz on the pharmacokinetics of an oral contraceptive containing ethinyl estradiol and norgestimate in healthy HIV-negative women. *Antivir Ther*. 2011;16(2):149-156. Available at http://www.ncbi.nlm.nih.gov/pubmed/21447863.

24. Vogler MA, Patterson K, Kamemoto L, et al. Contraceptive efficacy of oral and transdermal hormones when co-administered with protease inhibitors in HIV-1-infected women: pharmacokinetic results of ACTG trial A5188. *J Acquir Immune Defic Syndr*. 2010;55(4):473-482. Available at http://www.ncbi.nlm.nih.gov/pubmed/20842042.

25. Zhang J, Chung E, Yones C, et al. The effect of atazanavir/ritonavir on the pharmacokinetics of an oral contraceptive containing ethinyl estradiol and norgestimate in healthy women. *Antivir Ther*. 2011;16(2):157-164. Available at http://www.ncbi.nlm.nih.gov/pubmed/21447864.

26. Stuart GS, Moses A, Corbett A, et al. Combined oral contraceptives and antiretroviral PK/PD in Malawian women: pharmacokinetics and pharmacodynamics of a combined oral contraceptive and a generic combined formulation antiretroviral in Malawi. *J Acquir Immune Defic Syndr*. 2011;58(2):e40-43. Available at http://www.ncbi.nlm.nih.gov/pubmed/21921726.

27. Morrison CS, Nanda K. Hormonal contraception and HIV: an unanswered question. *Lancet Infect Dis*. 2012;12(1):2-3. Available at http://www.ncbi.nlm.nih.gov/pubmed/21975268.

28. Heffron R, Donnell D, Rees H, et al. Use of hormonal contraceptives and risk of HIV-1 transmission: a prospective cohort study. *Lancet Infect Dis*. 2012;12(1):19-26. Available at http://www.ncbi.nlm.nih.gov/pubmed/21975269.

29. Blish CA, Baeten JM. Hormonal contraception and HIV-1 transmission. *Am J Reprod Immunol*. 2011;65(3):302-307. Available at http://www.ncbi.nlm.nih.gov/pubmed/21087338.

30. Stringer EM, Kaseba C, Levy J, et al. A randomized trial of the intrauterine contraceptive device vs hormonal contraception in women who are infected with the human immunodeficiency virus. *Am J Obstet Gynecol.* 2007;197(2):144 e141-148. Available at http://www.ncbi.nlm.nih.gov/entrez/query.fcgi?cmd=Retrieve&db=PubMed&dopt=Citation&list_uids=17689627.

31. Heikinheimo O, Lehtovirta P, Aho I, Ristola M, Paavonen J. The levonorgestrel-releasing intrauterine system in human immunodeficiency virus-infected women: a 5-year follow-up study. *Am J Obstet Gynecol.* 2011;204(2):126 e121-124. Available at http://www.ncbi.nlm.nih.gov/pubmed/21035781.

32. Curtis KM, Nanda K, Kapp N. Safety of hormonal and intrauterine methods of contraception for women with HIV/AIDS: a systematic review. *AIDS.* 2009;(23)(1):S55-67. Available at http://www.ncbi.nlm.nih.gov/entrez/query.fcgi?cmd=Retrieve&db=PubMed&dopt=Citation&list_uids=20081389.

33. U.S. Medical Eligibility Criteria for Contraceptive Use. Recommendations and Reports June 18, 2010 / 59(RR04);1-6; Prepared by Division of Reproductive Health, National Center for Chronic Disease Prevention and Health Promotion. 2010. Available at http://www.cdc.gov/mmwr/preview/mmwrhtml/rr5904a1.htm?s_cid=rr5904a1_e.

34. Heikinheimo O, Lahteenmaki P. Contraception and HIV infection in women. *Hum Reprod Update.* 2009;15(2):165-176. Available at http://www.ncbi.nlm.nih.gov/pubmed/18978360.

35. Lehtovirta P, Paavonen J, Heikinheimo O. Experience with the levonorgestrel-releasing intrauterine system among HIV-infected women. *Contraception.* 2007;75(1):37-39. Available at http://www.ncbi.nlm.nih.gov/pubmed/17161122.

36. Ioannidis JP, Abrams EJ, Ammann A, et al. Perinatal transmission of human immunodeficiency virus type 1 by pregnant women with RNA virus loads <1000 copies/ml. *J Infect Dis.* 2001;183(4):539-545. Available at http://www.ncbi.nlm.nih.gov/entrez/query.fcgi?cmd=Retrieve&db=PubMed&dopt=Citation&list_uids=11170978.

37. Mofenson LM, Lambert JS, Stiehm ER, et al; for Pediatric AIDS Clinical Trials Group Study 185 Team. Risk factors for perinatal transmission of human immunodeficiency virus type 1 in women treated with zidovudine. *N Engl J Med.* 1999;341(6):385-393. Available at http://www.ncbi.nlm.nih.gov/entrez/query.fcgi?cmd=Retrieve&db=PubMed&dopt=Citation&list_uids=10432323.

38. Garcia PM, Kalish LA, Pitt J, et al; for the Women and Infants Transmission Study Group. Maternal levels of plasma human immunodeficiency virus type 1 RNA and the risk of perinatal transmission. *N Engl J Med.* 1999;341(6):394-402. Available at http://www.ncbi.nlm.nih.gov/entrez/query.fcgi?cmd=Retrieve&db=PubMed&dopt=Citation&list_uids=10432324.

39. Gaur AH, Freimanis-Hance L, Dominguez K, et al. Knowledge and practice of prechewing/prewarming food by HIV-infected women. *Pediatrics.* 2011;127(5):e1206-1211. Available at http://www.ncbi.nlm.nih.gov/entrez/query.fcgi?cmd=Retrieve&db=PubMed&dopt=Citation&list_uids=21482608.

40. Ickovics JR, Wilson TE, Royce RA, et al. Prenatal and postpartum zidovudine adherence among pregnant women with HIV: results of a MEMS substudy from the Perinatal Guidelines Evaluation Project. *J Acquir Immune Defic Syndr.* 2002;30(3):311-315. Available at http://www.ncbi.nlm.nih.gov/pubmed/12131568.

41. Bardeguez AD, Lindsey JC, Shannon M, et al. Adherence to antiretrovirals among US women during and after pregnancy. *J Acquir Immune Defic Syndr.* 2008;48(4):408-417. Available at http://www.ncbi.nlm.nih.gov/pubmed/18614923.

42. Mellins CA, Chu C, Malee K, et al. Adherence to antiretroviral treatment among pregnant and postpartum HIV-infected women. *AIDS Care.* 2008;20(8):958-968. Available at http://www.ncbi.nlm.nih.gov/pubmed/18608073.

43. Turner BJ, Newschaffer CJ, Zhang D, Cosler L, Hauck WW. Antiretroviral use and pharmacy-based measurement of adherence in postpartum HIV-infected women. *Med Care.* 2000;38(9):911-925. Available at http://www.ncbi.nlm.nih.gov/pubmed/10982113.

44. Rana AI, Gillani FS, Flanigan TP, Nash BT, Beckwith CG. Follow-up care among HIV-infected pregnant women in Mississippi. *J Womens Health (Larchmt).* 2010;19(10):1863-1867. Available at http://www.ncbi.nlm.nih.gov/entrez/query.fcgi?cmd=Retrieve&db=PubMed&dopt=Citation&list_uids=20831428.

HIV-2 Infection (Last updated January 10, 2011; last reviewed January 10, 2011)

HIV-2 infection is endemic in West Africa. Although HIV-2 has had only limited spread outside this area, it should be considered in persons of West African origin or those who have had sexual contact or shared needles with persons of West African origin. The prevalence of HIV-2 infection is also disproportionately high in countries with strong socioeconomic ties to West Africa (e.g., France; Spain; Portugal; and former Portuguese colonies such as Brazil, Angola, Mozambique, and parts of India near Goa).

The clinical course of HIV-2 infection is generally characterized by a longer asymptomatic stage, lower plasma HIV-2 viral loads, and lower mortality rates compared with HIV-1 infection.[1-2] However, HIV-2 infection can progress to AIDS, and thus antiretroviral therapy (ART) may become necessary during the course of infection. Concomitant HIV-1 and HIV-2 infection may occur and should be considered in patients from an area with high prevalence of HIV-2. In the appropriate epidemiologic setting, HIV-2 infection should be suspected in patients with clinical conditions suggestive of HIV infection but with atypical serologic results (e.g., a positive screening assay with an indeterminate HIV-1 Western blot).[3] The possibility of HIV-2 infection should also be considered in the appropriate epidemiologic setting in patients with serologically confirmed HIV infection but low or undetectable viral loads or in those with declining CD4 counts despite apparent virologic suppression on ART.

The Multispot HIV-1/HIV-2 Rapid Test (Bio-Rad Laboratories) is Food and Drug Administration (FDA) approved for differentiating HIV-1 from HIV-2 infection. Commercially available HIV-1 viral load assays do not reliably detect or quantify HIV-2, and no HIV-2 commercial viral load assays are currently available.[4-5] Most studies reporting HIV-2 viral loads use "in-house" assays that are not widely available, making it difficult to monitor virologic response in the clinical setting. In addition, no validated HIV-2 genotypic or phenotypic antiretroviral (ARV) resistance assays are available.

To date, there have been no randomized trials addressing the question of when to start ART or the choice of initial or second-line therapy for HIV-2 infection;[6] thus, the optimal treatment strategy has not been defined. HIV-2 appears intrinsically resistant to non-nucleoside reverse transcriptase inhibitors (NNRTIs)[7] and to enfuvirtide.[8] *In vitro* data suggest HIV-2 is sensitive to the currently available nucleoside reverse transcriptase inhibitors (NRTIs), although with a lower barrier to resistance than HIV-1.[9-10] Variable sensitivity among protease inhibitors (PIs) has been reported; lopinavir (LPV), saquinavir (SQV), and darunavir (DRV) are more active against HIV-2 than other approved PIs.[11-14] The integrase inhibitor, raltegravir (RAL),[15] and the CCR5 antagonist, maraviroc (MVC), appear active against some HIV-2 isolates, although no approved assays to determine HIV-2 coreceptor tropism exist and HIV-2 is known to utilize multiple minor coreceptors in addition to CCR5 and CXCR4.[16] Several small studies suggest poor responses among HIV-2 infected individuals treated with some ARV regimens, including dual-NRTI regimens, regimens containing two NRTIs + NNRTI, and some unboosted PI-based regimens including nelfinavir (NFV) or indinavir (IDV) plus zidovudine (ZDV) and lamivudine (3TC).[6, 17-19] Clinical data on the utility of triple-NRTI regimens are conflicting.[20-21] In general, boosted PI-containing regimens have resulted in more favorable virologic and immunologic responses.[21] One small study suggested satisfactory responses to lopinavir/ritonavir (LPV/r)-containing regimens in 17 of 29 (59%) of ARV-naive subjects.[22]

Resistance-associated mutations develop commonly in HIV-2 patients on therapy.[17, 21, 23] Genotypic algorithms used to predict drug resistance in HIV-1 may not be applicable to HIV-2, because pathways and mutational patterns leading to resistance may differ.[10, 21, 24] CD4 cell recovery on therapy may be poor,[25] suggesting that more reliable methods for monitoring disease progression and treatment efficacy in HIV-2 infection are needed.

Some groups have recommended specific preferred and alternative regimens for initial therapy of HIV-2 infection,[24] though as yet there are no controlled trial data to reliably predict their success. Until more definitive data are available in an ART-naive patient with HIV-2 mono-infection or with HIV-1/HIV-2 dual infection who requires treatment, clinicians should initiate a regimen containing two NRTIs and a boosted PI. Monitoring of virologic response in such patients is problematic because of the lack of a commercially available HIV-2 viral load assay; however, clinical and CD4 count improvement can be used to assess treatment response.

References

1. Matheron S, Pueyo S, Damond F, et al. Factors associated with clinical progression in HIV-2 infected-patients: the French ANRS cohort. *AIDS*. 2003;17(18):2593-2601.

2. Marlink R, Kanki P, Thior I, et al. Reduced rate of disease development after HIV-2 infection as compared to HIV-1. *Science*. 1994;265(5178):1587-1590.

3. O'Brien TR, George JR, Epstein JS, et al. Testing for antibodies to human immunodeficiency virus type 2 in the United States. *MMWR Recomm Rep*. 1992;41(RR-12):1-9.

4. Chan PA, Wakeman SE, Flanigan T, et al. HIV-2 diagnosis and quantification in high-risk patients. *AIDS Res Ther*. 2008;5:18.

5. Damond F, Benard A, Ruelle J, et al. Quality control assessment of human immunodeficiency virus type 2 (HIV-2) viral load quantification assays: results from an international collaboration on HIV-2 infection in 2006. *J Clin Microbiol*. 2008;46(6):2088-2091.

6. Gottlieb GS, Eholie SP, Nkengasong JN, et al. A call for randomized controlled trials of antiretroviral therapy for HIV-2 infection in West Africa. *AIDS*. 2008;22(16):2069-2072; discussion 2073-2064.

7. Tuaillon E, Gueudin M, Lemee V, et al. Phenotypic susceptibility to nonnucleoside inhibitors of virion-associated reverse transcriptase from different HIV types and groups. *J Acquir Immune Defic Syndr*. 2004;37(5):1543-1549.

8. Poveda E, Rodes B, Toro C, et al. Are fusion inhibitors active against all HIV variants? *AIDS Res Hum Retroviruses*. 2004;20(3):347-348.

9. Boyer PL, Sarafianos SG, Clark PK, et al. Why do HIV-1 and HIV-2 use different pathways to develop AZT resistance? *PLoS Pathog*. 2006;2(2):e10.

10. Smith RA, Anderson DJ, Pyrak CL, et al. Antiretroviral drug resistance in HIV-2: three amino acid changes are sufficient for classwide nucleoside analogue resistance. *J Infect Dis*. 2009;199(9):1323-1326.

11. Parkin NT, Schapiro JM. Antiretroviral drug resistance in non-subtype B HIV-1, HIV-2 and SIV. *Antivir Ther*. 2004;9(1):3-12.

12. Desbois D, Roquebert B, Peytavin G, et al. In vitro phenotypic susceptibility of human immunodeficiency virus type 2 clinical isolates to protease inhibitors. *Antimicrob Agents Chemother*. 2008;52(4):1545-1548.

13. Brower ET, Bacha UM, Kawasaki Y, et al. Inhibition of HIV-2 protease by HIV-1 protease inhibitors in clinical use. *Chem Biol Drug Des*. 2008;71(4):298-305.

14. Rodes B, Sheldon J, Toro C, et al. Susceptibility to protease inhibitors in HIV-2 primary isolates from patients failing antiretroviral therapy. *J Antimicrob Chemother*. 2006;57(4):709-713.

15. Roquebert B, Damond F, Collin G, et al. HIV-2 integrase gene polymorphism and phenotypic susceptibility of HIV-2 clinical isolates to the integrase inhibitors raltegravir and elvitegravir in vitro. *J Antimicrob Chemother*. 2008;62(5):914-920.

16. Owen SM, Ellenberger D, Rayfield M, et al. Genetically divergent strains of human immunodeficiency virus type 2 use multiple coreceptors for viral entry. *J Virol*. 1998;72(7):5425-5432.

17. Gottlieb GS, Badiane NM, Hawes SE, et al. Emergence of multiclass drug-resistance in HIV-2 in antiretroviral-treated individuals in Senegal: implications for HIV-2 treatment in resouce-limited West Africa. *Clin Infect Dis*. 2009;48(4):476-483.

18. Jallow S, Kaye S, Alabi A, et al. Virological and immunological response to Combivir and emergence of drug resistance mutations in a cohort of HIV-2 patients in The Gambia. *AIDS*. 2006;20(10):1455-1458.

19. Adje-Toure CA, Cheingsong R, Garcia-Lerma JG, et al. Antiretroviral therapy in HIV-2-infected patients: changes in plasma viral load, CD4+ cell counts, and drug resistance profiles of patients treated in Abidjan, Cote d'Ivoire. *AIDS*. 2003;17 Suppl 3:S49-54.

20. Matheron S, Damond F, Benard A, et al. CD4 cell recovery in treated HIV-2-infected adults is lower than expected: results from the French ANRS CO5 HIV-2 cohort. *AIDS*. 2006;20(3):459-462.

21. Ruelle J, Roman F, Vandenbroucke AT, et al. Transmitted drug resistance, selection of resistance mutations and moderate antiretroviral efficacy in HIV-2: analysis of the HIV-2 Belgium and Luxembourg database. *BMC Infect Dis*. 2008;8:21.

22. Benard A, Damond F, Campa P, et al. Good response to lopinavir/ritonavir-containing antiretroviral regimens in antiretroviral-naive HIV-2-infected patients. *AIDS*. 2009;23(9):1171-1173.

23. Damond F, Matheron S, Peytavin G, et al. Selection of K65R mutation in HIV-2-infected patients receiving tenofovir-containing regimen. *Antivir Ther*. 2004;9(4):635-636.

24. Gilleece Y, Chadwick DR, Breuer J, et al. British HIV Association guidelines for antiretroviral treatment of HIV-2-positive individuals 2010. *HIV Med*. 2010;11(10):611-619.

25. Drylewicz J, Matheron S, Lazaro E, et al. Comparison of viro-immunological marker changes between HIV-1 and HIV-2-infected patients in France. *AIDS*. 2008;22(4):457-468.

HIV and the Older Patient (Last updated March 27, 2012; last reviewed March 27, 2012)

Key Considerations When Caring for Older HIV-Infected Patients
• Antiretroviral therapy (ART) is recommended in patients >50 years of age, regardless of CD4 cell count **(BIII)**, because the risk of non-AIDS related complications may increase and the immunologic response to ART may be reduced in older HIV-infected patients.
• ART-associated adverse events may occur more frequently in older HIV-infected adults than in younger HIV-infected individuals. Therefore, the bone, kidney, metabolic, cardiovascular, and liver health of older HIV-infected adults should be monitored closely.
• The increased risk of drug-drug interactions between antiretroviral (ARV) drugs and other medications commonly used in older HIV-infected patients should be assessed regularly, especially when starting or switching ART and concomitant medications.
• HIV experts and primary care providers should work together to optimize the medical care of older HIV-infected patients with complex comorbidities.
• Counseling to prevent secondary transmission of HIV remains an important aspect of the care of the older HIV-infected patient.
Rating of Recommendations: A = Strong; B = Moderate; C = Optional *Rating of Evidence: I = Data from randomized controlled trials; II = Data from well-designed nonrandomized trials or observational cohort studies with long-term clinical outcomes; III = Expert opinion*

Effective antiretroviral therapy (ART) has increased survival in HIV-infected individuals, resulting in an increasing number of older individuals living with HIV infection. In the United States, approximately 30% of people currently living with HIV/AIDS are age 50 years or older and trends suggest that the proportion of older persons living with HIV/AIDS will increase steadily.[1] Care of HIV-infected patients increasingly will involve adults 60 to 80 years of age, a population for which data from clinical trials or pharmacokinetic studies are very limited.

There are several distinct areas of concern regarding the association between age and HIV disease.[2] First, older HIV-infected patients may suffer from aging-related comorbid illnesses that can complicate the management of HIV infection, as outlined in detail below. Second, HIV disease may affect the biology of aging, possibly resulting in early manifestations of many clinical syndromes generally associated with advanced age. Third, reduced mucosal and immunologic defenses (such as post-menopausal atrophic vaginitis) and changes in risk behaviors (for example, decrease in condom use because of less concern about pregnancy and increased use of erectile dysfunction drugs) in older adults could lead to increased risk of acquisition and transmission of HIV.[3-4] Finally, because older adults generally are perceived to be at low risk of HIV infection, screening for HIV in this population remains low. For these reasons, HIV infection in many older adults may not be diagnosed until late in the disease process. This section focuses on HIV diagnosis and treatment considerations in the older HIV-infected patient.

HIV Diagnosis and Prevention

Even though many older individuals are engaged in risk behaviors associated with acquisition of HIV, they may be perceived to be at low risk of infection and, as a result, they are less likely to be tested for HIV than younger persons.[5] According to one U.S. survey, 71% of men and 51% of women age 60 years and older continue to be sexually active,[6] with less concern about the possibility of pregnancy contributing to less condom use. Another national survey reported that among individuals age 50 years or older, condoms were not used during most recent intercourse with 91% of casual partners or 70% of new partners.[7] In addition, results from a CDC survey[8] show that in 2008 only 35% of adults age 45 to 64 years had ever been tested for HIV infection despite the 2006 CDC recommendation that individuals age 13 to 64 years be tested at least once and more often if sexually active.[9] Clinicians must be attuned to the possibility of HIV infection in older patients, including those older than 64 years of age who, based on CDC recommendations, would not be screened for HIV. Furthermore, sexual history taking, risk-reduction counseling, and screening for sexually transmitted diseases (STDs) (if indicated), are important components of general health care for HIV-infected and -uninfected older patients.

Failure to consider a diagnosis of HIV in older persons likely contributes to later disease presentation and initiation of ART.[10] One surveillance report showed that the proportion of patients who progressed to AIDS within 1 year of diagnosis was greater among patients >60 years of age (52%) than among patients younger than 25 years (16%).[1] When individuals >50 years of age present with severe illnesses, AIDS-related opportunistic infections (OIs) need to be considered in the differential diagnosis of the illness.

Initiating Antiretroviral Therapy

Concerns about decreased immune recovery and increased risk of serious non-AIDS events are factors that favor initiating ART in patients >50 years of age regardless of CD4 cell count (**BIII**). (See Initiating Antiretroviral Therapy in Treatment-Naive Patients.) Data that would favor use of any one of the Panel's recommended initial ART regimens (see What to Start) on the basis of age are not available. The choice of regimen should be informed by a comprehensive review of the patient's other medical conditions and medications. A noteworthy limitation of currently available information is lack of data on the long-term safety of specific antiretroviral (ARV) drugs in older patients, such as use of tenofovir disoproxil fumarate (TDF) in older patients with declining renal function. The recommendations on how frequently to monitor parameters of ART effectiveness and safety for adults age >50 years are similar to those for the general HIV-infected population; however, the recommendations for older adults focus particularly on the adverse events of ART pertaining to renal, liver, cardiovascular, metabolic, and bone health (see Table 13).

HIV, Aging, and Antiretroviral Therapy

The efficacy, pharmacokinetics, adverse effects, and drug interaction potentials of ART in the older adult have not been studied systematically. There is no evidence that the virologic response to ART is different in older patients than in younger patients. However, CD4 T-cell recovery after starting ART generally is less robust in older patients than in younger patients.[11-14] This observation suggests that starting ART at a younger age will result in better immunologic and possibly clinical outcomes.

Hepatic metabolism and renal elimination are the major routes of drug clearance, including the clearance of ARV drugs. Both liver and kidney function may decrease with age, which may result in impaired drug elimination and drug accumulation.[15] Current ARV drug doses are based on pharmacokinetic and pharmacodynamic data derived from studies conducted in subjects with normal organ function. Most clinical trials include only a small proportion of study participants >50 years of age. Whether drug accumulation in the older patient may lead to greater incidence and severity of adverse effects than seen in younger patients is unknown.

HIV-infected patients with aging-associated comorbidities may require additional pharmacologic intervention, making therapeutic management increasingly complex. In addition to taking medications to manage HIV infection and comorbid conditions, many older HIV-infected patients also are taking medications to ameliorate discomfort (e.g., pain medications, sedatives) or to manage adverse effects of medications (e.g., anti-emetics). They also may self-medicate with over-the-counter medicines or supplements. In the HIV-negative population, polypharmacy is a major cause of iatrogenic problems in geriatric patients.[16] This may be the result of medication errors (by prescribers or patients), nonadherence, additive drug toxicities, and drug-drug interactions. Older HIV-infected patients probably are at an even greater risk of polypharmacy and its attendant adverse consequences than younger HIV-infected or similarly aged HIV-uninfected patients.

Drug-drug interactions are common with ART and easily can be overlooked by prescribers.[17] The available drug interaction information on ARV agents is derived primarily from pharmacokinetic studies performed in a small number of relatively young, HIV-uninfected subjects with normal organ function (see Tables 14-16b). Data from these studies provide clinicians with a basis to assess whether a significant interaction may exist. However, the magnitude of the interaction may be different in older HIV-infected patients than in younger HIV-infected patients.

Nonadherence is the most common cause of treatment failure. Complex dosing requirements, high pill burden, inability to access medications because of cost or availability, limited health literacy including lack of numeracy skills, misunderstanding of instructions, depression, and neurocognitive impairment are among the key reasons for nonadherence.[18] Although many of these factors likely will be more prevalent in an aging HIV-infected population, some data suggest that older HIV-infected patients may be more adherent to ART than younger HIV-infected patients.[19-21] Clinicians should assess adherence regularly to identify any factors, such as neurocognitive deficits, that may make adherence a challenge. One or more interventions such as discontinuation of unnecessary medications; regimen simplification; or use of adherence tools, including pillboxes, daily calendars, and evidence-based behavioral approaches may be necessary to facilitate medication adherence (see Adherence to Antiretroviral Therapy).

Non-AIDS HIV-Related Complications and other Comorbidities

With the reduction in AIDS-related morbidity and mortality observed with effective use of ART, non-AIDS conditions constitute an increasing proportion of serious illnesses in ART-treated HIV-infected populations.[22-24] Heart disease and cancer are the leading causes of death in older Americans.[25] Similarly, for HIV-infected patients on ART, non-AIDS events such as heart disease, liver disease, and cancer have emerged as major causes of morbidity and mortality. Neurocognitive impairment, already a major health problem in aging patients, may be exacerbated by the effect of HIV infection on the brain.[26] That the presence of multiple non-AIDS comorbidities coupled with the immunologic effects of HIV infection could add to the disease burden of an aging HIV-infected person is a concern.[27-29] At present, primary care recommendations are the same for HIV-infected and HIV-uninfected adults and focus on identifying and managing risks of conditions such as heart, liver, and renal disease; cancer; and bone demineralization.[30-32]

Discontinuing Antiretroviral Therapy in Older Patients

Important issues to discuss with aging HIV-infected patients are living wills, advance directives, and long-term care planning including financial concerns. Health care cost sharing (e.g., co-pays, out-of-pocket costs), loss of employment, and other financial-related factors can cause interruptions in treatment. Clinic systems can minimize loss of treatment by helping patients maintain access to insurance.

For the severely debilitated or terminally ill HIV-infected patient, adding palliative care medications, while perhaps beneficial, further increases the complexity and risk of negative drug interactions. For such patients, a balanced consideration of both the expected benefits of ART and the toxicities and negative quality-of-life effects of ART is needed.

Few data exist on the use of ART in severely debilitated patients with chronic, severe, or non-AIDS terminal conditions.[33-34] Withdrawal of ART usually results in rebound viremia and a decline in CD4 cell count. Acute retroviral syndrome after abrupt discontinuation of ART has been reported. In very debilitated patients, if there are no significant adverse reactions to ART, most clinicians would continue therapy. In cases where ART negatively affects quality of life, the decision to continue therapy should be made together with the patient and/or family members after a discussion on the risks and benefits of continuing or withdrawing ART.

Conclusion

HIV infection may increase the risk of many major health conditions experienced by aging adults and possibly accelerate the aging process.[35] As HIV-infected adults age, their health problems become increasingly complex, placing additional demands on the health care system. This adds to the concern that outpatient clinics providing HIV care in the United States share the same financial problems as other chronic disease and primary care clinics and that reimbursement for care is not sufficient to maintain care at a sustainable level.[36] Continued involvement of HIV experts in the care of older HIV-infected patients is warranted. However, given that the current shortage of primary care providers and geriatricians is projected to continue, current HIV providers will need to adapt to the shifting need for expertise in geriatrics through continuing education and ongoing assessment of the evolving health needs of aging HIV-infected patients.[37] The aging of the HIV-infected population also signals a need for more information on long-term safety and efficacy of ARV drugs in older patients.

References

1. Centers for Disease Control and Prevention. HIV Surveillance Report http://www.cdc.gov/hiv/topics/surveillance/resources/reports/. Published February 2011. Accessed December 7, 2011.

2. Deeks SG, Phillips AN. HIV infection, antiretroviral treatment, ageing, and non-AIDS related morbidity. *BMJ*. 2009;338:a3172.

3. Levy JA, Ory MG, Crystal S. HIV/AIDS interventions for midlife and older adults: current status and challenges. *J Acquir Immune Defic Syndr*. Jun 1 2003;33(Suppl 2):S59-67.

4. Levy BR, Ding L, Lakra D, Kosteas J, Niccolai L. Older persons' exclusion from sexually transmitted disease risk-reduction clinical trials. *Sex Transm Dis*. Aug 2007;34(8):541-544.

5. Stone VE, Bounds BC, Muse VV, Ferry JA. Case records of the Massachusetts General Hospital. Case 29-2009. An 81-year-old man with weight loss, odynophagia, and failure to thrive. *N Engl J Med*. Sep 17 2009;361(12):1189-1198.

6. Zablotsky D, Kennedy M. Risk factors and HIV transmission to midlife and older women: knowledge, options, and the initiation of safer sexual practices. *J Acquir Immune Defic Syndr*. Jun 1 2003;33(Suppl 2):S122-130.

7. Schick V, Herbenick D, Reece M, et al. Sexual behaviors, condom use, and sexual health of Americans over 50: implications for sexual health promotion for older adults. *J Sex Med*. Oct 2010;7(Suppl 5):315-329.

8. Vital signs: HIV testing and diagnosis among adults—United States, 2001-2009. *MMWR Morb Mortal Wkly Rep*. Dec 3 2010;59(47):1550-1555.

9. Branson BM, Handsfield HH, Lampe MA, et al. Revised recommendations for HIV testing of adults, adolescents, and pregnant women in health-care settings. *MMWR Recomm Rep*. Sep 22 2006;55(RR-14):1-17.

10. Althoff KN, Gebo KA, Gange SJ, et al. CD4 count at presentation for HIV care in the United States and Canada: are those over 50 years more likely to have a delayed presentation? *AIDS Res Ther*. 2010;7:45.

11. Sabin CA, Smith CJ, d'Arminio Monforte A, et al. Response to combination antiretroviral therapy: variation by age. *AIDS*. Jul 31 2008;22(12):1463-1473.

12. Althoff KN, Justice AC, Gange SJ, et al. Virologic and immunologic response to HAART, by age and regimen class. *AIDS*. Oct 23 2010;24(16):2469-2479.

13. Bosch RJ, Bennett K, Collier AC, Zackin R, Benson CA. Pretreatment factors associated with 3-year (144-week) virologic and immunologic responses to potent antiretroviral therapy. *J Acquir Immune Defic Syndr*. Mar 1 2007;44(3):268-277.

14. Nogueras M, Navarro G, Anton E, et al. Epidemiological and clinical features, response to HAART, and survival in HIV-infected patients diagnosed at the age of 50 or more. *BMC Infect Dis*. 2006;6:159.

15. Sitar DS. Aging issues in drug disposition and efficacy. *Proc West Pharmacol Soc*. 2007;50:16-20.

16. Steinman MA, Hanlon JT. Managing medications in clinically complex elders: "There's got to be a happy medium." *JAMA*. Oct 13 2010;304(14):1592-1601.

17. Marzolini C, Back D, Weber R, et al. Ageing with HIV: medication use and risk for potential drug-drug interactions. *J Antimicrob Chemother*. Sep 2011;66(9):2107-2111.

18. Gellad WF, Grenard JL, Marcum ZA. A systematic review of barriers to medication adherence in the elderly: looking beyond cost and regimen complexity. *Am J Geriatr Pharmacother*. Feb 2011;9(1):11-23.

19. Wellons MF, Sanders L, Edwards LJ, Bartlett JA, Heald AE, Schmader KE. HIV infection: treatment outcomes in older and younger adults. *J Am Geriatr Soc*. Apr 2002;50(4):603-607.

20. Wutoh AK, Elekwachi O, Clarke-Tasker V, Daftary M, Powell NJ, Campusano G. Assessment and predictors of antiretroviral adherence in older HIV-infected patients. *J Acquir Immune Defic Syndr*. Jun 1 2003;33(Suppl 2):S106-114.

21. Silverberg MJ, Leyden W, Horberg MA, DeLorenze GN, Klein D, Quesenberry CP, Jr. Older age and the response to and tolerability of antiretroviral therapy. *Arch Intern Med*. Apr 9 2007;167(7):684-691.

22. Justice AC. HIV and aging: time for a new paradigm. *Curr HIV/AIDS Rep*. May 2010;7(2):69-76.

23. Palella FJ, Jr., Baker RK, Moorman AC, et al. Mortality in the highly active antiretroviral therapy era: changing causes of death and disease in the HIV outpatient study. *J Acquir Immune Defic Syndr*. Sep 2006;43(1):27-34.

24. Smit C, Geskus R, Walker S, et al. Effective therapy has altered the spectrum of cause-specific mortality following HIV seroconversion. *AIDS*. Mar 21 2006;20(5):741-749.

25. Kochanek KD, Xu J, Murphy SL, Minino AM, King HC. Deaths: Preliminary data for 2009. *National Vital Statistics Reports*. 2011;59(4):1-54.

26. Vance DE, Wadley VG, Crowe MG, Raper JL, Ball KK. Cognitive and everyday functioning in older and younger adults with and without HIV. *Clinical Gerontologists* 2011;34(5):413-426.

27. Guaraldi G, Orlando G, Zona S, et al. Premature age-related comorbidities among HIV-infected persons compared with the general population. *Clin Infect Dis*. Dec 2011;53(11):1120-1126.

28. Capeau J. Premature Aging and Premature Age-Related Comorbidities in HIV-Infected Patients: Facts and Hypotheses. *Clin Infect Dis*. Dec 2011;53(11):1127-1129.

29. Hasse B, Ledergerber B, Furrer H, et al. Morbidity and aging in HIV-infected persons: the Swiss HIV cohort study. *Clin Infect Dis*. Dec 2011;53(11):1130-1139.

30. Aberg JA, Kaplan JE, Libman H, et al. Primary care guidelines for the management of persons infected with human immunodeficiency virus: 2009 update by the HIV medicine Association of the Infectious Diseases Society of America. *Clin Infect Dis*. Sep 1 2009;49(5):651-681.

31. Henry K. Internal medicine/primary care reminder: what are the standards of care for HIV-positive patients aged 50 years and older? *Curr HIV/AIDS Rep*. Aug 2009;6(3):153-161.

32. American Academy of HIV Medicine. The HIV and Aging Consensus Project: Recommended treatment strategies for clinicians managing older patients with HIV. http://www.aahivm.org/Upload Module/upload/HIV and Aging/Aging report working document FINAL.pdf. 2011.

33. Selwyn PA. Chapter 75. In: Berger AM S, JL, Von Roenn JH, ed. Palliative care in HIV/AIDS. In Principles and Practice of Palliative Care and Supportive Oncology 3rd Edition. Philadelphia, PA: Lippincott Williams and Wilkins; 2007:833-848.

34. Harding R, Simms V, Krakauer E, et al. Quality HIV Care to the End of life. *Clin Infect Dis*. Feb 15 2011;52(4):553-554; author reply 554.

35. Martin J, Volberding P. HIV and premature aging: A field still in its infancy. *Ann Intern Med*. Oct 5 2010;153(7):477-479.

36. Chen RY, Accortt NA, Westfall AO, et al. Distribution of health care expenditures for HIV-infected patients. *Clin Infect Dis*. Apr 1 2006;42(7):1003-1010.

37. Martin CP, Fain MJ, Klotz SA. The older HIV-positive adult: a critical review of the medical literature. *Am J Med*. Dec 2008;121(12):1032-1037.

Considerations for Antiretroviral Use in Patients with Coinfections

HIV/Hepatitis B Virus (HBV) Coinfection (Last updated January 10, 2011; last reviewed January 10, 2011)

Panel's Recommendations

- Prior to initiation of antiretroviral therapy (ART), all patients who test positive for hepatitis B surface antigen (HBsAg) should be tested for hepatitis B virus (HBV) DNA using a quantitative assay to determine the level of HBV replication **(AIII)**.

- Because emtricitabine (FTC), lamivudine (3TC), and tenofovir (TDF) have activity against both HIV and HBV, if HBV or HIV treatment is needed, ART should be initiated with the combination of TDF + FTC or TDF + 3TC as the nucleoside reverse transcriptase inhibitor (NRTI) backbone of a fully suppressive antiretroviral (ARV) regimen **(AI)**.

- If HBV treatment is needed and TDF cannot safely be used, the alternative recommended HBV therapy is entecavir in addition to a fully suppressive ARV regimen **(BI)**. Other HBV treatment regimens include peginterferon alfa monotherapy or adefovir in combination with 3TC or FTC or telbivudine in addition to a fully suppressive ARV regimen **(BII)**.

- Entecavir has activity against HIV; its use for HBV treatment without ART in patients with dual infection may result in the selection of the M184V mutation that confers HIV resistance to 3TC and FTC. Therefore, entecavir must be used in addition to a fully suppressive ARV regimen when used in HIV/HBV-coinfected patients **(AII)**.

- Discontinuation of agents with anti-HBV activity may cause serious hepatocellular damage resulting from reactivation of HBV; patients should be advised against self-discontinuation and carefully monitored during interruptions in HBV treatment **(AII)**.

- If ART needs to be modified due to HIV virologic failure and the patient has adequate HBV suppression, the ARV drugs active against HBV should be continued for HBV treatment in combination with other suitable ARV agents to achieve HIV suppression **(AIII)**.

Rating of Recommendations: A = Strong; B = Moderate; C = Optional

Rating of Evidence: I = Data from randomized controlled trials; II = Data from well-designed nonrandomized trials or observational cohort studies with long-term clinical outcomes; III = Expert opinion

---

Approximately 5%–10% of HIV-infected persons also have chronic HBV infection, defined as testing positive for HBsAg for more than 6 months.[1] The progression of chronic HBV to cirrhosis, end-stage liver disease, and/or hepatocellular carcinoma is more rapid in HIV-infected persons than in persons with chronic HBV alone.[2] Conversely, chronic HBV does not substantially alter the progression of HIV infection and does not influence HIV suppression or CD4 cell responses following ART initiation.[3-4] However, several liver-associated complications that are ascribed to flares in HBV activity, discontinuation of dually active ARVs, or toxicity of ARVs can affect the treatment of HIV in patients with HBV coinfection.[5-7] These include the following:

- FTC, 3TC, and TDF are approved ARVs that also have antiviral activity against HBV. Discontinuation of these drugs may potentially cause serious hepatocellular damage resulting from reactivation of HBV.[8]

- Entecavir has activity against HIV; its use for HBV treatment without ART in patients with dual infection may result in the selection of the M184V mutation that confers HIV resistance to 3TC and FTC. Therefore, entecavir must be used in addition to a fully suppressive ARV regimen when used in HIV/HBV-coinfected patients **(AII)**.[9]

- 3TC-resistant HBV is observed in approximately 40% of patients after 2 years on 3TC for chronic HBV and in approximately 90% of patients after 4 years when 3TC is used as the only active drug for HBV in coinfected patients. Therefore, 3TC or FTC should be used in combination with other anti-HBV drugs **(AII)**.[10]

- Immune reconstitution after initiation of treatment for HIV and/or HBV can be associated with elevation in transaminases, possibly because HBV is primarily an immune-mediated disease.[11]

- Some ARV agents can cause increases in transaminase levels. The rate and magnitude of these increases are higher with HBV coinfection.[12-13] The etiology and consequences of these changes in liver function tests are unclear because continuation of ART may be accompanied by resolution of the changes. Nevertheless, some experts suspend the implicated agent(s) when the serum alanine transferase (ALT) level is increased to 5 10 times the upper limit of normal. However, in HIV/HBV-coinfected persons, increases in transaminase levels can herald hepatitis B e antigen (HBeAg) seroconversion due to immune reconstitution, so the cause of the elevations should be investigated prior to the decision to discontinue medications. In persons with transaminase increases, HBeAg seroconversion should be evaluated by testing for HBeAg and anti-HBe as well as HBV DNA levels.

Recommendations for HBV/HIV-Coinfected Patients

- All patients with chronic HBV should be advised to abstain from alcohol, assessed for immunity to hepatitis A virus (HAV) infection (anti-HAV antibody total) and vaccinated if nonimmune, advised on methods to prevent HBV transmission (methods that do not differ from those to prevent HIV transmission), and evaluated for the severity of HBV infection as outlined in the Guidelines for Prevention and Treatment of Opportunistic Infections in HIV-Infected Adults and Adolescents.[14]

- Prior to intiation of ART, all persons who test positive for HBsAg should be tested for HBV DNA using a quantitative assay to determine the level of HBV replication **(AIII)**. Persons with chronic HBV infection already receiving ART active against HBV should undergo quantitative HBV DNA testing every 6 12 months to determine the effectiveness of therapy in suppressing HBV replication. The goal of HBV therapy with NRTIs is to prevent liver disease complications by sustained suppression of HBV replication to the lowest achievable level.

- **If not yet on therapy and HBV or HIV treatment is needed:** In persons without HIV infection, the recommended anti-HBV drugs for the treatment of persons naive to HBV therapy are TDF and entecavir.[15-16] In HIV-infected patients, however, only TDF can be considered part of the ARV regimen; entecavir has weak anti-HIV activity and must not be considered part of an ARV regimen. In addition, only TDF is fully active for the treatment of persons with known or suspected 3TC-resistant HBV infection. To avoid selection of HBV-resistant variants, when possible, these agents should not be used as the only agent with anti-HBV activity in an ARV regimen **(AIII)**.

Preferred regimen. The combination of TDF + FTC or TDF + 3TC should be used as the NRTI backbone of a fully suppressive ARV regimen and for the treatment of HBV infection **(AII)**.[17-19]

Alternative regimens. If TDF cannot safely be used, entecavir should be used in addition to a fully suppressive ARV regimen **(AII)**; importantly, entecavir should not be considered to be a part of the ARV regimen[20] **(BII)**. Due to a partially overlapping HBV-resistance pathway, it is not known if the combination of entecavir + 3TC or FTC will provide additional virologic or clinical benefit compared with entecavir alone. In persons with known or suspected 3TC-resistant HBV infection, the entecavir dose should be increased from 0.5 mg/day to 1 mg/day. However, entecavir resistance may emerge rapidly in patients with 3TC-resistant HBV infection. Therefore, entecavir should be used with caution in such patients with frequent monitoring (~ every 3 months) of the HBV DNA level to detect viral breakthrough. Other HBV treatment regimens include peginterferon alfa monotherapy or adefovir in combination with 3TC or FTC or telbivudine in addition to a fully suppressive ARV regimen;[17, 21-22] however, data on these regimens in persons with HIV/HBV coinfection are limited **(BII)**. Due to safety concerns, peginterferon alfa should not be used in

HIV/HBV-coinfected persons with cirrhosis.

- **Need to discontinue medications active against HBV:** The patient's clinical course should be monitored with frequent liver function tests. The use of adefovir dipivoxil, entecavir, or telbivudine to prevent flares, especially in patients with marginal hepatic reserve such as persons with compensated or decompensated cirrhosis, can be considered.[8] These alternative HBV regimens should only be used in addition to a fully suppressive ARV regimen.

- **Need to change ART because of HIV resistance:** If the patient has adequate HBV suppression, the ARV drugs active against HBV should be continued for HBV treatment in combination with other suitable ARV agents to achieve HIV suppression **(AIII)**.

References

1. Spradling PR, Richardson JT, Buchacz K, et al. Prevalence of chronic hepatitis B virus infection among patients in the HIV Outpatient Study, 1996-2007. *J Viral Hepat.* 2010.

2. Thio CL, Seaberg EC, Skolasky R, Jr., et al. HIV-1, hepatitis B virus, and risk of liver-related mortality in the Multicenter Cohort Study (MACS). *Lancet.* 2002;360(9349):1921-1926.

3. Konopnicki D, Mocroft A, de Wit S, et al. Hepatitis B and HIV: prevalence, AIDS progression, response to highly active antiretroviral therapy and increased mortality in the EuroSIDA cohort. *AIDS.* 2005;19(6):593-601.

4. Hoffmann CJ, Seaberg EC, Young S, et al. Hepatitis B and long-term HIV outcomes in coinfected HAART recipients. *AIDS.* 2009;23(14):1881-1889.

5. Bellini C, Keiser O, Chave JP, et al. Liver enzyme elevation after lamivudine withdrawal in HIV-hepatitis B virus co-infected patients: the Swiss HIV Cohort Study. *HIV Med.* 2009;10(1):12-18.

6. Law WP, Dore GJ, Duncombe CJ, et al. Risk of severe hepatotoxicity associated with antiretroviral therapy in the HIV-NAT Cohort, Thailand, 1996-2001. *AIDS.* 2003;17(15):2191-2199.

7. Wit FW, Weverling GJ, Weel J, et al. Incidence of and risk factors for severe hepatotoxicity associated with antiretroviral combination therapy. *J Infect Dis.* 2002;186(1):23-31.

8. Dore GJ, Soriano V, Rockstroh J, et al. Frequent hepatitis B virus rebound among HIV-hepatitis B virus-coinfected patients following antiretroviral therapy interruption. *AIDS.* 2010;24(6):857-865.

9. McMahon MA, Jilek BL, Brennan TP, et al. The HBV drug entecavir - effects on HIV-1 replication and resistance. *N Engl J Med.* 2007;356(25):2614-2621.

10. Benhamou Y, Bochet M, Thibault V, et al. Long-term incidence of hepatitis B virus resistance to lamivudine in human immunodeficiency virus-infected patients. *Hepatology.* 1999;30(5):1302-1306.

11. Manegold C, Hannoun C, Wywiol A, et al. Reactivation of hepatitis B virus replication accompanied by acute hepatitis in patients receiving highly active antiretroviral therapy. *Clin Infect Dis.* 2001;32(1):144-148.

12. Sulkowski MS, Thomas DL, Chaisson RE, et al. Hepatotoxicity associated with antiretroviral therapy in adults infected with human immunodeficiency virus and the role of hepatitis C or B virus infection. *JAMA.* 2000;283(1):74-80.

13. den Brinker M, Wit FW, Wertheim-van Dillen PM, et al. Hepatitis B and C virus co-infection and the risk for hepatotoxicity of highly active antiretroviral therapy in HIV-1 infection. *AIDS.* 2000;14(18):2895-2902.

14. Centers for Disease Control and Prevention (CDC). Guidelines for prevention and treatment of opportunistic infections in HIV-infected adults and adolescents: recommendations from CDC, the National Institutes of Health, and the HIV Medicine Association of the Infectious Diseases Society of America. *MMWR Recomm Rep.* 2009;58(RR-4):1-207.

15. Lok AS, McMahon BJ. Chronic hepatitis B: update 2009. *Hepatology.* 2009;50(3):661-662.

16. Woo G, Tomlinson G, Nishikawa Y, et al. Tenofovir and entecavir are the most effective antiviral agents for chronic hepatitis B: a systematic review and Bayesian meta-analyses. *Gastroenterology.* 2010;139(4):1218-1229.

17. Peters MG, Andersen J, Lynch P, et al. Randomized controlled study of tenofovir and adefovir in chronic hepatitis B virus and HIV infection: ACTG A5127. *Hepatology*. 2006;44(5):1110-1116.

18. Matthews GV, Seaberg E, Dore GJ, et al. Combination HBV therapy is linked to greater HBV DNA suppression in a cohort of lamivudine-experienced HIV/HBV coinfected individuals. *AIDS*. 2009;23(13):1707-1715.

19. de Vries-Sluijs TE, Reijnders JG, Hansen BE, et al. Long-Term Therapy with Tenofovir is Effective for Patients Co-Infected with HIV and HBV. *Gastroenterology*. 2010.

20. Pessoa MG, Gazzard B, Huang AK, et al. Efficacy and safety of entecavir for chronic HBV in HIV/HBV coinfected patients receiving lamivudine as part of antiretroviral therapy. *AIDS*. 2008;22(14):1779-1787.

21. Benhamou Y, Bochet M, Thibault V, et al. Safety and efficacy of adefovir dipivoxil in patients co-infected with HIV-1 and lamivudine-resistant hepatitis B virus: an open-label pilot study. *Lancet*. 2001;358(9283):718-723.

22. Ingiliz P, Valantin MA, Thibault V, et al. Efficacy and safety of adefovir dipivoxil plus pegylated interferon-alpha2a for the treatment of lamivudine-resistant hepatitis B virus infection in HIV-infected patients. *Antivir Ther*. 2008;13(7):895-900.

HIV/Hepatitis C Virus (HCV) Coinfection (Last updated March 27, 2012; last reviewed March 27, 2012)

Key Considerations When Managing Patients Coinfected with HIV and Hepatitis C Virus
• All HIV-infected patients should be screened for hepatitis C virus (HCV) infection, preferably before starting antiretroviral therapy (ART).
• ART may slow the progression of liver disease by preserving or restoring immune function and reducing HIV-related immune activation and inflammation. For most HIV/HCV-coinfected patients, including those with cirrhosis, the benefits of ART outweigh concerns regarding drug-induced liver injury (DILI). Therefore, ART should be considered for HIV/HCV-coinfected patients, regardless of CD4 count **(BII)**.
• Initial ART combination regimens for most HIV/HCV-coinfected patients are the same as those for individuals without HCV infection. However, when treatment for both HIV and HCV is indicated, consideration of potential drug-drug interactions and overlapping toxicities should guide ART regimen selection or modification (see discussion in the text).
• Combined treatment of HIV and HCV can be complicated by large pill burden, drug interactions, and overlapping toxicities. Although ART should be initiated for most HIV/HCV-coinfected patients regardless of CD4 cell count, in ART-naive patients with CD4 counts >500 cells/mm^3 some clinicians may choose to defer ART until completion of HCV treatment.
• In patients with lower CD4 counts (e.g., <200 cells/mm^3), it may be preferable to initiate ART and delay HCV therapy until CD4 counts increase as a result of ART.
Rating of Recommendations: A = Strong; B = Moderate; C = Optional
Rating of Evidence: I = Data from randomized controlled trials; II = Data from well-designed nonrandomized trials or observational cohort studies with long-term clinical outcomes; III = Expert opinion

Approximately one-third of patients with chronic hepatitis C virus (HCV) infection progress to cirrhosis at a median time of less than 20 years.[1, 2] The rate of progression increases with older age, alcoholism, male sex, and HIV infection.[3-6] In a meta-analysis, individuals coinfected with HIV/HCV were found to have three times greater risk of progression to cirrhosis or decompensated liver disease than were HCV-monoinfected patients.[5] This accelerated rate is magnified in HIV/HCV-coinfected patients with low CD4 counts. Although ART appears to slow the rate of HCV disease progression in HIV/HCV-coinfected patients, several studies have demonstrated that the rate continues to exceed that observed in those without HIV infection.[7, 8] Whether HCV infection accelerates HIV progression, as measured by AIDS-related opportunistic infections (OIs) or death,[9] is unclear. If such an increased risk of HIV progression exists, it may reflect the impact of injection drug use, which is strongly linked to HCV infection.[10,11] The increased frequency of antiretroviral (ARV)-associated hepatotoxicity with chronic HCV infection also complicates HIV treatment.[12, 13]

A combination regimen of peginterferon and ribavirin (PegIFN/RBV) has been the mainstay of treatment for HCV infection. In HCV genotype 1-infected patients without HIV, addition of an HCV NS3/4A protease inhibitor (PI) boceprevir or telaprevir to PegIFN/RBV significantly improves the rate of sustained virologic response (SVR).[14, 15] Clinical trials of these HCV PIs in combination with PegIFN/RBV for the treatment of HCV genotype 1 infection in HIV-infected patients are currently under way. Both boceprevir and telaprevir are substrates and inhibitors of cytochrome P (CYP) 3A4/5 and p-glycoprotein (p-gp); boceprevir is also metabolized by aldo-keto reductase. These drugs have significant interactions with certain ARV drugs that are metabolized by the same pathways. As such, the presence of HCV infection and the treatment of HCV may influence HIV treatment as discussed below.

Assessment of HIV/Hepatitis C Virus Coinfection Before Initiation of Antiretroviral Therapy

• All HIV-infected patients should be screened for HCV infection using sensitive immunoassays licensed for detection of antibody to HCV in blood.[16] HCV-seronegative patients at risk for the acquistion of HCV infection should undergo repeat testing annually. HCV-seropositive patients should be tested for HCV RNA using a qualitative or quantitative assay to confirm the presence of active infection.[17]

- Patients with HIV/HCV coinfection should be counseled to avoid consuming alcohol and to use appropriate precautions to prevent transmission of HIV and/or HCV to others. HIV/HCV-coinfected patients who are susceptible to hepatitis A virus (HAV) or hepatitis B virus (HBV) infection should be vaccinated against these viruses.

- All patients with HIV/HCV coinfection should be evaluated for HCV therapy. HCV treatment is recommended according to standard guidelines.[18, 19] Strong preference should be given to commence HCV treatment in patients with higher CD4 counts. For patients with lower CD4 counts (e.g., <200 cells/mm^3), it may be preferable to initiate ART and delay HCV therapy until CD4 counts increase as a result of HIV treatment.[17, 20-22]

Antiretroviral Therapy in HIV/Hepatitis C Virus Coinfection

- When to start antiretroviral therapy: The rate of liver disease (liver fibrosis) progression is accelerated in HIV/HCV-coinfected patients, particularly in individuals with low CD4 counts (≤350 cells/mm^3). Data largely from retrospective cohort studies are inconsistent regarding the effect of ART on the natural history of HCV disease.[6, 23, 24] However, ART may slow the progression of liver disease by preserving or restoring immune function and reducing HIV-related immune activation and inflammation.[25-27] Thus, for most coinfected patients, including those with high CD4 counts and those with cirrhosis, the benefits of ART outweigh concerns regarding DILI. Therefore, ART should be initiated for most HIV/HCV-coinfected patients, regardless of CD4 count **(BII)**. However, in HIV treatment-naive patients with CD4 counts >500 cells/mm^3, some clinicians may choose to defer ART until completion of HCV treatment.

- What antiretroviral to start and what antiretroviral not to use: Initial ARV combination regimens for most HIV treatment-naive patients with HCV are the same as those for patients without HCV infection. Special considerations for ARV selection in HIV/HCV-coinfected patients include:

  - When both HIV and HCV treatments are indicated, the choice of ARV regimen should be guided by the HCV treatment regimen selected with careful consideration of potential drug-drug interactions and overlapping toxicities (as discussed below).

  - Cirrhotic patients should be carefully assessed for signs of liver decompensation according to the Child-Turcotte-Pugh classification system because hepatically metabolized ARV drugs may require dose modification or avoidance in patients with Child-Pugh class B and C disease. (See Appendix B, Table 7.)

- Hepatotoxicity: DILI following initiation of ART is more common in HIV/HCV-coinfected patients than in those with HIV monoinfection. The greatest risk of DILI may be observed in coinfected individuals with advanced liver disease (e.g., cirrhosis or end-stage liver disease).[28] Eradication of HCV infection with treatment may decrease the likelihood of ARV-associated DILI.[29]

  - Given the substantial heterogeneity in patient populations and drug regimens, comparison of DILI incidence rates for individual ARV agents across clinical trials is difficult. In such studies, the highest incidence rates of significant elevations in liver enzyme levels (>5 times the upper limit of the laboratory reference range) have been observed during therapy with ARV drugs that are no longer commonly used in clinical practice, including stavudine (d4T) (with or without didanosine [ddI]), nevirapine (NVP), or full-dose ritonavir (RTV) (600 mg twice daily).[30] Additionally, certain ARV agents should be avoided if possible because they have been associated with higher incidence of serious liver-associated adverse effects, such as fatty liver disease with nucleoside reverse transcriptase inhibitors (NRTIs) such as d4T, ddI, or zidovudine (ZDV);[31] noncirrhotic portal hypertension associated with ddI;[32] and hepatotoxicity associated with RTV-boosted tipranavir.[33]

- Alanine aminotransferase (ALT) and aspartate aminotransferase (AST) levels should be monitored at 1 month after initiation of ART and then every 3 to 6 months. Mild to moderate fluctuations in ALT and/or AST are typical in individuals with chronic HCV infection. In the absence of signs and/or symptoms of liver disease these fluctuations do not require interruption of ART. Significant ALT and/or AST elevation should prompt careful evaluation for signs and symptoms of liver insufficiency and for alternative causes of liver injury (e.g., acute HAV or HBV infection, hepatobiliary disease, or alcoholic hepatitis); short-term interruption of the ART regimen or of the specific drug suspected to be responsible for the DILI may be required.[34]

Treating Both HIV and Hepatitis C Virus Infection

Concurrent treatment of HIV and HCV is feasible but may be complicated by high pill burden, drug interactions, and overlapping drug toxicities. In this context, the decision to treat chronic HCV should also include consideration of the medical need for such treatment on the basis of an assessment of HCV disease stage. Some clinicians may choose to defer HCV therapy in HIV/HCV-coinfected patients with no or minimal liver fibrosis. If treatment with PegIFN/RBV alone or in combination with one of the HCV NS3/4A PIs (boceprevir or telaprevir) is initiated, the ART regimen may need to be modified to reduce the potential for drug interactions and/or toxicities that may develop during the period of concurrent HIV and HCV treatment.

Considerations for using certain nucleoside reverse transcriptase inhibitors and hepatitis C virus treatments:

- ddI **should not be given** with RBV because of the potential for drug-drug interactions leading to life-threatening ddI-associated mitochondrial toxicity including hepatomegaly/steatosis, pancreatitis, and lactic acidosis **(AII)**.[35]

- Combined use of ZDV and RBV is associated with increased rates of anemia, making RBV dose reduction necessary. Therefore, this combination should be avoided when possible.[36] Because the risk of anemia may further increase when boceprevir or telaprevir is combined with PegIFN/RBV, ZDV **should not be given** with this combination **(AIII)**.

- Abacavir (ABC) has been associated with decreased response to PegIFN/RBV in some, but not all, retrospective studies; current evidence is insufficient to recommend avoiding this combination.[37-39]

Considerations for the use of HCV NS3/4A protease inhibitors (boceprevir or telaprevir) and antiretroviral therapy:

- Boceprevir is approved for the treatment of HCV genotype 1 infection in patients without HIV infection. After 4 weeks of PegIFN/RBV therapy, boceprevir is added to the regimen for 24, 32, or 44 additional weeks of HCV therapy. Data on the use of an HCV regimen containing boceprevir together with ART in HIV/HCV-coinfected individuals are limited. In 1 small study of coinfected patients, higher HCV response was observed with boceprevir plus PegIFN/RBV (64 patients) than with PegIFN/RBV alone (34 patients). In this study, patients received ART that included HIV-1 ritonavir-boosted atazanavir (ATV/r), darunavir (DRV/r), or lopinavir (LPV/r) or raltegravir (RAL) plus dual NRTIs.[40]

  Boceprevir is primarily metabolized by aldo-keto reductase, but because the drug is also a substrate and inhibitor of CYP3A4/5 and p-gp enzymes, it may interact with ARVs metabolized by these pathways. Based on drug interaction studies in healthy volunteers, boceprevir can be co-administered with RAL.[41] However, co-administration of boceprevir with ATV/r, DRV/r, LPV/r, or efavirenz (EFV) is not recommended because of bidirectional drug interactions (see Table 15a and 15b).[42, 43] Importantly, the pharmacokinetic (PK) interactions of HIV PIs with boceprevir were not identified before the approval of boceprevir and before participant enrollment in the HIV/HCV-coinfection trial; consequently, some coinfected patients have received HIV PIs and boceprevir during HCV treatment. Patients who are currently receiving these drug combinations should be advised not to stop any medication until contacting their health care providers. If therapy with HIV PIs and boceprevir is continued, patients should be closely monitored for HIV and HCV responses and consideration should be given to switching the HIV PI or EFV to RAL during boceprevir therapy. Additional clinical trial data are needed to determine if other ARVs may be co-administered with boceprevir.

- Telaprevir is approved for the treatment of HCV genotype 1 infection in patients without HIV infection. Telaprevir is administered in combination with PegIFN/RBV for the initial 12 weeks of HCV therapy followed by 12 or 36 weeks of additional treatment with PegIFN/RBV. Data on the use of this regimen in HIV/HCV-coinfected individuals are limited. In 1 small study of coinfected patients, higher HCV response was observed with telaprevir plus PegIFN/RBV (38 patients) than with PegIFN/RBV alone (22 patients). In this study, patients received ART containing EFV or ATV/r plus tenofovir/emtricitabine (TDF/FTC) or no ART during the HCV therapy.[44]

  Because telaprevir is a substrate and an inhibitor of CYP3A4 and p-gp enzymes, the drug may interact with ARVs metabolized by these pathways. On the basis of drug interaction studies in healthy volunteers and data on responses in coinfected patients enrolled in the small clinical trial noted above, telaprevir can be co-administered with ATV/r[45] and RAL[46] at the standard recommended dose of telaprevir (750 mg every 7 9 hours) and with EFV at an increased dose of telaprevir (1125 mg every 7 9 hours) (see Table 15b); however, co-administration of telaprevir with DRV/r, fosamprenavir/ritonavir (FPV/r), or LPV/r is not recommended because of bidirectional drug interactions.[45] Data on PK interactions of telaprevir with other ARVs including non-nucleoside reverse transcriptase inhibitors (NNRTIs) other than EFV and with maraviroc (MVC) are not available; therefore, co-administration of telaprevir with other ARVs cannot be recommended.

Following are preliminary recommendations for the use of boceprevir or telaprevir in HIV patients coinfected with HCV genotype 1 based on current ART use. These recommendations may be modified as new drug interaction and clinical trial information become available.

Patients not on ART:	Use either boceprevir or telaprevir
Patients receiving RAL + 2-NRTI:	Use either boceprevir or telaprevir
Patients receiving ATV/r + 2-NRTI:	Use telaprevir at standard dose. Do not use boceprevir.
Patients receiving EFV + 2-NRTI:	Use telaprevir at increased dose of 1125 mg every 7 9 hours. Do not use boceprevir.

Patients receiving other ARV regimens:

- If HCV disease is minimal (i.e., no or mild portal fibrosis), consider deferring HCV treatment given rapidly evolving HCV drug development.

- If good prognostic factors for HCV treatment response are present   IL28B CC genotype or low HCV RNA level (<400,000 International Unit [IU]/mL)   consider use of PegIFN/RBV without HCV NS3/4A PI.

- On the basis of ART history and HIV genotype testing results, if possible, consider switching to the ART regimens listed above to permit the use of boceprevir or telaprevir.

- For patients with complex ART history or resistance to multiple classes of ART, consultation with experts regarding the optimal strategy to minimize the risk of HIV breakthrough may be needed. In such patients, telaprevir may be the preferred HCV NS3/4A PI because its duration of use (12 weeks) is shorter than that of boceprevir (24 to 44 weeks).

Summary:

In summary, HCV coinfection and use of PegIFN/RBV with or without HCV NS3/4A PIs (telaprevir or boceprevir) to treat HCV may impact the treatment of HIV because of increased pill burden, toxicities, and drug-drug interactions. Because ART may slow the progression of HCV-related liver disease, ART should be considered for most HIV/HCV-coinfected patients, regardless of CD4 count. If treatment with PegIFN/RBV alone or in combination with one of the HCV NS3/4A PIs (telaprevir or boceprevir) is initiated, the ART regimen may need to be modified to reduce the potential for drug-drug interactions and/or drug toxicities that may develop during the period of concurrent HIV and HCV treatment. The science of HCV drug development is evolving rapidly. As new clinical trial data on the management of HIV/HCV-coinfected patients with newer HCV drugs become available, the Panel will modify its recommendations accordingly.

References

1. Alter MJ, et al. The natural history of community-acquired hepatitis C in the United States. The Sentinel Counties Chronic non-A, non-B Hepatitis Study Team. *N Engl J Med*. 1992;327(27):1899-1905.

2. Thomas DL, et al. The natural history of hepatitis C virus infection: host, viral, and environmental factors. *JAMA*. 2000;284(4):450-456.

3. Poynard T, Bedossa B, Opolon P. Natural history of liver fibrosis progression in patients with chronic hepatitis C. The OBSVIRC, METAVIR, CLINIVIR, and DOSVIRC groups. *Lancet*. 1997;349(9055):825-832.

4. Wiley TE, et al. Impact of alcohol on the histological and clinical progression of hepatitis C infection. *Hepatology*. 1998;28(3):805-809.

5. Graham CS, et al. Influence of human immunodeficiency virus infection on the course of hepatitis C virus infection: a meta-analysis. *Clin Infect Dis*. 2001;33(4):562-569.

6. Thein HH, et al. Natural history of hepatitis C virus infection in HIV-infected individuals and the impact of HIV in the era of highly active antiretroviral therapy: a meta-analysis. *AIDS*. 2008;22(15):1979-1991.

7. Weber R, et al. Liver-related deaths in persons infected with the human immunodeficiency virus: the D:A:D study. *Arch Intern Med*. 2006;166(15):1632-1641.

8. Kitahata MM, et al. Effect of early versus deferred antiretroviral therapy for HIV on survival. *N Engl J Med*. 2009;360(18):1815-1826.

9. Greub G, et al. Clinical progression, survival, and immune recovery during antiretroviral therapy in patients with HIV-1 and hepatitis C virus coinfection: the Swiss HIV Cohort Study. *Lancet*. 2000;356(9244):1800-1805.

10. Vlahov D, et al. Prognostic indicators for AIDS and infectious disease death in HIV-infected injection drug users: plasma viral load and CD4+ cell count. *JAMA*. 1998; 279(1):35-40.

11. Celentano DD, et al. Self-reported antiretroviral therapy in injection drug users. *JAMA*. 1998;280(6):544-546.

12. Sulkowski MS, et al. Hepatotoxicity associated with antiretroviral therapy in adults infected with human immunodeficiency virus and the role of hepatitis C or B virus infection. *JAMA*. 2000;283(1):74-80.

13. Sulkowski MS, Thomas DL, Mehta SH, et al. Hepatotoxicity associated with nevirapine or efavirenz-containing antiretroviral therapy: role of hepatitis C and B infections. *Hepatology*. 2002;35(1):182-189.

14. Poordad F, et al. Boceprevir for untreated chronic HCV genotype 1 infection. *N Engl J Med*. 2011;364(13):1195-1206.

15. Jacobson IM, et al. Telaprevir for previously untreated chronic hepatitis C virus infection. *N Engl J Med*. 2011;364(25):2405-2416.

16. Centers for Disease Control and Prevention (CDC). Guidelines for prevention and treatment of opportunistic infections in HIV-infected adults and adolescents: recommendations from CDC, the National Institutes of Health, and the HIV Medicine Association of the Infectious Diseases Society of America. *MMWR Recomm Rep*. 2009;58(RR-4):1-207.

17. Ghany MG, et al. Diagnosis, management, and treatment of hepatitis C: an update. *Hepatology*. 2009;49(4):1335-1374.

18. Ghany MG, et al. An update on treatment of genotype 1 chronic hepatitis C virus infection: 2011 practice guideline by the American Association for the Study of Liver Diseases. *Hepatology*. 2011;54(4):1433-1444.

19. Panel on Antiretroviral Guidelines for Adults and Adolescents. Guidelines for the prevention and treatment of opportunistic infections in adults and adolescents with HIV/AIDS. Department of Health and Human Services. 2012 (In Press).

20. Soriano V, et al. Care of patients coinfected with HIV and hepatitis C virus: 2007 updated recommendations from the HCV-HIV International Panel. *AIDS*. 2007;21(9):1073-1089.

21. Tien PC. Management and treatment of hepatitis C virus infection in HIV-infected adults: recommendations from the Veterans Affairs Hepatitis C Resource Center Program and National Hepatitis C Program Office. *Am J Gastroenterol*. 2005;100(10):2338-2354.

22. Avidan NU, et al. Hepatitis C Viral Kinetics During Treatment With Peg IFN-alpha-2b in HIV/HCV Coinfected Patients as a Function of Baseline CD4+ T-Cell Counts. *J Acquir Immune Defic Syndr*. 2009;52(4):452-458.

23. Sulkowski MS, et al. Rapid fibrosis progression among HIV/hepatitis C virus-co-infected adults. *AIDS*. 2007;21(16): 2209-2216.

24. Brau N, et al. Slower fibrosis progression in HIV/HCV-coinfected patients with successful HIV suppression using antiretroviral therapy. *J Hepatol*. 2006;44(1):47-55.

25. Macias J, et al. Fast fibrosis progression between repeated liver biopsies in patients coinfected with human immunodeficiency virus/hepatitis C virus. *Hepatology*. 2009;50(4):1056-1063.

26. Verma S, Goldin RD, Main J. Hepatic steatosis in patients with HIV-Hepatitis C Virus coinfection: is it associated with antiretroviral therapy and more advanced hepatic fibrosis? *BMC Res Notes*. 2008;1:46.

27. Ragni MV, et al. Highly active antiretroviral therapy improves ESLD-free survival in HIV-HCV co-infection. *Haemophilia*. 2009;15(2):552-558.

28. Aranzabal L, et al. Influence of liver fibrosis on highly active antiretroviral therapy-associated hepatotoxicity in patients with HIV and hepatitis C virus coinfection. *Clin Infect Dis*. 2005;40(4):588-593.

29. Labarga P, et al. Hepatotoxicity of antiretroviral drugs is reduced after successful treatment of chronic hepatitis C in HIV-infected patients. *J Infect Dis*. 2007;196(5):670-676.

30. Nunez M. Hepatotoxicity of antiretrovirals: incidence, mechanisms and management. *J Hepatol*. 2006;44(1 Suppl):S132-S139.

31. McGovern BH, et al. Hepatic steatosis is associated with fibrosis, nucleoside analogue use, and hepatitis C virus genotype 3 infection in HIV-seropositive patients. *Clin Infect Dis*. 2006;43(3):365-372.

32. Kovari H, et al. Association of noncirrhotic portal hypertension in HIV-infected persons and antiretroviral therapy with didanosine: a nested case-control study. *Clin Infect Dis*. 2009;49(4):626-635.

33. Food and Drug Administration. Aptivus (package insert). http://www.accessdata.fda.gov/drugsatfda docs/label/2011/ 021814s011lbl.pdf. Accessed March 26, 2012.

34. Sulkowski MS, Thomas DL. Hepatitis C in the HIV-infected patient. *Clin Liver Dis*. 2003;7(1):179-194.

35. Fleischer R, Boxwell D, Sherman KE. Nucleoside analogues and mitochondrial toxicity. *Clin Infect Dis*. 2004;38(8):e79-e80.

36. Alvarez D, et al. Zidovudine use but not weight-based ribavirin dosing impacts anaemia during HCV treatment in HIV-infected persons. *J Viral Hepat*. 2006;13(10):683-689.

37. Vispo E, et al. Low response to pegylated interferon plus ribavirin in HIV-infected patients with chronic hepatitis C treated with abacavir. *Antivir Ther*. 2008;13(3):429-437.

38. Laufer N, et al. Abacavir does not influence the rate of virological response in HIV-HCV-coinfected patients treated with pegylated interferon and weight-adjusted ribavirin. *Antivir Ther*. 2008;13(7):953-957.

39. Mira JA, et al. Efficacy of pegylated interferon plus ribavirin treatment in HIV/hepatitis C virus co-infected patients receiving abacavir plus lamivudine or tenofovir plus either lamivudine or emtricitabine as nucleoside analogue backbone. *J Antimicrob Chemother*. 2008;62(6):1365-1373.

40. Sulkowski, M., S. Pol, et al. (2012). Boceprevir + pegylated interferon + ribavirin for the treatment of HCV/HIV coinfected patients: End of treatment (Week 48) interim results. 18th Conference on Retroviruses and Opportunistic Infections. Seattle, WA, Abs 47.

41. de Kanter CB, Blonk M, Colbers A, Fillekes Q, Schouwenberg B, Burger D. The Influence of the HCV Protease Inhibitor Bocepravir on the Pharmocokinetics of the HIV Integrase Inhibitor Raltegravir. Paper presented at: 19th Conference on Retroviruses and Opportunistic Infections (CROI);March 5-8, 2012; Seattle, WA.

42. Hulskotte E, Feng H-P, Xuan F, van Zutven M, O'Mara E, Youngberg S, Wagner J, Butterton J. Pharmacokinetic interaction between the HCV protease inhibitor bocepravir and ritonavir-boosted HIV-1 protease inhibitors atazanavir, lopinavir, and darunavir. Paper presented at: 19th Conference on Retroviruses and Opportunistic Infections (CROI); March 5-8, 2012; Seattle, WA.

43. Food and Drug Administration, Victrelis (package insert). http://www.accessdata.fda.gov/drugsatfda docs/label/2011/202258lbl.pdf. Accessed March 23, 2012.

44. Dieterich D., V. Soriano, et al. (2012). Telaprevir in combination with peginterferion a-2a + ribavirin in HCV/HIV-coinfected patients: a 24-week treatment interim analysis. 18th Conference on Retroviruses and Opportunistic Infections. Seattle, WA, Abs 46.

45. Food and Drug Administration, INCIVEK (package insert). Accessed March 23, 2012.

46. van Heeswijk R, et al. The pharmacokinetic interaction between telaprevir and raltegravir in healthy volunteers. Paper presented at:51st Interscience Conference on Antimicrobial Agents and Chemotherapy (ICAAC); September 17-20, 2011; Chicago, IL.

Mycobacterium Tuberculosis Disease with HIV Coinfection (Last updated March 27, 2012; last reviewed March 27, 2012)

Panel's Recommendations
• The principles for treatment of active tuberculosis (TB) disease in HIV-infected patients are the same as those for HIV-uninfected patients **(AI)**.
• All HIV-infected patients with diagnosed active TB should be started on TB treatment immediately **(AI)**.
• All HIV-infected patients with diagnosed active TB should be treated with antiretroviral therapy (ART) **(AI)**.
• In patients with CD4 counts <50 cells/mm^3, ART should be initiated within 2 weeks of starting TB treatment **(AI)**.

• In patients with CD4 counts ≥50 cells/mm^3 who present with clinical disease of major severity as indicated by clinical evaluation (including low Karnofsky score, low body mass index [BMI], low hemoglobin, low albumin, organ system dysfunction, or extent of disease), ART should be initiated within 2 to 4 weeks of starting TB treatment. The strength of this recommendation varies on the basis of CD4 cell count:
  • CD4 count 50 to 200 cells/mm^3 **(BI)**
  • CD4 count >200 cells/mm^3 **(BIII)**

• In patients with CD4 counts ≥50 cells/mm^3 who do not have severe clinical disease, ART can be delayed beyond 2 to 4 weeks of starting TB therapy but should be started within 8 to 12 weeks of TB therapy initiation. The strength of this recommendation also varies on the basis of CD4 cell count:
  • CD4 count 50 to 500 cells/mm^3 **(AI)**
  • CD4 count >500 cells/mm^3 **(BIII)**

• In all HIV-infected pregnant women with active TB, ART should be started as early as feasible, both for maternal health and for prevention of mother-to-child transmission (PMTCT) of HIV **(AIII)**.
• In HIV-infected patients with documented multidrug-resistant (MDR) and extensively drug-resistant (XDR) TB, ART should be initiated within 2 to 4 weeks of confirmation of TB drug resistance and initiation of second-line TB therapy **(BIII)**.
• Despite pharmacokinetic drug interactions, a rifamycin (rifampin or rifabutin) should be included in TB regimens for patients receiving ART, with dosage adjustment if necessary **(AII)**.
• Rifabutin is the preferred rifamycin to use in HIV-infected patients with active TB disease on a protease inhibitor (PI)-based regimen because the risk of substantial drug interactions with PIs is lower with rifabutin than with rifampin **(AII)**.
• Co-administration of rifampin and PIs (with or without ritonavir [RTV] boosting) is not recommended **(AII)**.
• Rifapentine (RPT) is NOT recommended in HIV-infected patients receiving ART for treatment of latent TB infection (LTBI) or active TB, unless in the context of a clinical trial **(AIII)**.
• Immune reconstitution inflammatory syndrome (IRIS) may occur after initiation of ART. Both ART and TB treatment should be continued while managing IRIS **(AIII)**.
• Treatment support, which can include directly observed therapy (DOT) of TB treatment, is strongly recommended for HIV-infected patients with active TB disease **(AII)**.
Rating of Recommendations: A = Strong; B = Moderate; C = Optional *Rating of Evidence: I = Data from randomized controlled trials; II = Data from well-designed nonrandomized trials or observational cohort studies with long-term clinical outcomes; III = Expert opinion*

Treatment of Active Tuberculosis in HIV-Infected Patients

HIV infection significantly increases the risk of progression from latent to active TB disease. The CD4 cell count influences both the frequency and severity of active TB disease.[1-2] Active TB also negatively affects

HIV disease. It may be associated with a higher HIV viral load and more rapid progression of HIV disease.[3]

Active pulmonary or extrapulmonary TB disease requires prompt initiation of TB treatment. The treatment of active TB disease in HIV-infected patients should follow the general principles guiding treatment for individuals without HIV **(AI)**. Treatment of drug-susceptible TB disease should include a standard regimen that consists of isoniazid (INH) + a rifamycin (rifampin or rifabutin) + pyrazinamide + ethambutol given for 2 months, followed by INH + a rifamycin for 4 to 7 months.[4] The Guidelines for Prevention and Treatment of Opportunistic Infections in HIV-Infected Adults and Adolescents[4] include a more complete discussion of the diagnosis and treatment of TB disease in HIV-infected patients.

All patients with HIV/TB disease should be treated with ART **(AI)**. Important issues related to the use of ART in patients with active TB disease include: (1) when to start ART, (2) significant pharmacokinetic drug-drug interactions between rifamycins and some antiretroviral (ARV) agents, (3) the additive toxicities associated with concomitant ARV and TB drug use, (4) the development of TB-associated IRIS after ART initiation, and (5) the need for treatment support including DOT and the integration of HIV and TB care and treatment.

Antiretroviral Therapy in Patients with Active Tuberculosis

Patients Diagnosed with Tuberculosis While Receiving Antiretroviral Therapy

When TB is diagnosed in a patient receiving ART, the patient's ARV regimen should be assessed with particular attention to potential pharmacokinetic interactions with rifamycins (discussed below). The patient's regimen may need to be modified to permit use of the optimal TB treatment regimen (see Tables 14 16 for dosing recommendations).

Patients Not Yet Receiving Antiretroviral Therapy

Until recently, when to start ART in patients with active TB has been a subject of debate. Survival is improved when ART is started early following initiation of TB therapy, but a delay in initiating ART often was favored because of the potential complications of high pill burden, additive toxicities, drug interactions, adherence, and the potential for development of IRIS.Recent studies primarily conducted in resource-limited settings, including three randomized controlled trials, have helped clarify the question of when to start ART in patients with active TB.[5-8]

The SAPiT study conducted in South Africa convincingly demonstrated that starting ART during rather than after concluding treatment for TB can significantly reduce mortality. In this study, ambulatory HIV-infected patients with smear-positive TB and CD4 counts <500 cells/mm^3 were randomized to one of three treatment arms: integrated therapy with ART initiated either during the first 4 weeks of TB therapy or after the first 8 weeks of TB treatment (i.e., during the continuation phase of TB therapy) or sequential therapy with ART initiated after the conclusion of standard TB therapy. The median CD4 cell count of participants at study entry was 150 cells/mm^3. The sequential therapy arm was stopped when an early analysis demonstrated that the mortality rate in the combined two integrated arms was 56% lower than the rate in the sequential therapy arm. Treatment was continued in the two integrated arms until study completion.[5]

With the completion of SAPiT and 2 other randomized controlled trials, CAMELIA and STRIDE, the question on the optimal time to initiate ART during TB therapy has been addressed. Findings from these trials now serve as the basis for the Panel's recommendations on when to start ART in patients with active TB.

In the final analysis of the SAPiT trial, there were no differences in rates of AIDS or death between the 2 integrated arms of the study (patients who started ART within 4 weeks after initiating TB treatment vs. those who started ART at 8 12 weeks [i.e., within 4 weeks after completing the intensive phase of TB treatment]).

However, in patients with baseline CD4 counts <50 cells/mm^3 (17% of the study population), the rate of AIDS or death was lower in the earlier therapy group than in the later therapy group (8.5 vs. 26.3 cases per 100 person-years, a strong trend favoring the earlier treatment arm, P 0.06). For all patients, regardless of CD4 cell count, earlier therapy was associated with a higher incidence of IRIS and of adverse events that required a switch in ARV drugs than later therapy. Two deaths were attributed to IRIS.[6]

In the CAMELIA study, which was conducted in Cambodia[7], patients who had CD4 counts <200 cells/mm^3 were randomized to initiate ART at 2 weeks or 8 weeks after initiation of TB treatment. Study participants had advanced HIV disease, with a median entry CD4 count of 25 cells/mm^3; low BMIs (median 16.8 kg/m^2), Karnofsky scores (87% <70), and hemoglobin levels (median 8.7 g/dl); and high rates of disseminated TB disease. Compared with therapy initiated at 8 weeks, ART initiated at 2 weeks resulted in a 38% reduction in mortality (P 0.006). A significant reduction in mortality was seen in patients with CD4 counts ≤50 cells/mm^3 and in patients with CD4 counts 51 to 200 cells/mm^3. Overall, 6 deaths associated with TB-IRIS were reported.

The ACTG 5221 (STRIDE) trial, a multinational study conducted at 28 sites, randomized ART-naive patients with confirmed or probable TB and CD4 counts <250 cells/mm^3 to earlier (<2 weeks) or later (8 12 weeks) ART.[8] At study entry, the participants' median CD4 count was 77 cells/mm^3. The rates of mortality and AIDS diagnoses were not different between the earlier and later arms, although higher rates of IRIS were seen in the earlier arm. However, a significant reduction in AIDS or death was seen in the subset of patients with CD4 counts <50 cells/mm^3 who were randomized to the earlier ART arm (P 0.02).

In each of these 3 studies, IRIS was more common in patients initiating ART earlier than in patients starting ART later, but the syndrome was infrequently associated with mortality. Collectively these 3 trials demonstrate that in patients with active TB and with very low CD4 cell counts (i.e., <50 cells/mm^3), early initiation of ART can reduce mortality and AIDS progression, albeit at the risk of increased IRIS. These findings strongly favor initiation of ART within the first 2 weeks of TB treatment in patients with CD4 cell counts <50 cells/mm^3 **(AI)**.

The question of when to start ART in patients with CD4 counts ≥50 cells/mm^3 is also informed by these studies. The STRIDE and SAPiT studies in which the patients with CD4 cell counts ≥50 cells/mm^3 were relatively healthy and with reasonable Karnofsky scores (note the SAPiT study excluded patients with Karnofsky scores <70) and BMIs demonstrated that ART initiation in these patients can be delayed until 8 to 12 weeks after initiation of TB therapy **(AI** for CD4 counts 51 500 cells/mm^3 and **BIII** for CD4 counts >500 cells/mm^3).

However, the CAMELIA study, which included more patients who were severely ill than the STRIDE and SAPiT studies, showed that early initiation of ART improved survival both in patients with CD4 counts ≤50 cells/mm^3 and in patients with CD4 counts from 51 to 200 cells/mm^3. In a multivariate analysis, age >40 years, low BMI (<16), low Karnofsky score (<40), elevated aspartate aminotransferase (AST) level (>1.25 x the upper limit of normal [ULN]), disseminated and MDR TB were independently associated with poor survival; whereas in a univariate analysis, hemoglobin <10g/dl also was associated with poor survival.

Thus, recently published results from the three clinical trials are complementary in defining the need for ART and use of CD4 count and clinical status to inform decisions on the optimal time to initiate ART in patients with HIV and TB disease. Earlier initiation of ART within 2 to 4 weeks of TB treatment should be strongly considered for patients with CD4 cell counts from 50 to 200 cells/mm^3 who have evidence of clinical disease of major severity as indicated by clinical evaluation, low Karnofsky score, low BMI, low hemoglobin, low albumin, or organ system dysfunction **(BI)**. Initiation of ART within 2 to 4 weeks also should be considered for patients with CD4 counts >200 cells/mm^3 who present with evidence of severe disease **(BIII)**.

Of additional importance, each of the above studies demonstrated excellent responses to ART, with 90% and >95% of participants achieving suppressed viremia (HIV RNA <400 copies/mL) at 12 months in the SAPiT and CAMELIA studies, respectively, and 74% of participants at 2 years in the STRIDE study.

Mortality rates in patients with MDR or XDR TB and HIV coinfection are very high.[9] Retrospective case control studies and case series provide growing evidence of better outcomes associated with receipt of ART in such coinfected patients,[10] but the optimal timing for initiation of ART is unknown. However, given the high rates and rapid mortality, most experts recommend that ART be initiated within 2 to 4 weeks after confirmation of the diagnosis of drug resistance and initiation of second-line TB therapy **(BIII)**.

All HIV-infected pregnant women with active TB should be started on ART as early as feasible, both for maternal health and to prevent perinatal transmission of HIV **(AIII)**. The choice of ART should be based on efficacy and safety in pregnancy and take into account potential drug-drug interactions between ARVs and rifamycins (see Perinatal Guidelines for more detailed discussions).[11]

TB meningitis often is associated with severe complications and high mortality rate. In a randomized study conducted in Vietnam, patients were randomized to immediate ART or to therapy deferred until 2 months after initiation of TB treatment. A higher rate of severe (Grade 4) adverse events was seen in patients who received immediate ART than in those who deferred therapy (80.3% vs. 69.1%, respectively; P 0.04).[12] In this study 59.8% of the immediate ART patients and 55.5% of the delayed ART patients died within 9 months. However, in the United States, where patients may be more closely monitored and treated for severe adverse events such as central nervous system (CNS) IRIS, many experts feel that ART should be initiated as for other HIV/TB-coinfected patients **(CIII)**.

Drug Interaction Considerations

A rifamycin is a crucial component in treatment of drug-sensitive TB. However, both rifampin and rifabutin are inducers of the hepatic cytochrome P (CYP) 450 and uridine diphosphate gluconyltransferase (UGT) 1A1 enzymes and are associated with significant interactions with most ARV agents including all PIs, non-nucleoside reverse transcriptase inhibitors (NNRTIs), maraviroc (MVC), and raltegravir (RAL). Rifampin is a potent enzyme inducer, leading to accelerated drug clearance and significant reduction in ARV drug exposure. Despite these interactions, some observational studies suggest that good virologic, immunologic, and clinical outcomes may be achieved with standard doses of efavirenz (EFV)[13-14] and, to a lesser extent, nevirapine (NVP)[15-16] when combined with rifampin. However, rifampin is not recommended in combination with all PIs and the NNRTIs etravirine (ETR) and rilpivirine (RPV). When rifampin is used with MVC or RAL, increased dosage of the ARV is generally recommended. Rifabutin, a weaker enzyme inducer, is an alternative to rifampin. Because rifabutin is a substrate of the CYP 450 enzyme system, its metabolism may be affected by the NNRTI or PI. Tables 14, 15a, 15b, 15d, and 15e outline the magnitude of these interactions and provide dosing recommendations when rifamycins and selected ARV drugs are used concomitantly. After determining the drugs and doses to use, clinicians should monitor patients closely to assure good control of both TB and HIV infections. Suboptimal HIV suppression or suboptimal response to TB treatment should prompt assessment of drug adherence, subtherapeutic drug levels (consider therapeutic drug monitoring [TDM]), and acquired drug resistance.

Rifapentine is a long-acting rifamycin that can be given once weekly with INH for the treatment of active or latent TB infection. Similar to rifampin and rifabutin, rifapentine is also a CYP3A4 inducer. No systematic study has been performed to assess the magnitude of the enzyme induction effect of rifapentine on the metabolism of ARV drugs and other concomitant drugs. Significant enzyme induction can result in reduced ARV drug exposure, which may compromise virologic efficacy. Rifapentine is **not recommended** for treatment of latent or active TB infection in patients receiving ART, unless given in the context of a clinical trial **(AIII)**.

Anti-Tuberculosis/Antiretroviral Drug Toxicities

ARV agents and TB drugs, particularly INH, rifamycin, and pyrazinamide, can cause drug-induced hepatitis. These first-line TB drugs should be used for treatment of active TB disease, even with co-administration of other potentially hepatotoxic drugs or when baseline liver disease is present (AIII). Patients receiving potentially hepatotoxic drugs should be monitored frequently for clinical symptoms and signs of hepatitis and have laboratory monitoring for hepatotoxicity. Peripheral neuropathy can occur with administration of INH, didanosine (ddI), or stavudine (d4T) or may be a manifestation of HIV infection. All patients receiving INH also should receive supplemental pyridoxine to reduce peripheral neuropathy. Patients should be monitored closely for signs of drug-related toxicities and receive alternative ARVs to ddI or d4T.

Immune Reconstitution Inflammatory Syndrome with Tuberculosis and Antiretroviral Agents

IRIS occurs in two forms: unmasking and paradoxical. The mechanism of the syndrome is the same for both forms: restoration of immune competence by administration of ART, resulting in an exuberant host response to TB bacilli and/or antigens. Unmasking IRIS refers to the initial clinical manifestations of active TB that occurs soon after ART is started. Paradoxical IRIS refers to the worsening of TB clinical symptoms after ART is started in patients who are receiving TB treatment. Severity of IRIS ranges from mild to severe to life threatening. IRIS has been reported in 8% to more than 40% of patients starting ART after TB is diagnosed, although the incidence depends on the definition of IRIS and the intensity of monitoring.[17-18]

Predictors of IRIS include CD4 count <50 cells/mm^3; higher on-ART CD4 counts; high pre-ART and lower on-ART HIV viral loads; severity of TB disease, especially high pathogen burden; and less than 30-day interval between initiation of TB and HIV treatments.[19-22] Most IRIS in HIV/TB disease occurs within 3 months of the start of TB treatment. Delaying initiation of ART for 2 to 8 weeks may reduce the incidence and severity of IRIS. However, this possible advantage of delayed ART must be weighed against the potential benefit of earlier ART in improving immune function and preventing progression of HIV disease and mortality.

Patients with mild or moderately severe IRIS can be managed symptomatically or treated with nonsteroidal anti-inflammatory agents. Patients with more severe IRIS can be treated successfully with corticosteroids. A recent randomized, placebo-controlled trial demonstrated benefit of corticosteroids in the management of IRIS symptoms (as measured by decreasing days of hospitalization and Karnofsky performance score) without adverse consequences.[23] In the presence of IRIS, neither TB therapy nor ART should be stopped because both therapies are necessary for the long-term health of the patient (AIII).

Immune Reconstitution with Antiretroviral Therapy: Conversion to Positive Tuberculin Skin Test and Interferon-Gamma Release Assay

Immune reconstitution with ART may result in unmasking LTBI (i.e., conversion of a previously negative tuberculin skin test [TST] to a positive TST or a positive interferon-gamma [IFN-γ] release assay [IGRA] for *Mycobacterium tuberculosis*-specific proteins). A positive IGRA, similar to a positive TST, is indicative of LTBI in the absence of evidence of active TB disease.[24] Because treatment for LTBI is indicated in the absence of evidence of active TB disease, clinicians should be aware of this phenomenon. Patients with a negative TST or IGRA and advanced HIV disease (i.e., CD4 count <200 cells/mm^3) should have a repeat TST or IGRA after initiation of ART and CD4 count increase to >200 cells/mm^3 (BII).[25]

Caring for Patients with HIV and Tuberculosis

Close collaboration among clinicians, health care institutions, and public health programs involved in the diagnosis and treatment of HIV-infected patients with active TB disease is necessary in order to integrate care and improve medication adherence and TB treatment completion rates, reduce drug toxicities, and maximize HIV outcomes. HIV-infected patients with active TB disease should receive treatment support, including adherence counseling and DOT, corresponding to their needs **(AII)**. ART simplification or use of coformulated fixed-dose combinations also may help to improve drug adherence.

References

1. Jones BE, Young SM, Antoniskis D, Davidson PT, Kramer F, Barnes PF. Relationship of the manifestations of tuberculosis to CD4 cell counts in patients with human immunodeficiency virus infection. *Am Rev Respir Dis.* Nov 1993;148(5):1292-1297.

2. Perlman DC, el-Sadr WM, Nelson ET, et al. Variation of chest radiographic patterns in pulmonary tuberculosis by degree of human immunodeficiency virus-related immunosuppression. The Terry Beirn Community Programs for Clinical Research on AIDS (CPCRA). The AIDS Clinical Trials Group (ACTG). *Clin Infect Dis.* Aug 1997;25(2):242-246.

3. Whalen C, Horsburgh CR, Hom D, Lahart C, Simberkoff M, Ellner J. Accelerated course of human immunodeficiency virus infection after tuberculosis. *Am J Respir Crit Care Med.* Jan 1995;151(1):129-135.

4. Kaplan JE, Benson C, Holmes KH, Brooks JT, Pau A, Masur H. Guidelines for prevention and treatment of opportunistic infections in HIV-infected adults and adolescents: recommendations from CDC, the National Institutes of Health, and the HIV Medicine Association of the Infectious Diseases Society of America. *MMWR Recomm Rep.* Apr 10 2009;58(RR-4):1-207; quiz CE201-204.

5. Abdool Karim SS, Naidoo K, Grobler A, et al. Timing of initiation of antiretroviral drugs during tuberculosis therapy. *N Engl J Med.* Feb 25 2010;362(8):697-706.

6. Abdool Karim SS, Naidoo K, Grobler A, et al. Integration of antiretroviral therapy with tuberculosis treatment. *N Engl J Med.* Oct 20 2011;365(16):1492-1501.

7. Blanc FX, Sok T, Laureillard D, et al. Earlier versus later start of antiretroviral therapy in HIV-infected adults with tuberculosis. *N Engl J Med.* Oct 20 2011;365(16):1471-1481.

8. Havlir DV, Kendall MA, Ive P, et al. Timing of antiretroviral therapy for HIV-1 infection and tuberculosis. *N Engl J Med.* Oct 20 2011;365(16):1482-1491.

9. Gandhi NR, Shah NS, Andrews JR, et al. HIV coinfection in multidrug- and extensively drug-resistant tuberculosis results in high early mortality. *Am J Respir Crit Care Med.* Jan 1 2010;181(1):80-86.

10. Dheda K, Shean K, Zumla A, et al. Early treatment outcomes and HIV status of patients with extensively drug-resistant tuberculosis in South Africa: a retrospective cohort study. *Lancet.* May 22 2010;375(9728):1798-1807.

11. Panel on Treatment of HIV-Infected Pregnant Women and Prevention of Perinatal Transmission. Recommendations for Use of Antiretroviral Drugs in Pregnant HIV-1-Infected Women for Maternal Health and Interventions to Reduce Perinatal HIV Transmission in the United States, Sep. 14, 2011; pp 1-207. Available at http://aidsinfo.nih.gov/contentfiles/PerinatalGL.pdf. 2011.

12. Torok ME, Yen NT, Chau TT, et al. Timing of initiation of antiretroviral therapy in human immunodeficiency virus (HIV)—associated tuberculous meningitis. *Clin Infect Dis.* Jun 2011;52(11):1374-1383.

13. Friedland G, Khoo S, Jack C, Lalloo U. Administration of efavirenz (600 mg/day) with rifampicin results in highly variable levels but excellent clinical outcomes in patients treated for tuberculosis and HIV. *J Antimicrob Chemother.* Dec 2006;58(6):1299-1302.

14. Manosuthi W, Kiertiburanakul S, Sungkanuparph S, et al. Efavirenz 600 mg/day versus efavirenz 800 mg/day in HIV-

infected patients with tuberculosis receiving rifampicin: 48 weeks results. *AIDS*. Jan 2 2006;20(1):131-132.

15. Moses M, Zachariah R, Tayler-Smith K, et al. Outcomes and safety of concomitant nevirapine and rifampicin treatment under programme conditions in Malawi. *Int J Tuberc Lung Dis*. Feb 2010;14(2):197-202.

16. Shipton LK, Wester CW, Stock S, et al. Safety and efficacy of nevirapine- and efavirenz-based antiretroviral treatment in adults treated for TB-HIV co-infection in Botswana. *Int J Tuberc Lung Dis*. Mar 2009;13(3):360-366.

17. Haddow LJ, Moosa MY, Easterbrook PJ. Validation of a published case definition for tuberculosis-associated immune reconstitution inflammatory syndrome. *AIDS*. Jan 2 2010;24(1):103-108.

18. Meintjes G, Lawn SD, Scano F, et al. Tuberculosis-associated immune reconstitution inflammatory syndrome: case definitions for use in resource-limited settings. *Lancet Infect Dis*. Aug 2008;8(8):516-523.

19. Manosuthi W, Kiertiburanakul S, Phoorisri T, Sungkanuparph S. Immune reconstitution inflammatory syndrome of tuberculosis among HIV-infected patients receiving antituberculous and antiretroviral therapy. *J Infect*. Dec 2006;53(6):357-363.

20. Colebunders R, John L, Huyst V, Kambugu A, Scano F, Lynen L. Tuberculosis immune reconstitution inflammatory syndrome in countries with limited resources. *Int J Tuberc Lung Dis*. Sep 2006;10(9):946-953.

21. Michailidis C, Pozniak AL, Mandalia S, Basnayake S, Nelson MR, Gazzard BG. Clinical characteristics of IRIS syndrome in patients with HIV and tuberculosis. *Antivir Ther*. 2005;10(3):417-422.

22. Lawn SD, Myer L, Bekker LG, Wood R. Tuberculosis-associated immune reconstitution disease: incidence, risk factors and impact in an antiretroviral treatment service in South Africa. *AIDS*. Jan 30 2007;21(3):335-341.

23. Meintjes, G., R. J. Wilkinson, et al. (2010). Randomized placebo-controlled trial of prednisone for paradoxical tuberculosis-associated immune reconstitution inflammatory syndrome. *AIDS* 24(15): 2381-2390.

24. Menzies D, Pai M, Comstock G. Meta-analysis: new tests for the diagnosis of latent tuberculosis infection: areas of uncertainty and recommendations for research. *Ann Intern Med*. Mar 6 2007;146(5):340-354.

25. Girardi E, Palmieri F, Zaccarelli M, et al. High incidence of tuberculin skin test conversion among HIV-infected individuals who have a favourable immunological response to highly active antiretroviral therapy. *AIDS*. Sep 27 2002;16(14):1976-1979.

Limitations to Treatment Safety and Efficacy

Adherence to Antiretroviral Therapy (Last updated March 27, 2012; last reviewed March 27, 2012)

Adherence to antiretroviral therapy (ART) has been correlated strongly with HIV viral suppression, reduced rates of resistance, an increase in survival, and improved quality of life.[1-2] In the past few years, ART regimens have been greatly simplified. Although newer regimens include more fixed-dose combination products and offer once-daily dosing, adherence remains a challenge. Because HIV treatment is a lifelong endeavor, and because many patients will initiate therapy when they are generally in good health, feel well, and demonstrate no obvious signs or symptoms of HIV disease, adherence poses a special challenge and requires commitment from the patient and the health care team.

Adherence remains a challenging and complicated topic. This section provides clinicians with some guidance in their approaches to assist patients in maintaining adherence.

Factors Associated with Nonadherence

Adherence to ART can be influenced by characteristics of the patient, the regimen, the clinical setting, and the provider/patient relationship.[3] To assure adherence, it is critical that the patient receive and understand information about HIV disease, the goal of therapy, and the specific regimen prescribed. A number of factors have been associated with poor adherence, including the following:

- low levels of health literacy[4] or numeracy (ability to understand numerical-related health information);[5]
- certain age-related challenges (e.g., polypharmacy, vision loss, cognitive impairment)[6];
- younger age;
- psychosocial issues (e.g., depression, homelessness, low social support, stressful life events, or psychosis);[7]
- nondisclosure of HIV serostatus[8]
- neurocognitive issues (e.g., cognitive impairment, dementia)
- active (but not history of) substance abuse, particularly for patients who have experienced recent relapse;
- stigma[9];
- difficulty with taking medication (e.g., trouble swallowing pills, daily schedule issues);
- complex regimens (e.g., high pill burden, high-frequency dosing, food requirements);
- adverse drug effects;
- nonadherence to clinic appointments[10]
- cost and insurance coverage issues; and
- treatment fatigue.

Adherence studies conducted in the early era of combination ART with unboosted protease inhibitors (PIs) found that virologic failure is much less likely to occur in patients who adhere to more than 95% of their prescribed doses than in those who are less adherent.[11] More recent adherence studies were conducted using boosted PIs and non-nucleoside reverse transcriptase inhibitors (NNRTIs). These studies suggest that the longer half-lives of boosted PIs and efavirenz may make the drugs more forgiving of lapses in adherence.[12-13] Nonetheless, clinicians should encourage patients to adhere as closely as possible to the prescribed doses and schedules for all ART regimens.

Measurement of Adherence

There is no gold standard for the assessment of adherence,[1] but there are many validated tools and strategies to choose from. Although patient self-report of adherence predictably overestimates adherence by as much as 20%,[14] this measure still is associated with viral load responses.[15] Thus, a patient's report of suboptimal adherence is a strong indicator of nonadherence and should be taken seriously.

When ascertained in a simple, nonjudgmental, routine, and structured format that normalizes less-than-perfect adherence and minimizes socially desirable responses, patient self-report remains the most useful method for the assessment and longitudinal monitoring of a patient's adherence in the clinical setting. A survey of all doses missed during the past 3 days or the past week accurately reflects longitudinal adherence and is the most practical and readily available tool for adherence assessments in clinical trials and in clinical practice.[1] Other strategies also may be effective. One study found that asking patients to rate their adherence on a six-point scale during 1 month was more accurate than asking them about the frequency of missed doses or to estimate the percentage of doses taken during the previous 3 or 7 days.[16] Pharmacy records and pill counts also can be used in addition to simply asking the patient about adherence.[17] Other methods of assessing adherence include the use of electronic measurement devices (e.g., bottle caps, dispensing systems). However, these methods may not be feasible in some clinical settings.

Interventions to Improve Adherence

Before writing the first prescriptions, the clinician should assess the patient's readiness to take medication, including information such as factors that may limit adherence (psychiatric illness, active drug use, etc.) and make additional support necessary; the patient's understanding of the disease and the regimen; and the patient's social support, housing, work and home situation, and daily schedules.

During the past several years, a number of advances have simplified many regimens dramatically, particularly those for treatment-naive patients. Prescribing regimens that are simple to take, have a low pill burden and low-frequency dosing, have no food requirements, and have low incidence and severity of adverse effects will facilitate adherence.[18] The Panel considered both regimen simplicity and effectiveness when making current treatment recommendations (see What to Start).

Patients should understand that their first regimen usually offers the best chance for a simple regimen that affords long-term treatment success and prevention of drug resistance. Given that effective response to ART is dependent on good adherence, clinicians should identify barriers to adherence such as a patient's schedule, competing psychosocial needs, learning needs, and literacy level before treatment is initiated. As appropriate, resources and strategies that will help the patient to achieve and maintain good adherence should be employed.

Individualizing treatment with involvement of the patient in decision making is the cornerstone of any treatment plan.[17] The first principle of successful treatment is negotiation of an understandable plan to which the patient can commit.[19-20] Establishing a trusting relationship over time and maintaining good communication will help to improve adherence and long-term outcomes.

An increasing number of interventions have demonstrated efficacy in improving adherence to ART. A meta-analysis of 19 randomized controlled trials of ART adherence interventions found that intervention participants were 1.5 times as likely to report 95% adherence and 1.25 times as likely to achieve an undetectable viral load as participants in comparison conditions.[21]

In a more recent synthesis, CDC provides new guidance to assist providers in selecting from among the many possible adherence interventions. According to efficacy criteria described by the CDC HIV/AIDS Prevention Research Synthesis (PRS) project, CDC has identified a subset of best-evidence medication adherence interventions. In December 2010, CDC published a new online Medication Adherence chapter of the Compendium of Evidence-Based HIV Behavioral Interventions that includes eight medication adherence behavioral interventions identified from the scientific literature published or in press from January 1996 through December 2009. For descriptions of the interventions, see: http://www.cdc.gov/hiv/topics/research/prs/ma-good-evidence-interventions.htm.[22] Since these reviews have been conducted, additional evidence also has accumulated regarding the efficacy and benefits of motivational interviewing.[23]

In summary, effective adherence interventions vary in their modality and duration, providing clinics, providers, and patients with options to suit a range of needs and settings. Some effective interventions identified include multiple nurse home visits, five-session group intervention, pager messaging, and couples-based interventions. Substance abuse therapy and strengthening social support also can improve adherence. All health care team members, including nurses, nurse practitioners, pharmacists, medication managers, and social workers, have integral roles in successful adherence programs.[24-27] Directly observed therapy (DOT) has been shown to be effective in provision of ART to active drug users.[28] However, the benefits cannot be sustained after transitioning the drug users out of the methadone clinics and halting the provision of ART by DOT.[29]

To routinely determine whether such additional adherence intervention is warranted, assessments should be done at each clinical encounter and should be the responsibility of the entire health care team. Routine monitoring of HIV viral load and pharmacy records are useful determinants for the need of intensified efforts.

Conclusion

Significant progress has been made regarding determinants, measurements, and interventions to improve adherence to ART. Given the various assessment strategies and potential interventions available, the challenge for the treatment team is to select the techniques that provide the best fit for the treatment setting, resources available, and patient population. The complexity and the importance of adherence encourage clinicians to continue to seek novel, patient-centered ways to improve adherence and to tailor adherence interventions. Early detection of nonadherence and prompt intervention can reduce greatly the development of viral resistance and the likelihood of virologic failure.

Table 12. Strategies to Improve Adherence to Antiretroviral Therapy

Strategies	Examples
Use a multidisciplinary team approach Provide an accessible, trusting health care team	• Nurses, social workers, pharmacists, and medications managers
Establish a trusting relationship with the patient	
Establish patient readiness to start ART	
Assess and simplify the regimen, if possible	
Identify potential barriers to adherence before starting ART	• Psychosocial issues • Active substance abuse or at high risk of relapse • Low literacy • Low numeracy • Busy daily schedule and/or travel away from home • Nondisclosure of HIV diagnosis • Skepticism about ART • Lack of prescription drug coverage • Lack of continuous access to medications
Provide resources for the patient	• Referrals for mental health and/or substance abuse treatment • Resources to obtain prescription drug coverage • Pillboxes
Involve the patient in ARV regimen selection	• For each option, review regimen potency, potential side effects, dosing frequency, pill burden, storage requirements, food requirements, and consequences of nonadherence
Assess adherence at every clinic visit	• Use a simple checklist that the patient can complete in the waiting room • Ensure that other members of the health care team also assess adherence • Ask the patient open-ended questions (e.g., *In the last 3 days, please tell me how you took your medicines.*)
Identify the type of nonadherence	• Failure to fill the prescription(s) • Failure to take the right dose(s) at the right time(s) • Nonadherence to food requirements
Identify reasons for nonadherence	• Adverse effects from medications • Complexity of regimen (pill burden, dosing frequency, etc.) • Difficulty swallowing large pills • Forgetfulness • Failure to understand dosing instructions • Inadequate understanding of drug resistance and its relationship to adherence • Pill fatigue • Other potential barriers
If resources allow, select from among available effective interventions	• See http://www.cdc.gov/hiv/topics/research/prs/ma-good-evidence-interventions.htm

Key to Abbreviations: ART = antiretroviral therapy; ARV = antiretroviral

References

1. Chesney MA. The elusive gold standard. Future perspectives for HIV adherence assessment and intervention. *J Acquir Immune Defic Syndr*. Dec 1 2006;43(Suppl 1):S149-155.

2. World Heath Organization (WHO). Adherence to long term therapies – evidence for action. 2003. http://www.who.int/chp/knowledge/publications/adherence_full_report.pdf.

3. Schneider J, Kaplan SH, Greenfield S, Li W, Wilson IB. Better physician-patient relationships are associated with higher reported adherence to antiretroviral therapy in patients with HIV infection. *J Gen Intern Med*. Nov 2004;19(11):1096-1103.

4. Marcus EN. The silent epidemic—the health effects of illiteracy. *N Engl J Med*. Jul 27 2006;355(4):339-341.

5. Moore JO, Boyer EW, Safren S, et al. Designing interventions to overcome poor numeracy and improve medication adherence in chronic illness, including HIV/AIDS. *J Med Toxicol*. Jun 2011;7(2):133-138.

6. van Eijken M, Tsang S, Wensing M, de Smet PA, Grol RP. Interventions to improve medication compliance in older patients living in the community: a systematic review of the literature. *Drugs Aging*. 2003;20(3):229-240.

7. Halkitis PN, Shrem MT, Zade DD, Wilton L. The physical, emotional and interpersonal impact of HAART: exploring the realities of HIV seropositive individuals on combination therapy. *J Health Psychol*. May 2005;10(3):345-358.

8. Stirratt MJ, Remien RH, Smith A, et al. The role of HIV serostatus disclosure in antiretroviral medication adherence. *AIDS Behav*. Sep 2006;10(5):483-493.

9. Carr RL, Gramling LF. Stigma: a health barrier for women with HIV/AIDS. *J Assoc Nurses AIDS Care*. Sep-Oct 2004;15(5):30-39.

10. Mugavero MJ, Lin HY, Allison JJ, et al. Racial disparities in HIV virologic failure: do missed visits matter? *J Acquir Immune Defic Syndr*. Jan 1 2009;50(1):100-108.

11. Paterson DL, Swindells S, Mohr J, et al. Adherence to protease inhibitor therapy and outcomes in patients with HIV infection. *Ann Intern Med*. Jul 4 2000;133(1):21-30.

12. Bangsberg DR. Less than 95% adherence to nonnucleoside reverse-transcriptase inhibitor therapy can lead to viral suppression. *Clin Infect Dis*. Oct 1 2006;43(7):939-941.

13. Raffa JD, Tossonian HK, Grebely J, Petkau AJ, DeVlaming S, Conway B. Intermediate highly active antiretroviral therapy adherence thresholds and empirical models for the development of drug resistance mutations. *J Acquir Immune Defic Syndr*. Mar 1 2008;47(3):397-399.

14. Arnsten JH, Demas PA, Farzadegan H, et al. Antiretroviral therapy adherence and viral suppression in HIV-infected drug users: comparison of self-report and electronic monitoring. *Clin Infect Dis*. Oct 15 2001;33(8):1417-1423.

15. Simoni JM, Kurth AE, Pearson CR, Pantalone DW, Merrill JO, Frick PA. Self-report measures of antiretroviral therapy adherence: A review with recommendations for HIV research and clinical management. *AIDS Behav*. May 2006;10(3):227-245.

16. Lu M, Safren SA, Skolnik PR, et al. Optimal recall period and response task for self-reported HIV medication adherence. *AIDS Behav*. Jan 2008;12(1):86-94.

17. Bieszk N, Patel R, Heaberlin A, Wlasuk K, Zarowitz B. Detection of medication nonadherence through review of pharmacy claims data. *Am J Health Syst Pharm*. Feb 15 2003;60(4):360-366.

18. Raboud J, Li M, Walmsley S, et al. Once daily dosing improves adherence to antiretroviral therapy. *AIDS Behav*. Oct 2011;15(7):1397-1409.

19. Vermeire E, Hearnshaw H, Van Royen P, Denekens J. Patient adherence to treatment: three decades of research. A comprehensive review. *J Clin Pharm Ther*. Oct 2001;26(5):331-342.

20. Williams A, Friedland G. Adherence, compliance, and HAART. *AIDS Clin Care*. 1997;9(7):51-54, 58.

21. Simoni JM, Pearson CR, Pantalone DW, Marks G, Crepaz N. Efficacy of interventions in improving highly active antiretroviral therapy adherence and HIV-1 RNA viral load. A meta-analytic review of randomized controlled trials. *J*

Acquir Immune Defic Syndr. Dec 1 2006;43(Suppl 1):S23-35.

22. Centers for Disease Control and Prevention PRSP. Compendium of Evidence-Based HIV Behavioral Interventions: Medication Adherence Chapter. Retrieved from Compendium of Evidence-Based HIV Behavioral Interventions website: http://www.cdc.gov/hiv/topics/research/prs/ma-chapter.htm. 2011.

23. Krummenacher I, Cavassini M, Bugnon O, Schneider MP. An interdisciplinary HIV-adherence program combining motivational interviewing and electronic antiretroviral drug monitoring. *AIDS Care*. May 2011;23(5):550-561.

24. McPherson-Baker S, Malow RM, Penedo F, Jones DL, Schneiderman N, Klimas NG. Enhancing adherence to combination antiretroviral therapy in non-adherent HIV-positive men. *AIDS Care*. Aug 2000;12(4):399-404.

25. Kalichman SC, Cherry J, Cain D. Nurse-delivered antiretroviral treatment adherence intervention for people with low literacy skills and living with HIV/AIDS. *J Assoc Nurses AIDS Care*. Sep-Oct 2005;16(5):3-15.

26. Remien RH, Stirratt MJ, Dognin J, Day E, El-Bassel N, Warne P. Moving from theory to research to practice. Implementing an effective dyadic intervention to improve antiretroviral adherence for clinic patients. *J Acquir Immune Defic Syndr*. Dec 1 2006;43(Suppl 1):S69-78.

27. Mannheimer SB, Morse E, Matts JP, et al. Sustained benefit from a long-term antiretroviral adherence intervention. Results of a large randomized clinical trial. *J Acquir Immune Defic Syndr*. Dec 1 2006;43(Suppl 1):S41-47.

28. Altice FL, Maru DS, Bruce RD, Springer SA, Friedland GH. Superiority of directly administered antiretroviral therapy over self-administered therapy among HIV-infected drug users: a prospective, randomized, controlled trial. *Clin Infect Dis*. Sep 15 2007;45(6):770-778.

29. Berg KM, Litwin AH, Li X, Heo M, Arnsten JH. Lack of sustained improvement in adherence or viral load following a directly observed antiretroviral therapy intervention. *Clin Infect Dis*. Nov 2011;53(9):936-943.

Adverse Effects of Antiretroviral Agents (Last updated February 12, 2013; last reviewed February 12, 2013)

Adverse effects have been reported with use of all antiretroviral (ARV) drugs; they are among the most common reasons for switching or discontinuing therapy and for medication nonadherence.[1] However, with the use of newer ARV regimens, rates of treatment-limiting adverse events in antiretroviral therapy (ART)-naive patients enrolled in randomized trials appear to be declining and are generally now occurring in less than 10% of study participants. However, because most clinical trials have a relatively short follow-up duration, the longer term complications of ART can be underestimated. In the Swiss Cohort study, during 6 years of follow-up, the presence of laboratory adverse events was associated with higher rates of mortality, which highlights the importance of adverse events in overall patient management.[2]

Several factors may predispose individuals to adverse effects of ARV medications. For example, compared with men, women (especially ART-naive women with CD4 counts >250 cells/mm^3) seem to have a higher propensity to develop Stevens-Johnson syndrome, rashes, and hepatotoxicity from nevirapine (NVP)[3-5] and have higher rates of lactic acidosis due to nucleoside reverse transcriptase inhibitors (NRTIs).[6-8] Other factors may also contribute to the development of adverse events:

- Concomitant use of medications with overlapping and additive toxicities;
- Comorbid conditions that may increase the risk of or exacerbate adverse effects (e.g., alcoholism[9] or coinfection with viral hepatitis[10-12] may increase the risk of hepatotoxicity);
- Drug-drug interactions that may lead to an increase in drug toxicities (e.g., interactions that result from concomitant use of statins with protease inhibitors [PIs]); or
- Genetic factors that predispose patients to abacavir (ABC) hypersensitivity reaction (HSR).[13, 14]

The therapeutic goals of ART include achieving and maintaining viral suppression and improving immune function, but an overarching goal should be to select a regimen that is not only effective but also safe. This requires consideration of the toxicity potential of an ARV regimen, as well as the individual patient's underlying conditions, concomitant medications, and prior history of drug intolerances.

In addition, it should be appreciated that, in general, the overall benefits of ART outweigh its risks and that some conditions (e.g., anemia, cardiovascular disease [CVD], renal impairment), may be more likely in the absence of ART.[15, 16]

Information on adverse events of ARVs is outlined in several tables in the guidelines. Table 13 provides clinicians with a list of the most common and/or severe known ARV-associated adverse events by drug class. The most common adverse effects of individual ARV agents are summarized in Appendix B, Tables 1 6.

Table 13. Antiretroviral Therapy-Associated Common and/or Severe Adverse Effects (page 1 of 5)

(See Appendix B for additional information listed by drug. Empty spaces in the table may mean no reported cases for the particular side effect or no data are available for the specific ARV drug class)

Adverse Effects	NRTIs	NNRTIs	PIs	INSTI	EI
Bleeding events			**All PIs:** Increased spontaneous bleeding, hematuria in patients with hemophilia **TPV:** Reports of intracranial hemorrhage. Risks include CNS lesions, trauma, surgery, hypertension, alcohol abuse, coagulopathy, and concomitant use of anti-coagulant or anti-platelet agents, including vitamin E		
Bone marrow suppression	**ZDV:** Anemia, neutropenia				
Cardiovascular disease (CVD)	**ABC and ddI:** Associated with an increased risk of MI in some, but not all, cohort studies. Absolute risk greatest in patients with traditional CVD risk factors.		**PIs:** Associated with MI and stroke in some cohort studies. Data on newer PIs (**ATV, DRV, and TPV**) are limited. **SQV/r, ATV/r,** and **LPV/r:** PR interval prolongation. Risks include structural heart disease, conduction system abnormalities, cardiomyopathy, ischemic heart disease, and coadministration with drugs that prolong PR interval. **SQV/r:** QT interval prolongation in patients in a healthy volunteer study. Risks include underlying heart conditions, pre-existing prolonged QT or arrhythmia, or use with other QT-prolonging drugs. ECG is recommended before SQV initiation and should be considered during therapy.		
Central nervous system (CNS) effects	**d4T:** Associated with rapidly progressive, ascending neuromuscular weakness resembling Guillain-Barré syndrome (rare)	**EFV:** Somnolence, insomnia, abnormal dreams, dizziness, impaired concentration, depression, psychosis, and suicidal ideation. Symptoms usually subside or diminish after 2–4 weeks. Bedtime dosing may reduce symptoms. Risks include history of psychiatric illness, concomitant use of agents with neuropsychiatric effects, and increased plasma EFV concentrations due to genetic factors or increased absorption with food.		**RAL:** Depression (uncommon)	

Table 13. Antiretroviral Therapy-Associated Common and/or Severe Adverse Effects (page 2 of 5)

Adverse Effects	NRTIs	NNRTIs	PIs	INSTI	EI
Cholelithiasis			**ATV:** • History of kidney stones increases risk and patients may present with cholelithiasis and kidney stones concurrently • Typically presents as abdominal pain • Reported complications include cholecystitis, pancreatitis, choledocholithiasis, and cholangitis • Median time to onset is 42 months (range 1–90 months)		
Diabetes mellitus (DM)/insulin resistance	ZDV, d4T, and ddI		• Reported for some **PIs** (**IDV**, **LPV/r**), but not all **PIs**		
Dyslipidemia	**d4T > ZDV > ABC:** • ↑LDL and TG	**EFV** • ↑TG • ↑LDL • ↑HDL	↑LDL, ↑TG, ↑HDL: **All RTV-boosted PIs** ↑TG: **LPV/r = FPV/r and LPV/r > DRV/r and ATV/r**		
Gastrointestinal (GI) effects	**Nausea and vomiting:** ddI and **ZDV** > other **NRTIs** **Pancreatitis: ddI**		GI intolerance (e.g., diarrhea, nausea, vomiting) **Diarrhea:** Common with **NFV**; **LPV/r > DRV/r and ATV/r**	**Nausea and diarrhea:** EVG/COBI/TDF/FTC	

Guidelines for the Use of Antiretroviral Agents in HIV-1-Infected Adults and Adolescents

Table 13. Antiretroviral Therapy-Associated Common and/or Severe Adverse Effects (page 3 of 5)

Adverse Effects	NRTIs	NNRTIs	PIs	INSTI	EI
Hepatic effects	Reported for most **NRTIs** **ddI:** Prolonged exposure linked to non-cirrhotic portal hypertension, some cases with esophageal varicees **Steatosis:** Most commonly seen with **ZDV, d4T,** or **ddI** **Flares:** HIV/HBV-co-infected patients may develop severe hepatic flares when **TDF, 3TC,** and **FTC** are withdrawn or when HBV resistance develops.	**NVP > other NNRTIs** **NVP:** • Severe hepatic toxicity with **NVP** is often associated with skin rash or symptoms of hypersensitivity. • In ARV-naive patients, risk is greater for women with pre-**NVP** CD4 count >250 cells/mm^3 and men with pre-**NVP** CD4 count >400 cells/mm^3. Overall risk is higher for women than men. • Risk is greatest in the first few months of treatment. • 2-week dose escalation of **NVP** reduces risk of rash and possibly hepatotoxicity if related to hypersensitivity. • **NVP** is contraindicated in patients with moderate to severe hepatic insufficiency (Child-Pugh classification B or C). • Liver failure observed in HIV-uninfected individuals receiving **NVP** for post-exposure prophylaxis. **NVP** should <u>never</u> be used for this indication.	**All PIs:** Drug-induced hepatitis and hepatic decompensation (and rare cases of fatalities) have been reported with all **PIs** to varying degrees. The frequency of hepatic events is higher with **TPV/r** than with other PIs. **IDV, ATV:** Jaundice due to indirect hyperbilirubinemia **TPV/r:** Contraindicated in patients with moderate to severe hepatic insufficiency (Child-Pugh classification B or C)		**MVC:** Hepatotoxicity with or without rash or HSRs reported

Table 13. Antiretroviral Therapy-Associated Common and/or Severe Adverse Effects (page 4 of 5)

Adverse Effects	NRTIs	NNRTIs	PIs	INSTI	EI
Hypersensitivity reaction (HSR) (excluding rash alone or Stevens-Johnson syndrome [SJS])	**ABC:** • HLA-B*5701 screening should be performed before initiation of **ABC. ABC** should not be started if the HLA-B*5701 test result is positive. • Symptoms of HSR include (in descending frequency): fever, skin rash, malaise, nausea, headache, myalgia, chills, diarrhea, vomiting, abdominal pain, dyspnea, arthralgia, and respiratory symptoms. • Symptoms worsen with continuation of **ABC.** • Median onset of reactions is 9 days; approximately 90% of reactions occur within the first 6 weeks of treatment. • The onset of re-challenge reactions is within hours of re-challenge dose • Patients, regardless of HLA-B*5701 status, should not be re-challenged with **ABC** if HSR is suspected.	**NVP:** • Hypersensitivity syndrome of hepatic toxicity and rash that may be accompanied by fever, general malaise, fatigue, myalgias, arthralgias, blisters, oral lesions, conjunctivitis, facial edema, eosinophilia, granulocytopenia, lymphadenopathy, or renal dysfunction. • In ARV-naive patients, risk is greater for women with pre-**NVP** CD4 count >250 cells/mm^3 and men with pre-**NVP** CD4 count >400 cells/mm^3. Overall, risk is higher for women than men. • 2-week dose escalation of **NVP** reduces risk.		RAL	**MVC:** Reported as part of a syndrome related to hepatotoxicity
Lactic acidosis	**NRTIs, especially d4T, ZDV, and ddI:** • Insidious onset with GI prodrome, weight loss, and fatigue. May be rapidly progressive with tachycardia, tachypnea, jaundice, muscular weakness, mental status changes, respiratory distress, pancreatitis, and organ failure. • Mortality up to 50% in some case series, especially in patients with serum lactate >10 mmol/L • Females and obese patients at increased risk Laboratory findings: • ↑ lactate (often >5 mmol/L), anion gap, AST, ALT, PT, bilirubin • ↑ amylase and lipase in patients with pancreatitis • ↓ arterial pH, serum bicarbonate, serum albumin				

Table 13. Antiretroviral Therapy-Associated Common and/or Severe Adverse Effects (page 5 of 5)

Adverse Effects	NRTIs	NNRTIs	PIs	INSTI	EI
Lipodystrophy	**Lipoatrophy: Thymidine analogs (d4T > ZDV).** May be more likely when NRTIs combined with **EFV** than with a **RTV-boosted PI.**	<u>Lipohypertrophy:</u> Trunk fat increase observed with **EFV**-, **PI**-, and **RAL**-containing regimens; however, causal relationship has not been established.			
Myopathy/elevated creatine phosphokinase (CPK)	ZDV: Myopathy			**RAL:** ↑ CPK Muscle weakness and rhabdomyolysis	
Nephrotoxicity/urolithiasis	**TDF:** ↑ serum creatinine, proteinuria, hypophosphatemia, urinary phosphate wasting, glycosuria, hypokalemia, non-anion gap metabolic acidosis. Concurrent use with **PI** appears to increase risk.		**IDV:** ↑ serum creatinine, pyuria; hydronephrosis or renal atrophy. **IDV, ATV:** Stone, crystal formation; adequate hydration may reduce risk.	**EVG/COBI/TDF/FTC:** • **COBI** can cause non-pathologic decrease in CrCl. • May increase risk of **TDF**-related nephrotoxicity	
Osteopenia/osteoporosis	**TDF:** Associated with greater loss of BMD than with **ZDV, d4T,** and **ABC.**	Decreases in BMD observed in studies of regimens containing different **NRTIs** or **PIs.**			
Peripheral neuropathy	<u>Peripheral neuropathy</u> (pain and/or paresthesias, lower extremities > upper extremities): **d4T > ddI** and **ddC** (can be irreversible)				
Rash		All **NNRTIs**	ATV, DRV, FPV	RAL, EVG/COBI/TDF/FTC: Uncommon	MVC
Stevens-Johnson syndrome (SJS)/ toxic epidermal necrosis (TEN)	ddI, ZDV: Reported cases	NVP > DLV, EFV, ETR, RPV	FPV, DRV, IDV, LPV/r, ATV: Reported cases	RAL	

Key to Abbreviations: 3TC = lamivudine, ABC = abacavir, ALT = alanine aminotransferase, ARV = antiretroviral, AST = aspartate aminotransferase, ATV = atazanavir, ATV/r = atazanavir + ritonavir, BMD = bone mineral density, CrCl = creatinine clearance, CNS = central nervous system, COBI = cobicistat, CPK = creatine phosphokinase, CVD = cardiovascular disease, d4T = stavudine, ddC = zalcitabine, ddI = didanosine, DLV = delavirdine, DM = diabetes mellitus, DRV = darunavir, DRV/r = darunavir + ritonavir, ECG = electrocardiogram, EFV = efavirenz, EI = entry inhibitor, ETR = etravirine, EVG = elvitegravir, FPV = fosamprenavir, FPV/r = fosamprenavir + ritonavir, FTC = emtricitabine, GI = gastrointestinal, HBV = hepatitis B virus, HDL = high-density lipoprotein, HSR = hypersensitivity reaction, IDV = indinavir, INSTI = integrase strand transfer inhibitor, LDL = low-density lipoprotein, LPV/r = lopinavir + ritonavir, MI = myocardial infarction, MVC = maraviroc, NFV = nelfinavir, NNRTI = non-nucleoside reverse transcriptase inhibitor, NRTI = nucleoside reverse transcriptase inhibitor, NVP = nevirapine, PI = protease inhibitor, PT = prothrombin time, RAL = raltegravir, RPV = rilpivirine, RTV = ritonavir, SJS = Stevens-Johnson syndrome, SQV = saquinavir, SQV/r = saquinavir + ritonavir, TDF = tenofovir disoproxil fumarate, TEN = toxic epidermal necrosis, TG = triglyceride, TPV = tipranavir, TPV/r = tipranavir + ritonavir, ZDV = zidovudine

Guidelines for the Use of Antiretroviral Agents in HIV-1-Infected Adults and Adolescents

References

1. O'Brien ME, Clark RA, Besch CL, et al. Patterns and correlates of discontinuation of the initial HAART regimen in an urban outpatient cohort. *J Acquir Immune Defic Syndr*. 2003;34(4):407-414. Available at http://www.ncbi.nlm.nih.gov/entrez/query.fcgi?cmd=Retrieve&db=pubmed&dopt=Abstract&list_uids=14615659.

2. Keiser O, Fellay J, Opravil M, et al. Adverse events to antiretrovirals in the Swiss HIV Cohort Study: Effect on mortality and treatment modification. *Antivir Ther*. 2007;12(8):1157-1164. Available at http://www.ncbi.nlm.nih.gov/entrez/query.fcgi?cmd=Retrieve&db=pubmed&dopt=Abstract&list_uids=18240856.

3. Baylor MS, Johann-Liang R. Hepatotoxicity associated with nevirapine use. *J Acquir Immune Defic Syndr*. 2004;35(5):538-539. Available at http://www.ncbi.nlm.nih.gov/entrez/query.fcgi?cmd=Retrieve&db=pubmed&dopt=Abstract&list_uids=15021321.

4. Bersoff-Matcha SJ, Miller WC, Aberg JA, al. e. Sex differences in nevirapine rash. *Clin Infect Dis*. 2001;32(1):124-129. Available at http://www.ncbi.nlm.nih.gov/entrez/query.fcgi?cmd=Retrieve&db=PubMed&list_uids=11118391&dopt=Abstract.

5. Fagot JP, Mockenhaupt M, Bouwes-Bavinck JN, et al; for EuroSCAR Study Group. Nevirapine and the risk of Stevens-Johnson syndrome or toxic epidermal necrolysis. *AIDS*. 2001;15(14):1843-1848. Available at http://www.ncbi.nlm.nih.gov/entrez/query.fcgi?cmd=Retrieve&db=PubMed&list_uids=11579247&dopt=Abstract.

6. Moyle GJ, Datta D, Mandalia S, et al. Hyperlactataemia and lactic acidosis during antiretroviral therapy: relevance, reproducibility and possible risk factors. *AIDS*. 2002;16(10):1341-1349. Available at http://www.ncbi.nlm.nih.gov/entrez/query.fcgi?cmd=Retrieve&db=PubMed&list_uids=12131210&dopt=Abstract.

7. Bolhaar MG, Karstaedt AS. A high incidence of lactic acidosis and symptomatic hyperlactatemia in women receiving highly active antiretroviral therapy in Soweto, South Africa. *Clin Infect Dis*. 2007;45(2):254-260. Available at http://www.ncbi.nlm.nih.gov/entrez/query.fcgi?cmd=Retrieve&db=pubmed&dopt=Abstract&list_uids=17578788.

8. Geddes R, Knight S, Moosa MY, Reddi A, Uebel K, H S. A high incidence of nucleoside reverse transcriptase inhibitor (NRTI)-induced lactic acidosis in HIV-infected patients in a South African context. *S Afr Med J*. 2006;96(8):722-724. Available at http://www.ncbi.nlm.nih.gov/entrez/query.fcgi?cmd=Retrieve&db=pubmed&dopt=Abstract&list_uids=17019496.

9. Dieterich DT, Robinson PA, Love J, Stern JO. Drug-induced liver injury associated with the use of nonnucleoside reverse-transcriptase inhibitors. *Clin Infect Dis*. 2004;38(Suppl 2):S80-89. Available at http://www.ncbi.nlm.nih.gov/entrez/query.fcgi?cmd=Retrieve&db=pubmed&dopt=Abstract&list_uids=14986279.

10. denBrinker M, Wit FW, Wertheim-van Dillen PM, et al. Hepatitis B and C virus co-infection and the risk for hepatotoxicity of highly active antiretroviral therapy in HIV-1 infection. *AIDS*. 2000;14(18):2895-2902. Available at http://www.ncbi.nlm.nih.gov/entrez/query.fcgi?cmd=Retrieve&db=PubMed&list_uids=11153671&dopt=Abstract.

11. Sulkowski MS, Thomas DL, Chaisson RE, Moore RD. Hepatotoxicity associated with antiretroviral therapy in adults infected with human immunodeficiency virus and the role of hepatitis C or B virus infection. *JAMA*. 2000;283(1):74-80. Available at http://www.ncbi.nlm.nih.gov/entrez/query.fcgi?cmd=Retrieve&db=PubMed&list_uids=10632283&dopt=Abstract.

12. Saves M, Raffi F, Clevenbergh P, et al; and APROCO Study Group. Hepatitis B or hepatitis C virus infection is a risk factor for severe hepatic cytolysis after initiation of a protease inhibitor-containing antiretroviral regimen in human immunodeficiency virus-infected patients. *Antimicrob Agents Chemother*. 2000;44(12):3451-3455. Available at http://www.ncbi.nlm.nih.gov/entrez/query.fcgi?cmd=Retrieve&db=PubMed&list_uids=11083658&dopt=Abstract.

13. Mallal S, Phillips E, Carosi G, et al. HLA-B*5701 screening for hypersensitivity to abacavir. *N Engl J Med*. 2008;358(6):568-579. Available at http://www.ncbi.nlm.nih.gov/entrez/query.fcgi?cmd=Retrieve&db=pubmed&dopt=Abstract&list_uids=18256392.

14. Saag M, Balu R, Phillips E, et al. High sensitivity of human leukocyte antigen-b*5701 as a marker for immunologically confirmed abacavir hypersensitivity in white and black patients. *Clin Infect Dis*. 2008;46(7):1111-1118. Available at http://www.ncbi.nlm.nih.gov/entrez/query.fcgi?cmd=Retrieve&db=pubmed&dopt=Abstract&list_uids=18444831.

15. El-Sadr WM, Lundgren JD, Neaton JD, et al. CD4+ count-guided interruption of antiretroviral treatment. *N Engl J Med*. Nov 30 2006;355(22):2283-2296. Available at http://www.ncbi.nlm.nih.gov/entrez/query.fcgi?cmd=Retrieve&db=PubMed&dopt=Citation&list_uids=17135583.

16. Lichtenstein KA, Armon C, Buchacz K, et al. Initiation of antiretroviral therapy at CD4 cell counts ≥ 350 cells/mm^3 does not increase incidence or risk of peripheral neuropathy, anemia, or renal insufficiency. *J Acquir Immune Defic Syndr*. Jan 1 2008;47(1):27-35. Available at http://www.ncbi.nlm.nih.gov/entrez/query.fcgi?cmd=Retrieve&db=PubMed&dopt=Citation&list_uids=17971714.

Overview

Potential drug-drug and/or drug-food interactions should be taken into consideration when selecting an antiretroviral (ARV) regimen. A thorough review of concomitant medications can help in designing a regimen that minimizes undesirable interactions. In addition, the potential for drug interactions should be assessed when any new drug (including over-the-counter agents), is added to an existing ARV combination. Most drug interactions with ARV drugs are mediated through inhibition or induction of hepatic drug metabolism.[1] The mechanisms of drug interactions with each ARV drug class are briefly summarized below. Tables 14 16c list significant drug interactions with different ARV agents and recommendations on contraindications, dose modifications, and alternative agents.

Non-Nucleoside Reverse Transcriptase Inhibitors (NNRTIs)

All NNRTIs are metabolized in the liver by cytochrome P450 (CYP) 3A isoenzymes. In addition, efavirenz (EFV) and nevirapine (NVP) are substrates of CYP2B6 enzymes, and etravirine (ETR) is a substrate of CYP2C9 and 2C19 enzymes. Concomitantly administered drugs that induce or inhibit these enzymes can alter NNRTI drug concentrations, resulting in virologic failure or adverse effects. All NNRTIs, except rilpivirine (RPV), induce or inhibit CYP isoenzymes. EFV acts as a mixed inducer and inhibitor, but like NVP, it primarily induces CYP3A and 2B6 enzymes. ETR also induces CYP3A but inhibits CYP2C9 and 2C19 enzymes. The inducing effects of NNRTIs can result in sub-therapeutic concentrations of concomitantly administered drugs that are metabolized by CYP enzymes. Examples of such interacting medications include azole antifungals, rifamycins, benzodiazepines, hepatitis C virus (HCV) protease inhibitors, HMG-CoA reductase inhibitors (statins), and methadone. See Table 15b for dosing recommendations.

Protease Inhibitors (PIs)

All PIs are metabolized in the liver by CYP3A isoenzymes; consequently their metabolic rates may be altered in the presence of CYP inducers or inhibitors. Co-administration of PIs with ritonavir (RTV), a potent CYP3A inhibitor, intentionally increases PI exposure (see Pharmacokinetic Enhancing below). Co-administration of PIs with a potent CYP3A inducer may lead to suboptimal drug concentrations and reduced therapeutic effects of the PI. These drug combinations should be avoided if alternative agents can be used. If this is not possible, close monitoring of plasma HIV RNA, with or without ARV dosage adjustment and therapeutic drug monitoring (TDM), may be warranted. For example, the rifamycins (i.e., rifampin and, to a lesser extent, rifabutin) are CYP3A4 inducers that can significantly reduce plasma concentrations of most PIs.[2, 3] Rifabutin is a less potent CYP3A4 inducer than rifampin. Therefore, despite wider experience with rifampin use, rifabutin is generally considered a reasonable alternative to rifampin for the treatment of tuberculosis when used with a PI-based regimen.[4, 5] Table 15a lists dosage recommendations for concomitant use of rifamycins and other CYP3A4 inducers with PIs.

Some PIs may also induce or inhibit CYP isoenzymes, P-glycoprotein, or other transporters in the gut and elsewhere. Tipranavir (TPV), for example, is a potent inducer of CYP3A4 and P-glycoprotein. The net effect of ritonavir-boosted tipranavir (TPV/r) on CYP3A *in vivo*, however, appears to be enzyme inhibition. Thus, concentrations of drugs that are substrates for only CYP3A are most likely to be increased if the drugs are given with TPV/r. The net effect of TPV/r on a drug that is a substrate of both CYP3A and P-glycoprotein (P-gp) cannot be confidently predicted. Significant decreases in saquinavir (SQV), amprenavir (APV), and lopinavir (LPV) concentrations have been observed *in vivo* when the PIs were given with TPV/r.

The use of a CYP3A substrate that has a narrow margin of safety in the presence of a potent CYP3A inhibitor, such as the PIs, may lead to markedly prolonged elimination half-life ($t_{1/2}$) and toxic drug accumulation. Avoidance of concomitant use or dose reduction of the affected drug, with close monitoring for dose-related toxicities, may be warranted.

The list of drugs that may have significant interactions with PIs is extensive and is continuously expanding. Some examples of these drugs include lipid-lowering agents (e.g., statins), benzodiazepines, calcium channel blockers, immunosuppressants (e.g., cyclosporine, tacrolimus), anticonvulsants, rifamycins, erectile dysfunction agents (e.g., sildenafil), ergot derivatives, azole antifungals, macrolides, oral contraceptives, methadone, and HCV protease inhibitors. Herbal products, such as St. John's wort, can also cause interactions that risk adverse clinical effects. See Table 15a for dosage recommendations.

Integrase Strand Transfer Inhibitors (INSTIs)

Raltegravir (RAL) is primarily eliminated by glucuronidation mediated by the uridine diphosphate (UDP)-glucuronosyltransferase (UGT) 1A1 enzymes. Strong inducers of UGT1A1 enzymes (e.g., rifampin) can significantly reduce the concentration of RAL.[6] See Table 15e for dosage recommendations. Raltegravir does not appear to affect CYP or UGT enzymes or P-glycoprotein-mediated transport.

Elvitegravir (EVG) is available only as a fixed dose combination with cobicistat (COBI), tenofovir (TDF), and emtricitabine (FTC). EVG is metabolized largely by CYP3A enzymes but also undergoes glucuronidation by UGT 1A1/3 enzymes. Co-administration of EVG with COBI, a CYP3A inhibitor, increases EVG exposure (see Pharmacokinetic Enhancing below). Drugs that induce or inhibit CYP3A enzymes can alter concentrations of EVG. The co-formulation of EVG/COBI/TDF/FTC should not be co-administered with other ARVs because of potential drug interactions that may alter drug levels of EVG, COBI, or the concomitant drug. Examples of interacting drugs include those listed above for NNRTIs and PIs. See Table 15e for dosage recommendations.

Nucleoside Reverse Transcriptase Inhibitors (NRTIs)

Unlike PIs, NNRTIs, EVG, and maraviroc (MVC), NRTIs do not undergo hepatic transformation through the CYP metabolic pathway. Significant pharmacodynamic interactions of NRTIs and other drugs, such as additive bone marrow suppressive effects of zidovudine (ZDV) and ganciclovir, have been reported. Pharmacokinetic (PK) interactions have also been reported; for example, atazanavir (ATV) concentration can be reduced when it is co-administered with TDF.[7] However, the mechanisms underlying some of these interactions are still unclear. Table 15c lists significant interactions with NRTIs.

CCR5 Antagonist

MVC is a substrate of CYP3A enzymes and P-glycoprotein. As a consequence, the concentrations of MVC can be significantly increased in the presence of strong CYP3A inhibitors (such as RTV and other PIs, except for TPV/r) and are reduced when MVC is used with CYP3A inducers (such as EFV or rifampin). Dose adjustment is necessary when MVC is used in combination with these agents (see Table 16b or Appendix B, Table 6 for dosage recommendations). MVC is neither an inducer nor an inhibitor of the CYP3A system and does not alter the PKs of the drugs evaluated in interaction studies to date.

Fusion Inhibitor

The fusion inhibitor enfuvirtide (T20) is a 36-amino-acid peptide that does not enter human cells. It is expected to undergo catabolism to its constituent amino acids with subsequent recycling of the amino acids in the body pool. No clinically significant drug-drug interaction with T20 has been identified to date.

Pharmacokinetic (PK) Enhancing

PK enhancing is a strategy used in ARV treatment to increase the exposure of an ARV by concomitantly administering a drug that inhibits the specific drug metabolizing enzymes for which the ARV is a substrate.

Currently two agents are used in clinical practice as PK enhancers: RTV and COBI.

RTV is an HIV PI that is primarily used in clinical practice at a lower than approved dose (100 to 400 mg per day) as a PK enhancer for other PIs because of its inhibitory effects on CYP450, predominately CYP3A4 and P-glycoprotein (P-gp). RTV increases the trough concentration (C_{min}) and prolongs the half-life of the active PIs.[8] The higher C_{min} allows for a greater C_{min}: inhibitory concentration ratio, which reduces the risk that drug resistance will develop as a result of suboptimal drug exposure. The longer half-life of the PI allows for less frequent dosing, which may enhance medication adherence. Because RTV is a potent inhibitor, it may result in complex drug-drug interactions when used with PIs and with other ARVs or non ARVs. Tables 15a and 16a_c list interactions between RTV-containing PI regimens and other medications, as well as comments on the clinical management of these interactions.

COBI is a specific, potent CYP3A inhibitor that has a weak to no effect on other CYP450 isoforms. COBI has no ARV activity. The high water solubility of COBI allows for its co-formulation with other agents.[9] COBI is currently available only as part of a fixed dose combination of EVG/COBI/TDF/FTC. COBI is used to increase the plasma concentrations of EVG, an INSTI. Like RTV, COBI has a complex drug-drug interaction profile. COBI also is an inhibitor of P-gp-mediated transport, which appears to be the mechanism by which COBI increases the systemic exposure to TDF. Table 15e lists interactions with COBI identified in PK studies conducted to date, projected interactions, and drugs that should not be co-administered with COBI.

When using RTV- or COBI-containing regimens, clinicians should be vigilant in assessing the potential for adverse drug-drug interactions. This is especially important when prescribing CYP3A substrates for which no PK data are available.

References

1. Piscitelli SC, Gallicano KD. Interactions among drugs for HIV and opportunistic infections. *N Engl J Med.* 2001;344(13):984-996. Available at http://www.ncbi.nlm.nih.gov/entrez/query.fcgi?cmd=Retrieve&db=PubMed&dopt=Citation&list_uids=11274626.

2. Baciewicz AM, Chrisman CR, Finch CK, Self TH. Update on rifampin and rifabutin drug interactions. *Am J Med Sci.* 2008;335(2):126-136. Available at http://www.ncbi.nlm.nih.gov/entrez/query.fcgi?cmd=Retrieve&db=PubMed&dopt=Citation&list_uids=18277121.

3. Spradling P, Drociuk D, McLaughlin S, et al. Drug-drug interactions in inmates treated for human immunodeficiency virus and Mycobacterium tuberculosis infection or disease: an institutional tuberculosis outbreak. *Clin Infect Dis.* 2002;35(9):1106-1112. Available at http://www.ncbi.nlm.nih.gov/entrez/query.fcgi?cmd=Retrieve&db=PubMed&dopt=Citation&list_uids=12384845.

4. Singh R, Marshall N, Smith CJ, et al. No impact of rifamycin selection on tuberculosis treatment outcome in HIV coinfected patients. *AIDS.* 2013;27(3):481-484. Available at http://www.ncbi.nlm.nih.gov/pubmed/23014518.

5. Blumberg HM, Burman WJ, Chaisson RE, et al. American Thoracic Society/Centers for Disease Control and Prevention/Infectious Diseases Society of America: treatment of tuberculosis. *Am J Respir Crit Care Med.* 2003;167(4):603-662. Available at http://www.ncbi.nlm.nih.gov/entrez/query.fcgi?cmd=Retrieve&db=PubMed&dopt=Citation&list_uids=12588714.

6. Wenning LA, Hanley WD, Brainard DM, et al. Effect of rifampin, a potent inducer of drug-metabolizing enzymes, on the pharmacokinetics of raltegravir. *Antimicrob Agents Chemother.* 2009;53(7):2852-2856. Available at http://www.ncbi.nlm.nih.gov/entrez/query.fcgi?cmd=Retrieve&db=PubMed&dopt=Citation&list_uids=19433563.

7. Taburet AM, Piketty C, Chazallon C, et al. Interactions between atazanavir-ritonavir and tenofovir in heavily pretreated human immunodeficiency virus-infected patients. *Antimicrob Agents Chemother.* 2004;48(6):2091-2096. Available at http://www.ncbi.nlm.nih.gov/entrez/query.fcgi?cmd=Retrieve&db=PubMed&dopt=Citation&list_uids=15155205.

8. Kempf DJ, Marsh KC, Kumar G, et al. Pharmacokinetic enhancement of inhibitors of the human immunodeficiency virus protease by co-administration with ritonavir. *Antimicrob Agents Chemother*. 1997;41(3):654-660. Available at http://www.ncbi.nlm.nih.gov/entrez/query.fcgi?cmd=Retrieve&db=PubMed&dopt=Citation&list_uids=9056009.

9. Xu L, Desai MC. Pharmacokinetic enhancers for HIV drugs. *Curr Opin Investig Drugs*. 2009;10(8):775-786. Available at http://www.ncbi.nlm.nih.gov/pubmed/19649922.

Table 14. Drugs That Should Not Be Used With Antiretroviral Agents (Last updated February 12, 2013; last reviewed February 12, 2013) (page 1 of 2)

This table only lists drugs that should not be co-administered at any dose and regardless of ritonavir (RTV) boosting. See Tables 15 and 16 for more detailed pharmacokinetic (PK) interaction data.

Antiretroviral Agents[a,b]	Cardiac Agents	Lipid-Lowering Agents	Antimyco-bacterials	Gastro-intestinal Drugs	Neuro-leptics	Psycho-tropics	Ergot Derivatives (vasoconstrictors)	Herbs	Anti-retroviral Agents	Others
							Drug Categories			
ATV +/– RTV	amiodarone dronedarone	lovastatin simvastatin	rifampin rifapentine[c]	cisapride[e]	pimozide	midazolam[f] triazolam	dihydroergotamine ergonovine ergotamine methylergonovine	St. John's wort	ETR NVP	alfuzosin irinotecan salmeterol sildenafil for PAH
DRV/r	amiodarone dronedarone	lovastatin simvastatin	rifampin rifapentine[c]	cisapride[e]	pimozide	midazolam[f] triazolam	dihydroergotamine ergonovine ergotamine methylergonovine	St. John's wort	none	alfuzosin salmeterol sildenafil for PAH
FPV +/– RTV	amiodarone dronedarone flecainide propafenone	lovastatin simvastatin	rifampin rifapentine[c]	cisapride[e]	pimozide	midazolam[f] triazolam	dihydroergotamine ergonovine ergotamine methylergonovine	St. John's wort	ETR	alfuzosin salmeterol sildenafil for PAH
LPV/r	amiodarone dronedarone	lovastatin simvastatin	rifampin[d] rifapentine[c]	cisapride[e]	pimozide	midazolam[f] triazolam	dihydroergotamine ergonovine ergotamine methylergonovine	St. John's wort	none	alfuzosin salmeterol sildenafil for PAH
SQV/r	amiodarone dronedarone dofetilide flecainide lidocaine propafenone quinidine	lovastatin simvastatin	rifampin[d] rifapentine[c]	cisapride[e]	pimozide	midazolam[f] triazolam trazodone	dihydroergotamine ergonovine ergotamine methylergonovine	St. John's wort garlic supple-ments	none	alfuzosin salmeterol sildenafil for PAH
TPV/r	amiodarone dronedarone flecainide propafenone quinidine	lovastatin simvastatin	rifampin rifapentine[c]	cisapride[e]	pimozide	midazolam[f] triazolam	dihydroergotamine ergonovine ergotamine methylergonovine	St. John's wort	ETR	alfuzosin salmeterol sildenafil for PAH
EFV	none	none	rifapentine[c]	cisapride[e]	pimozide	midazolam[f] triazolam	dihydroergotamine ergonovine ergotamine methylergonovine	St. John's wort	other NNRTIs	none
ETR	none	none	rifampin rifapentine[c]	none	none	none	none	St John's wort	unboosted PIs ATV/r, FPV/r, or TPV/r other NNRTIs	carbamazepine phenobarbital phenytoin clopidogrel

Table 14. Drugs That Should Not Be Used With Antiretroviral Agents (Last updated February 12, 2013; last reviewed February 12, 2013) (page 2 of 2)

					Drug Categories					
Antiretroviral Agents[a,b]	Cardiac Agents	Lipid-Lowering Agents	Antimyco-bacterials	Gastro-intestinal Drugs	Neuro-leptics	Psycho-tropics	Ergot Derivatives (vasoconstrictors)	Herbs	Anti-retroviral Agents	Others
NVP	none	none	rifapentine[c]	none	none	none	none	St. John's wort	ATV +/− RTV other NNRTIs	ketoconazole
RPV	none	none	rifabutin rifampin rifapentine[c]	proton pump inhibitors	none	none	none	St. John's wort	other NNRTIs	carbamazepine oxcarbazepine phenobarbital phenytoin
MVC	none	none	rifapentine[c]	none	none	none	none	St. John's wort	none	none
EVG/COBI/ TDF/FTC	none	lovastatin simvastatin	rifabutin rifampin rifapentine[c]	cisapride[e]	pimozide	midazolam[f] triazolam	dihydroergotamine ergotamine methylergonovine	St. John's wort	All other ARVs	alfuzosin sildenafil for PAH

[a] DLV, IDV, NFV, and RTV (as sole PI) are not included in this table. Refer to the appropriate FDA package insert for information regarding DLV-, IDV-, NFV-, and RTV (as sole PI)-related drug interactions.

[b] Certain listed drugs are contraindicated on the basis of theoretical considerations. Thus, drugs with narrow therapeutic indices and suspected metabolic involvement with CYP450 3A, 2D6, or unknown pathways are included in this table. Actual interactions may or may not occur in patients.

[c] HIV-infected patients treated with rifapentine have a higher rate of tuberculosis (TB) relapse than those treated with other rifamycin-based regimens. Therefore an alternative agent to rifapentine is recommended.

[d] A high rate of Grade 4 serum transaminase elevation was seen when a higher dose of RTV was added to LPV/r or SQV or when double-dose LPV/r was used with rifampin to compensate for rifampin's induction effect and therefore, these dosing strategies should not be used.

[e] The manufacturer of cisapride has a limited-access protocol for patients who meet specific clinical eligibility criteria.

[f] Use of oral midazolam is contraindicated. Parenteral midazolam can be used with caution as a single dose and can be given in a monitored situation for procedural sedation.

Suggested alternatives to:

• **Lovastatin, simvastatin:** Fluvastatin, pitavastatin, and pravastatin (except for pravastatin with DRV/r) have the least potential for drug-drug interactions (see Table 15a). Use atorvastatin and rosuvastatin with caution; start with the lowest possible dose and titrate based on tolerance and lipid-lowering efficacy.

• **Rifampin:** Rifabutin (with dosage adjustment, see Tables 15a and 15b)

• **Midazolam, triazolam:** temazepam, lorazepam, oxazepam

Key to Abbreviations: ATV +/- RTV = atazanavir +/- ritonavir, ATV/r = atazanavir/ritonavir, COBI = cobicistat, CYP = cytochrome P, DLV = delavirdine, DRV/r = darunavir/ritonavir, EFV = efavirenz, ETR = etravirine, EVG = elvitegravir, FDA = Food and Drug Administration, FPV +/- RTV = fosamprenavir +/- ritonavir, FPV/r = fosamprenavir/ritonavir, IDV = indinavir, LPV/r = lopinavir/ritonavir, MVC = maraviroc, NFV = nelfinavir, NNRTI = non-nucleoside reverse transcriptase inhibitor, NVP = nevirapine, PAH = pulmonary arterial hypertension, PI = protease inhibitor, PK = pharmacokinetic, RPV = rilpivirine, RTV = ritonavir, SQV = saquinavir, SQV/r = saquinavir/ritonavir, TB = tuberculosis, TPV/r = tipranavir/ritonavir

Table 15a. Drug Interactions between Protease Inhibitors (PI)* and Other Drugs (Last updated February 12, 2013; last reviewed February 12, 2013) (page 1 of 10)

This table provides information relating to pharmacokinetic (PK) interactions between PIs and non-antiretroviral (ARV) drugs. When information is available, interactions with boosted and unboosted PIs are listed separately. For interactions between ARV agents and for dosing recommendations, refer to Table 16a.

* Nelfinavir (NFV) and indinavir (IDV) are not included in this table. Please refer to the NFV and IDV FDA package inserts for information regarding drug interactions with these PIs.

Concomitant Drug	PI	Effect on PI or Concomitant Drug Concentrations	Dosing Recommendations and Clinical Comments
Acid Reducers			
Antacids	ATV, ATV/r	When given simultaneously, ↓ ATV expected	Give ATV at least 2 hours before or 1 hour after antacids or buffered medications.
	FPV	APV AUC ↓ 18%; no significant change in APV C$_{min}$	Give FPV simultaneously with (or at least 2 hours before or 1 hour after) antacids.
	TPV/r	TPV AUC ↓ 27%	Give TPV at least 2 hours before or 1 hour after antacids.
H2 Receptor Antagonists	**RTV-boosted PIs**		
	ATV/r	↓ ATV	H2 receptor antagonist dose should not exceed a dose equivalent to famotidine 40 mg BID in ART-naive patients or 20 mg BID in ART-experienced patients. Give ATV 300 mg + RTV 100 mg simultaneously with and/or ≥10 hours after the H2 receptor antagonist. If using TDF and H2 receptor antagonist in ART-experienced patients, use ATV 400 mg + RTV 100 mg.
	DRV/r, LPV/r	No significant effect	No dosage adjustment necessary.
	PIs without RTV		
	ATV	↓ ATV	H2 receptor antagonist single dose should not exceed a dose equivalent of famotidine 20 mg or total daily dose equivalent of famotidine 20 mg BID in ART-naive patients. Give ATV at least 2 hours before and at least 10 hours after the H2 receptor antagonist.
	FPV	APV AUC ↓ 30%; no significant change in APV C$_{min}$	If concomitant use is necessary, give FPV at least 2 hours before H2 receptor antagonist. Consider boosting FPV with RTV.
Proton Pump Inhibitors (PPIs)	ATV	↓ ATV	**PPIs are not recommended in patients receiving unboosted ATV.** In these patients, consider alternative acid-reducing agents, RTV boosting, or alternative PIs.
	ATV/r	↓ ATV	PPIs should not exceed a dose equivalent to omeprazole 20 mg daily in PI-naive patients. PPIs should be administered at least 12 hours before ATV/r. **PPIs are not recommended in PI-experienced patients.**
	DRV/r, TPV/r	↓ omeprazole PI: no significant effect	May need to increase omeprazole dose when using TPV/r.
	FPV, FPV/r, LPV/r	No significant effect	No dosage adjustment necessary.
	SQV/r	SQV AUC ↑ 82%	Monitor for SQV toxicities.

Table 15a. Drug Interactions between Protease Inhibitors (PI)* and Other Drugs (Last updated February 12, 2013; last reviewed February 12, 2013) (page 2 of 10)

Concomitant Drug	PI	Effect on PI or Concomitant Drug Concentrations	Dosing Recommendations and Clinical Comments
Anticoagulants			
Warfarin	ATV, ATV/r, DRV/r, FPV, FPV/r, LPV/r, SQV/r, TPV/r	↑ or ↓ warfarin possible DRV/r ↓ S-warfarin AUC 21%	Monitor INR closely when stopping or starting PI and adjust warfarin dose accordingly.
Rivaroxaban	All PIs	↑ rivaroxaban	Avoid concomitant use. Co-administration is expected to result in increased exposure of rivaroxaban which may lead to risk of increased bleeding.
Anticonvulsants			
Carbamazepine	**RTV-boosted PIs**		
	ATV/r, FPV/r, LPV/r, SQV/r, TPV/r	↑ carbamazepine possible TPV/r ↑ carbamazepine AUC 26% May ↓ PI levels substantially	Consider alternative anticonvulsant or monitor levels of both drugs and assess virologic response. **Do not co-administer with LPV/r once daily.**
	DRV/r	carbamazepine AUC ↑ 45% DRV: no significant change	Monitor anticonvulsant level and adjust dose accordingly.
	PIs without RTV		
	ATV, FPV	May ↓ PI levels substantially	Monitor anticonvulsant level and virologic response. Consider alternative anticonvulsant, RTV boosting for ATV and FPV, and/or monitoring PI level.
Lamotrigine	LPV/r	lamotrigine AUC ↓ 50% LPV: no significant change	A dose increase of lamotrigine may be needed and therapeutic concentration monitoring for lamotrigine may be indicated; particularly during dosage adjustment or consider alternative anticonvulsant. A similar interaction is possible with other RTV-boosted PIs.
Phenobarbital	All PIs	May ↓ PI levels substantially	Consider alternative anticonvulsant or monitor levels of both drugs and assess virologic response. **Do not co-administer with LPV/r once daily.**
Phenytoin	**RTV-boosted PIs**		
	ATV/r, DRV/r, SQV/r, TPV/r	↓ phenytoin possible ↓ PI possible	Consider alternative anticonvulsant or monitor levels of both drugs and assess virologic response.
	FPV/r	phenytoin AUC ↓ 22% APV AUC ↑ 20%	Monitor phenytoin level and adjust dose accordingly. No change in FPV/r dose recommended.
	LPV/r	phenytoin AUC ↓ 31% LPV/r AUC ↓ 33%	Consider alternative anticonvulsant or monitor levels of both drugs and assess virologic response. **Do not co-administer with LPV/r once daily.**
	PIs without RTV		
	ATV, FPV	May ↓ PI levels substantially	Consider alternative anticonvulsant, RTV boosting for ATV and FPV, and/or monitoring PI level. Monitor anticonvulsant level and virologic response.
Valproic Acid (VPA)	LPV/r	↓ or ⇔ VPA possible LPV AUC ↑ 75%	Monitor VPA levels and virologic response. Monitor for LPV-related toxicities.

Table 15a. Drug Interactions between Protease Inhibitors (PI)* and Other Drugs (Last updated February 12, 2013; last reviewed February 12, 2013) (page 3 of 10)

Concomitant Drug	PI	Effect on PI or Concomitant Drug Concentrations	Dosing Recommendations and Clinical Comments
Antidepressants			
Bupropion	LPV/r	bupropion AUC ↓ 57%	Titrate bupropion dose based on clinical response.
	TPV/r	bupropion AUC ↓ 46%	
Paroxetine	DRV/r	paroxetine AUC ↓ 39%	Titrate paroxetine dose based on clinical response.
	FPV/r	paroxetine AUC ↓ 55%	
Sertraline	DRV/r	sertraline AUC ↓ 49%	Titrate sertraline dose based on clinical response.
Trazodone	ATV/r, ATV, DRV/r, FPV/r, FPV, LPV/r, TPV/r	RTV 200 mg BID (for 2 days) ↑ trazodone AUC 240%	Use lowest dose of trazodone and monitor for CNS and cardiovascular adverse effects.
	SQV/r	↑ trazodone expected	**Contraindicated. Do not co-administer.**
Tricyclic Antidepressants (TCAs) (Amitriptyline, Desipramine, Imipramine, Nortriptyline)	All RTV-boosted PIs	↑ TCA expected	Use lowest possible TCA dose and titrate based on clinical assessment and/or drug levels.
Antifungals			
Fluconazole	**RTV-boosted PIs**		
	ATV/r	No significant effect	No dosage adjustment necessary.
	SQV/r	No data with RTV boosting SQV (1200 mg TID) AUC ↑ 50%	No dosage adjustment necessary.
	TPV/r	TPV AUC ↑ 50%	Fluconazole >200 mg daily is not recommended. If high-dose fluconazole is indicated, consider alternative PI or another class of ARV drug.
Itraconazole	**RTV-boosted PIs**		
	ATV/r, DRV/r, FPV/r, TPV/r	↑ itraconazole possible ↑ PI possible	Consider monitoring itraconazole level to guide dosage adjustments. High doses (>200 mg/day) are not recommended unless dose is guided by itraconazole levels.
	LPV/r	↑ itraconazole	Consider monitoring itraconazole level to guide dosage adjustments. High doses (>200 mg/day) are not recommended unless dose is guided by itraconazole levels
	SQV/r	Bidirectional interaction has been observed	Dose not established, but decreased itraconazole dosage may be warranted. Consider monitoring itraconazole level.
	PIs without RTV		
	ATV, FPV	↑ itraconazole possible ↑ PI possible	Consider monitoring itraconazole level to guide dosage adjustments.

Guidelines for the Use of Antiretroviral Agents in HIV-1-Infected Adults and Adolescents

Concomitant Drug	PI	Effect on PI or Concomitant Drug Concentrations	Dosing Recommendations and Clinical Comments
Antifungals, continued			
Posaconazole	ATV/r	ATV AUC ↑ 146%	Monitor for adverse effects of ATV.
	ATV	ATV AUC ↑ 268%	Monitor for adverse effects of ATV.
	FPV	FPV (1400 mg BID) ↓ posaconazole AUC 23%; (compared with FPV/RTV 700 mg/100 mg) APV AUC ↓ 65%	**Do not co-administer.**
Voriconazole	**RTV-boosted PIs**		
	All RTV-boosted PIs	RTV 400 mg BID ↓ voriconazole AUC 82% RTV 100 mg BID ↓ voriconazole AUC 39%	**Do not co-administer** voriconazole and RTV unless benefit outweighs risk. If administered, consider monitoring voriconazole level and adjust dose accordingly.
	PIs without RTV		
	ATV, FPV	↑ voriconazole possible ↑ PI possible	Monitor for toxicities.
Antimycobacterials			
Clarithromycin	ATV/r, ATV	clarithromycin AUC ↑ 94%	May cause QTc prolongation. Reduce clarithromycin dose by 50%. Consider alternative therapy (e.g., azithromycin).
	DRV/r, FPV/r, LPV/r, SQV/r, TPV/r	DRV/r ↑ clarithromycin AUC 57% FPV/r ↑ clarithromycin possible LPV/r ↑ clarithromycin expected RTV 500 mg BID ↑ clarithromycin 77% SQV unboosted ↑ clarithromycin 45% TPV/r ↑ clarithromycin 19% clarithromycin ↑ unboosted SQV 177% clarithromycin ↑ TPV 66%	Monitor for clarithromycin-related toxicities or consider alternative macrolide (e.g., azithromycin). Reduce clarithromycin dose by 50% in patients with CrCl 30–60 mL/min. Reduce clarithromycin dose by 75% in patients with CrCl <30 mL/min.
	FPV	APV AUC ↑ 18%	No dosage adjustment necessary.
Rifabutin	**RTV-boosted PIs**		
	ATV/r	rifabutin (150 mg once daily) AUC ↑ 110% and metabolite AUC ↑ 2,101% compared with rifabutin (300 mg daily) administered alone	Rifabutin 150 mg once daily or 300 mg three times a week. Monitor for antimycobacterial activity and consider therapeutic drug monitoring. PK data reported in this table are results from healthy volunteer studies. Lower rifabutin exposure has been reported in HIV-infected patients than in the healthy study participants.
	DRV/r	rifabutin (150 mg every other day) AUC not significantly changed and metabolite AUC ↑ 881% compared with rifabutin (300 mg once daily) administered alone	
	FPV/r	rifabutin (150 mg every other day) and metabolite AUC ↑ 64% compared with rifabutin (300 mg once daily) administered alone	
	LPV/r	rifabutin (150 mg once daily) and metabolite AUC ↑ 473% compared with rifabutin (300 mg daily) administered alone	
	SQV/r	↑ rifabutin with unboosted SQV	
	TPV/r	rifabutin (150 mg x 1 dose) and metabolite AUC ↑ 333%	

Concomitant Drug	PI	Effect on PI or Concomitant Drug Concentrations	Dosing Recommendations and Clinical Comments
Antimycobacterials, continued			
Rifabutin, continued	**PIs without RTV**		
	ATV, FPV	↑ rifabutin AUC expected	Rifabutin 150 mg daily or 300 mg three times a week
Rifampin	All PIs	↓ PI conc. by >75%	**Do not co-administer rifampin and PIs.** Additional RTV does not overcome this interaction and increases hepatotoxicity.
Rifapentine	All PIs	↓ PI expected	**Do not co-administer rifapentine and PIs.**
Benzodiazepines			
Alprazolam Diazepam	All PIs	↑ benzodiazepine possible RTV (200 mg BID for 2 days) ↑ alprazolam half-life 222% and AUC 248%	Consider alternative benzodiazepines such as lorazepam, oxazepam, or temazepam.
Lorazepam Oxazepam Temazepam	All PIs	No data	These benzodiazepines are metabolized via non-CYP450 pathways; there is less interaction potential than with other benzodiazepines.
Midazolam	All PIs	↑ midazolam expected SQV/r ↑ midazolam (oral) AUC 1,144% and C$_{max}$ 327%	**Do not co-administer oral midazolam and PIs.** Parenteral midazolam can be used with caution when given as a single dose in a monitored situation for procedural sedation.
Triazolam	All PIs	↑ triazolam expected RTV (200 mg BID) ↑ triazolam half-life 1,200% and AUC 2,000%	**Do not co-administer triazolam and PIs.**
Cardiac Medications			
Bosentan	All PIs	LPV/r ↑ bosentan 48-fold (day 4) and 5-fold (day 10) ↓ ATV expected	**Do not co-administer bosentan and ATV without RTV.** In patients on a PI (other than unboosted ATV) >10 days: Start bosentan at 62.5 mg once daily or every other day. In patients on bosentan who require a PI (other than unboosted ATV): Stop bosentan ≥36 hours before PI initiation and restart 10 days after PI initiation at 62.5 mg once daily or every other day.
Digoxin	RTV, SQV/r	RTV (200 mg BID) ↑ digoxin AUC 29% and half-life 43% SQV/r ↑ digoxin AUC 49%	Use with caution. Monitor digoxin levels. Digoxin dose may need to be decreased.
Dihydropyridine Calcium Channel Blockers (CCBs)	All PIs	↑ dihydropyridine possible	Use with caution. Titrate CCB dose and monitor closely. ECG monitoring is recommended when CCB used with ATV.
Diltiazem	ATV/r, ATV	diltiazem AUC ↑ 125%	Decrease diltiazem dose by 50%. ECG monitoring is recommended.
	DRV/r, FPV/r, FPV LPV/r, SQV/r, TPV/r	↑ diltiazem possible	Use with caution. Adjust diltiazem according to clinical response and toxicities.

Concomitant Drug	PI	Effect on PI or Concomitant Drug Concentrations	Dosing Recommendations and Clinical Comments
Corticosteroids			
Budesonide (systemic)	All PIs	↓ PI levels possible ↑ glucocorticoids	Use with caution. Co-administration can result in adrenal insufficiency, including Cushing's syndrome. **Do not co-administer unless potential benefits of systemic budesonide outweigh the risks of systemic corticosteroid adverse effects.**
Budesonide (inhaled or intranasal)	All RTV-boosted PIs	↑ glucocorticoids	Use with caution. Co-administration can result in adrenal insufficiency, including Cushing's syndrome. **Do not co-administer unless potential benefits of inhaled or intranasal budesonide outweigh the risks of systemic corticosteroid adverse effects.**
Dexamethasone	All PIs	↓ PI levels possible	Use systemic dexamethasone with caution or consider alternative corticosteroid for long-term use.
Fluticasone (inhaled or intranasal)	All RTV-boosted PIs	RTV 100 mg BID ↑ fluticasone AUC 350-fold and ↑ C_{max} 25-fold	Co-administration can result in adrenal insufficiency, including Cushing's syndrome. **Do not co-administer unless potential benefits of inhaled fluticasone outweigh the risks of systemic corticosteroid adverse effects.**
Prednisone	LPV/r	↑ prednisolone AUC 31% ↓ lopinavir	Use with caution. Co-administration can result in adrenal insufficiency, including Cushing's syndrome. **Do not co-administer unless potential benefits of prednisone outweigh the risks of systemic corticosteroid adverse effects.**
Hepatitis C NS3/4A Protease Inhibitors			
Boceprevir	ATV/r	ATV AUC ↓ 35%, C_{min} ↓ 49% RTV AUC ↓ 36% boceprevir AUC ⇔	**Co-administration is not recommended.**
	DRV/r	DRV AUC ↓ 44%, C_{min} ↓ 59% RTV AUC ↓ 26% boceprevir AUC ↓ 32%, C_{min} ↓ 35%	**Co-administration is not recommended.**
	LPV/r	LPV AUC ↓ 34%, C_{min} ↓ 43% RTV AUC ↓ 22% boceprevir AUC ↓ 45%, C_{min} ↓ 57%	**Co-administration is not recommended.**
Telaprevir	ATV/r	telaprevir AUC ↓ 20%	No dose adjustment necessary.
	DRV/r	telaprevir AUC ↓ 35% DRV AUC ↓ 40%	**Co-administration is not recommended.**
	FPV/r	telaprevir AUC ↓ 32% APV AUC ↓ 47%	**Co-administration is not recommended.**
	LPV/r	telaprevir AUC ↓ 54% LPV: no significant change	**Co-administration is not recommended.**

Concomitant Drug	PI	Effect on PI or Concomitant Drug Concentrations	Dosing Recommendations and Clinical Comments
Herbal Products			
St. John's Wort	All PIs	↓ PI expected	**Do not co-administer.**
Hormonal Contraceptives			
Hormonal Contraceptives	**RTV-boosted PIs**		
	ATV/r	ethinyl estradiol AUC ↓ 19% and C_{min} ↓ 37% norgestimate ↑ 85%	Oral contraceptive should contain at least 35 mcg of ethinyl estradiol. Oral contraceptives containing progestins other than norethindrone or norgestimate have not been studied.[a]
	DRV/r	ethinyl estradiol AUC ↓ 44% norethindrone AUC ↓ 14%	Use alternative or additional contraceptive method.
	FPV/r	ethinyl estradiol AUC ↓ 37% norethindrone AUC ↓ 34%	Use alternative or additional contraceptive method.
	LPV/r	ethinyl estradiol AUC ↓ 42% norethindrone AUC ↓ 17%	Use alternative or additional contraceptive method.
	SQV/r	↓ ethinyl estradiol	Use alternative or additional contraceptive method.
	TPV/r	ethinyl estradiol AUC ↓ 48% norethindrone: no significant change	Use alternative or additional contraceptive method.
	PIs without RTV		
	ATV	ethinyl estradiol AUC ↑ 48% norethindrone AUC ↑ 110%	Use oral contraceptive that contains no more than 30 mcg of ethinyl estradiol or use alternative contraceptive method. Oral contraceptives containing less than 25 mcg of ethinyl estradiol or progestins other than norethindrone or norgestimate have not been studied.[b]
	FPV	With APV: ↑ ethinyl estradiol and ↑ norethindrone C_{min}; APV C_{min} ↓ 20%	Use alternative contraceptive method.
HMG-CoA Reductase Inhibitors			
Atorvastatin	ATV/r, ATV	↑ atorvastatin possible	Titrate atorvastatin dose carefully and use lowest dose necessary.
	DRV/r FPV/r, FPV, SQV/r	DRV/r + atorvastatin 10 mg similar to atorvastatin 40 mg administered alone; FPV +/– RTV ↑ atorvastatin AUC 130%–153%; SQV/r ↑ atorvastatin AUC 79%	Titrate atorvastatin dose carefully and use the lowest necessary dose. Do not exceed 20 mg atorvastatin daily.
	LPV/r	LPV/r ↑ atorvastatin AUC 488%	Use with caution and use the lowest atorvastatin dose necessary.
	TPV/r	↑ atorvastatin AUC 836%	**Do not co-administer.**
Lovastatin	All PIs	Significant ↑ lovastatin expected	**Contraindicated. Do not co-administer.**
Pitavastatin	All PIs	ATV ↑ pitavastatin AUC 31% and C_{max} ↑ 60% ATV: no significant effect LPV/r ↓ pitavastatin AUC 20% LPV: no significant effect	No dose adjustment necessary.

Concomitant Drug	PI	Effect on PI or Concomitant Drug Concentrations	Dosing Recommendations and Clinical Comments
HMG-CoA Reductase Inhibitors, continued			
Pravastatin	DRV/r	pravastatin AUC ↑ 81%	Use lowest possible starting dose of pravastatin with careful monitoring.
	LPV/r	pravastatin AUC ↑ 33%	No dose adjustment necessary.
	SQV/r	pravastatin AUC ↓ 47%–50%	No dose adjustment necessary.
Rosuvastatin	ATV/r, LPV/r	ATV/r ↑ rosuvastatin AUC 3-fold and C_{max} ↑ 7-fold LPV/r ↑ rosuvastatin AUC 108% and C_{max} ↑ 366%	Titrate rosuvastatin dose carefully and use the lowest necessary dose. Do not exceed 10 mg rosuvastatin daily.
	DRV/r	rosuvastatin AUC ↑ 48% and C_{max} ↑ 139%	Titrate rosuvastatin dose carefully and use the lowest necessary dose while monitoring for toxicities.
	FPV +/- RTV	No significant effect on rosuvastatin	No dosage adjustment necessary.
	SQV/r	No data available	Titrate rosuvastatin dose carefully and use the lowest necessary dose while monitoring for toxicities.
	TPV/r	rosuvastatin AUC ↑ 26% and C_{max} ↑ 123%	No dosage adjustment necessary.
Simvastatin	All PIs	Significant ↑ simvastatin level; SQV/r 400 mg/400 mg BID ↑ simvastatin AUC 3,059%	**Contraindicated. Do not co-administer.**
Immunosuppressants			
Cyclosporine Sirolimus Tacrolimus	All PIs	↑ immunosuppressant possible	Initiate with an adjusted dose of immunosuppressant to account for potential increased concentrations of the immunosuppressant and monitor for toxicities. Therapeutic drug monitoring of immunosuppressant is recommended. Consult with specialist as necessary.
Narcotics/Treatment for Opioid Dependence			
Buprenorphine	ATV	buprenorphine AUC ↑ 93% norbuprenorphine[c] AUC ↑ 76% ↓ ATV possible	**Do not co-administer buprenorphine with unboosted ATV.**
	ATV/r	buprenorphine AUC ↑ 66% norbuprenorphine[c] AUC ↑ 105%	Monitor for sedation. Buprenorphine dose reduction may be necessary.
	DRV/r	buprenorphine: no significant effect norbuprenorphine[c] AUC ↑ 46% and C_{min} ↑ 71%	No dosage adjustment necessary. Clinical monitoring is recommended.
	FPV/r	buprenorphine: no significant effect norbuprenorphine[c] AUC ↓ 15%	No dosage adjustment necessary. Clinical monitoring is recommended.
	LPV/r	No significant effect	No dosage adjustment necessary.
	TPV/r	buprenorphine: no significant effect norbuprenorphine[c] AUC, C_{max}, and C_{min} ↓ 80% TPV C_{min} ↓ 19%–40%	Consider monitoring TPV level.

Concomitant Drug	PI	Effect on PI or Concomitant Drug Concentrations	Dosing Recommendations and Clinical Comments
Narcotics/Treatment for Opioid Dependence, continued			
Oxycodone	LPV/r	oxycodone AUC ↑ 2.6 fold	Monitor for opioid-related adverse effects. Oxycodone dose reduction may be necessary.
Methadone	**RTV-boosted PIs**		
	ATV/r, DRV/r, FPV/r, LPV/r, SQV/r, TPV/r	ATV/r, DRV/r, FPV/r ↓ R-methadone[d] AUC 16%–18%; LPV/r ↓ methadone AUC 26%–53%; SQV/r 1000/100 mg BID ↓ R-methadone[d] AUC 19%; TPV/r ↓ R-methadone[d] AUC 48%	Opioid withdrawal unlikely but may occur. Dosage adjustment of methadone is not usually required, but monitor for opioid withdrawal and increase methadone dose as clinically indicated.
	PIs without RTV		
	ATV	No significant effect	No dosage adjustment necessary.
	FPV	No data with unboosted FPV APV ↓ R-methadone[d] C_{min} 21%, AUC no significant change	Monitor and titrate methadone as clinically indicated. The interaction with FPV is presumed to be similar.
Phosphodiesterase Type 5 (PDE5) Inhibitors			
Avanafil	ATV, ATV/r, DRV/r, FPV/r, SQV/r, LPV/r	RTV (600 mg BID x 5 days) ↑ avanafil AUC 13-fold, C_{max} 2.4-fold	**Co-administration is not recommended.**
	FPV	No data	Avanafil dose should not exceed 50 mg once every 24 hours.
Sildenafil	All PIs	DRV/r + sildenafil 25 mg similar to sildenafil 100 mg alone; RTV 500 mg BID ↑ sildenafil AUC 1,000%; SQV unboosted ↑ sildenafil AUC 210%	<u>For treatment of erectile dysfunction</u> Start with sildenafil 25 mg every 48 hours and monitor for adverse effects of sildenafil. <u>For treatment of PAH</u> **Contraindicated**
Tadalafil	All PIs	RTV 200 mg BID ↑ tadalafil AUC 124%; TPV/r (1st dose) ↑ tadalafil AUC 133%; TPV/r steady state: no significant effect	<u>For treatment of erectile dysfunction</u> Start with tadalafil 5-mg dose and do not exceed a single dose of 10 mg every 72 hours. Monitor for adverse effects of tadalafil. <u>For treatment of PAH</u> *In patients on a PI >7 days:* Start with tadalafil 20 mg once daily and increase to 40 mg once daily based on tolerability. *In patients on tadalafil who require a PI:* Stop tadalafil ≥24 hours prior to PI initiation, restart 7 days after PI initiation at 20 mg once daily, and increase to 40 mg once daily based on tolerability. <u>For treatment of benign prostatic hyperplasia</u> Maximum recommended daily dose is 2.5 mg per day

Concomitant Drug	PI	Effect on PI or Concomitant Drug Concentrations	Dosing Recommendations and Clinical Comments
Phosphodiesterase Type 5 (PDE5) Inhibitors, continued			
Vardenafil	All PIs	RTV 600 mg BID ↑ vardenafil AUC 49-fold	Start with vardenafil 2.5 mg every 72 hours and monitor for adverse effects of vardenafil.
Miscellaneous Interactions			
Colchicine	All PIs	RTV 100 mg BID ↑ colchicine AUC 296%, C_{max} 184% With all PIs: significant ↑ in colchicine AUC expected	<u>For treatment of gout flares</u> Colchicine 0.6 mg x 1 dose, followed by 0.3 mg 1 hour later. Do not repeat dose for at least 3 days. *With FPV without RTV:* 1.2 mg x 1 dose and no repeat dose for at least 3 days <u>For prophylaxis of gout flares</u> Colchicine 0.3 mg once daily or every other day *With FPV without RTV:* colchicine 0.3 mg BID or 0.6 mg once daily or 0.3 mg once daily <u>For treatment of familial Mediterranean fever</u> Do not exceed colchicine 0.6 mg once daily or 0.3 mg BID. *With FPV without RTV:* Do not exceed 1.2 mg once daily or 0.6 mg BID. **Do not co-administer in patients with hepatic or renal impairment.**
Salmeterol	All PIs	↑ salmeterol possible	**Do not co-administer** because of potential increased risk of salmeterol-associated cardiovascular events.
Atovaquone/ proguanil	ATV/r, LPV/r	ATV/r ↓ atovaquone AUC 46% and ↓ proguanil AUC 41% LPV/r ↓ atovaquone AUC 74% and ↓ proguanil AUC 38%	No dosage recommendation. Consider alternative drug for malaria prophylaxis, if possible.

[a] The following products contain at least 35 mcg of ethinyl estradiol combined with norethindrone or norgestimate (generic formulation may also be available): Ovcon 35, 50; Femcon Fe; Brevicon; Modicon; Ortho-Novum 1/35, 10/11, 7/7/7; Norinyl 1/35; Tri-Norinyl; Ortho-Cyclen; Ortho Tri-Cyclen.

[b] The following products contain no more than 30 mcg of ethinyl estradiol combined with norethindrone or norgestimate (generic formulation may also be available): Loestrin 1/20, 1.5/30; Loestrin Fe 1/20, 1.5/30; Loestrin 24 Fe; Ortho Tri-Cyclen Lo.

[c] Norbuprenorphine is an active metabolite of buprenorphine.

[d] R-methadone is the active form of methadone.

Acronyms: APV = amprenavir, ART = antiretroviral therapy, ARV = antiretroviral, ATV = atazanavir, ATV/r = atazanavir + ritonavir, AUC = area under the curve, BID = twice daily, CCB = calcium channel blocker, C_{max} = maximum plasma concentration, C_{min} = minimum plasma concentration, CNS = central nervous system, CrCl = creatinine clearance, CYP = cytochrome P, DRV = darunavir, DRV/r = darunavir + ritonavir, ECG = electrocardiogram, FDA = Food and Drug Administration, FPV = fosamprenavir (FPV is a pro-drug of APV), FPV/r = fosamprenavir + ritonavir, IDV = indinavir, INR = international normalized ratio, LPV = lopinavir, LPV/r = lopinavir + ritonavir, NFV = nelfinavir, PAH = pulmonary arterial hypertension, PDE5 = phosphodiesterase type 5, PI = protease inhibitor, PK = pharmacokinetic, PPI = proton pump inhibitor, RTV = ritonavir, SQV = saquinavir, SQV/r = saquinavir + ritonavir, TCA = tricyclic antidepressant, TDF = tenofovir disoproxil fumarate, TID = three times a day, TPV = tipranavir, TPV/r = tipranavir + ritonavir, VPA = valproic acid

This table provides information relating to pharmacokinetic (PK) interactions between non-nucleoside reverse transcriptase inhibitors (NNRTIs) and non-antiretroviral (ARV) drugs. For interactions between ARV agents and for dosing recommendations, refer to Table 16b.

* Delavirdine (DLV) is not included in this table. Please refer to the DLV Food and Drug Administration package insert for information regarding drug interactions.

Concomitant Drug Class/Name	NNRTI[a]	Effect on NNRTI or Concomitant Drug Concentrations	Dosing Recommendations and Clinical Comments
Acid Reducers			
Antacids	RPV	↓ RPV expected when given simultaneously	Give antacids at least 2 hours before or at least 4 hours after RPV.
H2-Receptor Antagonists	RPV	↓ RPV	Give H2-receptor antagonists at least 12 hours before or at least 4 hours after RPV.
Proton Pump Inhibitors (PPI)	RPV	↓ RPV	**Contraindicated. Do not co-administer.**
Anticoagulants/Antiplatelets			
Warfarin	EFV, NVP	↑ or ↓ warfarin possible	Monitor INR and adjust warfarin dose accordingly.
	ETR	↑ warfarin possible	Monitor INR and adjust warfarin dose accordingly.
Clopidogrel	ETR	↓ activation of clopidogrel possible	ETR may prevent metabolism of clopidogrel (inactive) to its active metabolite. Avoid co-administration, if possible.
Anticonvulsants			
Carbamazepine Phenobarbital Phenytoin	EFV	carbamazepine + EFV: carbamazepine AUC ↓ 27% and EFV AUC ↓ 36% phenytoin + EFV: ↓ EFV and ↓ phenytoin possible	Monitor anticonvulsant and EFV levels or, if possible, use alternative anticonvulsant to those listed.
	ETR	↓ anticonvulsant and ETR possible	**Do not co-administer.** Consider alternative anticonvulsant.
	NVP	↓ anticonvulsant and NVP possible	Monitor anticonvulsant and NVP levels and virologic responses or consider alternative anticonvulsant.
	RPV	↓ RPV possible	**Contraindicated. Do not co-administer.** Consider alternative anticonvulsant.
Antidepressants			
Bupropion	EFV	bupropion AUC ↓ 55%	Titrate bupropion dose based on clinical response.
Paroxetine	EFV, ETR	No significant effect	No dosage adjustment necessary.
Sertraline	EFV	sertraline AUC ↓ 39%	Titrate sertraline dose based on clinical response.

Concomitant Drug Class/Name	NNRTI[a]	Effect on NNRTI or Concomitant Drug Concentrations	Dosing Recommendations and Clinical Comments
Antifungals			
Fluconazole	EFV	No significant effect	No dosage adjustment necessary.
	ETR	ETR AUC ↑ 86%	No dosage adjustment necessary. Use with caution.
	NVP	NVP AUC ↑ 110%	Increased risk of hepatotoxicity possible with this combination. Monitor NVP toxicity or use alternative ARV agent.
	RPV	↑ RPV possible	No dosage adjustment necessary. Clinically monitor for breakthrough fungal infection (RPV 150 mg/day reduces ketoconazole exposure; no data on interaction with fluconazole).
Itraconazole	EFV	itraconazole and OH-itraconazole AUC, C_{max}, and C_{min} ↓ 35%–44%	Failure to achieve therapeutic itraconazole concentrations has been reported. Avoid this combination if possible. If co-administered, closely monitor itraconazole concentration and adjust dose accordingly.
	ETR	↓ itraconazole possible ↑ ETR possible	Dose adjustments for itraconazole may be necessary. Monitor itraconazole level and antifungal response.
	NVP	↓ itraconazole possible ↑ NVP possible	Avoid combination if possible. If co-administered, monitor itraconazole concentration and adjust dose accordingly.
	RPV	↑ RPV possible	No dosage adjustment necessary. Clinically monitor for breakthrough fungal infection. (RPV 150 mg/day reduces ketoconazole exposure; no data on interaction with itraconazole.)
Posaconazole	EFV	posaconazole AUC ↓ 50% ↔ EFV	Avoid concomitant use unless the benefit outweighs the risk. If co-administered, monitor posaconazole concentration and adjust dose accordingly.
	ETR	↑ ETR possible	No dosage adjustment necessary.
	RPV	↑ RPV possible	No dosage adjustment necessary. Clinically monitor for breakthrough fungal infection. (RPV 150 mg/day reduces ketoconazole exposure; no data on interaction with posaconazole.)

Concomitant Drug Class/Name	NNRTI[a]	Effect on NNRTI or Concomitant Drug Concentrations	Dosing Recommendations and Clinical Comments
Antifungals, continued			
Voriconazole	EFV	voriconazole AUC ↓ 77% EFV AUC ↑ 44%	**Contraindicated at standard doses.** Dose: voriconazole 400 mg BID, EFV 300 mg daily.
	ETR	voriconazole AUC ↑ 14% ETR AUC ↑ 36%	No dosage adjustment necessary; use with caution. Consider monitoring voriconazole level.
	NVP	↓ voriconazole possible ↑ NVP possible	Monitor for toxicity and antifungal response and/or voriconazole level.
	RPV	↑ RPV possible	No dosage adjustment necessary. Clinically monitor for breakthrough fungal infection (RPV 150 mg/day reduces ketoconazole exposure; no data on interaction with voriconazole).
Antimycobacterials			
Clarithromycin	EFV	clarithromycin AUC ↓ 39%	Monitor for effectiveness or consider alternative agent, such as azithromycin, for MAC prophylaxis and treatment.
	ETR	clarithromycin AUC ↓ 39% ETR AUC ↑ 42%	Consider alternative agent, such as azithromycin, for MAC prophylaxis and treatment.
	NVP	clarithromycin AUC ↓ 31%	Monitor for effectiveness or use alternative agent, such as azithromycin, for MAC prophylaxis and treatment.
	RPV	↔ clarithromycin expected ↑ RPV possible	Consider alternative macrolide, such as azithromycin, for MAC prophylaxis and treatment.
Rifabutin	EFV	rifabutin ↓ 38%	Dose: rifabutin 450–600 mg once daily or 600 mg three times a week if EFV is not co-administered with a PI.
	ETR	rifabutin and metabolite AUC ↓ 17% ETR AUC ↓ 37%	**If ETR is used with an RTV-boosted PI, rifabutin should not be co-administered.** Dose: rifabutin 300 mg once daily **if** ETR is not co-administered with an RTV-boosted PI.
	NVP	rifabutin AUC ↑ 17% and metabolite AUC ↑ 24% NVP C$_{min}$ ↓ 16%	No dosage adjustment necessary. Use with caution.
	RPV	RPV AUC ↓ 46%	**Contraindicated. Do not co-administer.**
Rifampin	EFV	EFV AUC ↓ 26%	Maintain EFV dose at 600 mg once daily and monitor for virologic response. Consider therapeutic drug monitoring. Some clinicians suggest EFV 800 mg dose in patients who weigh more than 60 kg.
	ETR	Significant ↓ ETR possible	**Do not co-administer.**
	NVP	NVP ↓ 20%–58%	**Do not co-administer.**
	RPV	RPV AUC ↓ 80%	**Contraindicated. Do not co-administer.**

Table 15b. Drug Interactions between Non-Nucleoside Reverse Transcriptase Inhibitors* and Other Drugs (Last updated February 12, 2013; last reviewed February 12, 2013) (page 4 of 7)

Concomitant Drug Class/Name	NNRTI[a]	Effect on NNRTI or Concomitant Drug Concentrations	Dosing Recommendations and Clinical Comments
Antimycobacterials, continued			
Rifapentine	EFV, ETR, NVP, RPV	↓ NNRTI expected	**Do not co-administer.**
Benzodiazepines			
Alprazolam	EFV, ETR, NVP, RPV	No data	Monitor for therapeutic effectiveness of alprazolam.
Diazepam	ETR	↑ diazepam possible	Decreased dose of diazepam may be necessary.
Lorazepam	EFV	lorazepam C_{max} ↑ 16%, AUC ↔	No dosage adjustment necessary.
Midazolam	EFV	Significant ↑ midazolam expected	**Do not co-administer with oral midazolam.** Parenteral midazolam can be used with caution as a single dose and can be given in a monitored situation for procedural sedation.
Triazolam	EFV	Significant ↑ triazolam expected	**Do not co-administer.**
Cardiac Medications			
Dihydropyridine calcium channel blockers (CCBs)	EFV, NVP	↓ CCBs possible	Titrate CCB dose based on clinical response.
Diltiazem Verapamil	EFV	diltiazem AUC ↓ 69% ↓ verapamil possible	Titrate diltiazem or verapamil dose based on clinical response.
	NVP	↓ diltiazem or verapamil possible	
Corticosteroids			
Dexamethasone	EFV, ETR, NVP	↓ EFV, ETR, NVP possible	Consider alternative corticosteroid for long-term use. If dexamethasone is used with NNRTI, monitor virologic response.
	RPV	Significant ↓ RPV possible	**Contraindicated with more than a single dose of dexamethasone.**

Concomitant Drug Class/Name	NNRTI[a]	Effect on NNRTI or Concomitant Drug Concentrations	Dosing Recommendations and Clinical Comments
Hepatitis C NS3/4A - Protease Inhibitors			
Boceprevir	EFV	EFV AUC ↑ 20% boceprevir AUC ↓ 19%, C_{min} ↓ 44%	**Co-administration is not recommended.**
	ETR	ETR AUC ↓ 23% boceprevir AUC, C_{max} ↑ 10%	No dosage adjustment necessary.
Telaprevir	EFV	EFV AUC ↔ telaprevir AUC ↓ 26%, C_{min} ↓ 47% <u>With TDF</u>: EFV AUC ↓ 15%–18%, telaprevir AUC ↓ 18%–20%	Increase telaprevir dose to 1125 mg q8h.
Herbal Products			
St. John's wort	EFV, ETR, NVP, RPV	↓ NNRTI	**Do not co-administer.**
Hormonal Contraceptives			
Hormonal contraceptives	EFV	ethinyl estradiol ↔ levonorgestrel AUC ↓ 83% norelgestromin AUC ↓ 64% ↓ etonogestrel (implant) possible	Use alternative or additional contraceptive methods. Norelgestromin and levonorgestrel are active metabolites of norgestimate.
	ETR	ethinyl estradiol AUC ↑ 22% norethindrone: no significant effect	No dosage adjustment necessary.
	NVP	ethinyl estradiol AUC ↓ 20% norethindrone AUC ↓ 19%	Use alternative or additional contraceptive methods.
		DMPA: no significant change	No dosage adjustment necessary.
	RPV	ethinyl estradiol AUC ↑ 14% norethindrone: no significant change	No dosage adjustment necessary.
Levonorgestrel (for emergency contraception)	EFV	levonorgestrel AUC ↓ 58%	Effectiveness of emergency post-coital contraception may be diminished.
HMG-CoA Reductase Inhibitors			
Atorvastatin	EFV, ETR	atorvastatin AUC ↓ 32%–43%	Adjust atorvastatin according to lipid responses, not to exceed the maximum recommended dose.
	RPV	atorvastatin AUC ↔ atorvastatin metabolites ↑	No dosage adjustment necessary.

Concomitant Drug Class/Name	NNRTIª	Effect on NNRTI or Concomitant Drug Concentrations	Dosing Recommendations and Clinical Comments
HMG-CoA Reductase Inhibitors, continued			
Fluvastatin	ETR	↑ fluvastatin possible	Dose adjustments for fluvastatin may be necessary.
Lovastatin Simvastatin	EFV	simvastatin AUC ↓ 68%	Adjust simvastatin dose according to lipid responses, not to exceed the maximum recommended dose. If EFV used with RTV-boosted PI, simvastatin and lovastatin should be avoided.
	ETR, NVP	↓ lovastatin possible ↓ simvastatin possible	Adjust lovastatin or simvastatin dose according to lipid responses, not to exceed the maximum recommended dose. If ETR or NVP used with RTV-boosted PI, simvastatin and lovastatin should be avoided.
Pitavastatin	EFV, ETR, NVP, RPV	No data	No dosage recommendation.
Pravastatin Rosuvastatin	EFV	pravastatin AUC ↓ 44% rosuvatatin: no data	Adjust statin dose according to lipid responses, not to exceed the maximum recommended dose.
	ETR	No significant effect expected	No dosage adjustment necessary.
Immunosuppressants			
Cyclosporine Sirolimus Tacrolimus	EFV, ETR, NVP	↓ immunosuppressant possible	Increase in immunosuppressant dose may be necessary. Therapeutic drug monitoring of immunosuppressant is recommended. Consult with specialist as necessary.
Narcotics/Treatment for Opioid Dependence			
Buprenorphine	EFV	buprenorphine AUC ↓ 50% norbuprenorphineᵇ AUC ↓ 71%	No dosage adjustment recommended; monitor for withdrawal symptoms.
	ETR	buprenorphine AUC ↓ 25%	No dosage adjustment necessary.
	NVP	No significant effect	No dosage adjustment necessary.
Methadone	EFV	methadone AUC ↓ 52%	Opioid withdrawal common; increased methadone dose often necessary.
	ETR	No significant effect	No dosage adjustment necessary.
	NVP	methadone AUC ↓ 37%–51% NVP: no significant effect	Opioid withdrawal common; increased methadone dose often necessary.
	RPV	R-methadonec AUC ↓ 16%	No dosage adjustment necessary, but monitor for withdrawal symptoms.

Table 15b. Drug Interactions between Non-Nucleoside Reverse Transcriptase Inhibitors* and Other Drugs (Last updated February 12, 2013; last reviewed February 12, 2013) (page 7 of 7)

Concomitant Drug Class/Name	NNRTI[a]	Effect on NNRTI or Concomitant Drug Concentrations	Dosing Recommendations and Clinical Comments
Phosphodiesterase Type 5 (PDE5) Inhibitors			
Avanafil	EFV, ETR, NVP, RPV	No data	**Co-administration is not recommended.**
Sildenafil	ETR	sildenafil AUC ↓ 57%	May need to increase sildenafil dose based on clinical effect.
	RPV	sildenafil ↔	No dosage adjustment necessary.
Tadalafil	ETR	↓ tadalafil possible	May need to increase tadalafil dose based on clinical effect.
Vardenafil	ETR	↓ vardenafil possible	May need to increase vardenafil dose based on clinical effect.
Miscellaneous Interactions			
Atovaquone/ proguanil	EFV	↓ atovaquone AUC 75% ↓ proguanil AUC 43%	No dosage recommendation. Consider alternative drug for malaria prophylaxis, if possible.

[a] Approved dose for RPV is 25 mg once daily. Most PK interaction studies were performed using 75 to 150 mg per dose.

[b] Norbuprenorphine is an active metabolite of buprenorphine.

[c] R-methadone is the active form of methadone.

Key to Abbreviations: ARV = antiretroviral, AUC = area under the curve, BID = twice daily, CCB = calcium channel blocker, C_{max} = maximum plasma concentration, C_{min} = minimum plasma concentration, DLV = delavirdine, DMPA = depot medroxyprogesterone acetate, EFV = efavirenz, ETR = etravirine, FDA = Food and Drug Administration, INR = international normalized ratio, MAC = *Mycobacterium avium* complex, NNRTI = non-nucleoside reverse transcriptase inhibitor, NVP = nevirapine, OH-clarithromycin = active metabolite of clarithromycin, PDE5 = phosphodiesterase type 5, PI = protease inhibitor, PPI = proton pump inhibitor, RPV = rilpivirine, RTV = ritonavir, TDF = tenofovir disoproxil fumarate

Table 15c. Drug Interactions between Nucleoside Reverse Transcriptase Inhibitors and Other Drugs (Including Antiretroviral Agents) (Last updated February 12, 2013; last reviewed February 12, 2013) (page 1 of 2)

Concomitant Drug Class/Name	NRTI	Effect on NRTI or Concomitant Drug Concentrations	Dosage Recommendations and Clinical Comments
Antivirals			
Adefovir	TDF	No data	**Do not co-administer.** Serum concentrations of TDF and/or other renally eliminated drugs may be increased.
Boceprevir	TDF	No significant PK effects	No dose adjustment necessary.
Ganciclovir Valganciclovir	TDF	No data	Serum concentrations of these drugs and/or TDF may be increased. Monitor for dose-related toxicities.
	ZDV	No significant PK effects	Potential increase in hematologic toxicities
Ribavirin	ddl	↑ intracellular ddl	**Contraindicated. Do not co-administer.** Fatal hepatic failure and other ddl-related toxicities have been reported with co-administration.
	ZDV	Ribavirin inhibits phosphorylation of ZDV.	Avoid co-administration if possible, or closely monitor virologic response and hematologic toxicities.
Telaprevir	TDF	TDF AUC ↑ 30%, C_{min} ↑ 6%–41%	Monitor for TDF-associated toxicity.
Integrase Inhibitor			
RAL	TDF	RAL AUC ↑ 49%, C_{max} ↑ 64%	No dosage adjustment necessary.
Narcotics/Treatment for Opioid Dependence			
Buprenorphine	3TC, ddl, TDF, ZDV	No significant effect	No dosage adjustment necessary.
Methadone	ABC	methadone clearance ↑ 22%	No dosage adjustment necessary.
	d4T	d4T AUC ↓ 23%, C_{max} ↓ 44%	No dosage adjustment necessary.
	ZDV	ZDV AUC ↑ 29%–43%	Monitor for ZDV-related adverse effects.
NRTIs			
ddl	d4T	No significant PK interaction	**Do not co-administer.** Additive toxicities of peripheral neuropathy, lactic acidosis, and pancreatitis seen with this combination.
	TDF	ddl-EC AUC and C_{max} ↑ 48%–60%	**Avoid co-administration.**
Other			
Allopurinol	ddl	ddl AUC ↑ 113% <u>In patients with renal impairment</u>: ddl AUC ↑ 312%	**Contraindicated.** Potential for increased ddl-associated toxicities.

Guidelines for the Use of Antiretroviral Agents in HIV-1-Infected Adults and Adolescents

Table 15c. Drug Interactions between Nucleoside Reverse Transcriptase Inhibitors and Other Drugs (Including Antiretroviral Agents) (Last updated February 12, 2013; last reviewed February 12, 2013) (page 2 of 2)

Concomitant Drug Class/Name	NRTI	Effect on NRTI or Concomitant Drug Concentrations	Dosage Recommendations and Clinical Comments
PIs			
ATV	ddI	With ddI-EC + ATV (with food): ddI AUC ↓ 34%; ATV no change	Administer ATV with food 2 hours before or 1 hour after ddI.
	TDF	ATV AUC ↓ 25% and C_{min} ↓ 23%–40% (higher C_{min} with RTV than without RTV) TDF AUC ↑ 24%–37%	Dose: ATV/r 300/100 mg daily co-administered with TDF 300 mg daily. Avoid concomitant use without RTV. If using TDF and H2 receptor antagonist in ART-experienced patients, use ATV/r 400 mg/100 mg daily. Monitor for TDF-associated toxicity.
	ZDV	ZDV C_{min} ↓ 30%, no change in AUC	Clinical significance unknown.
DRV/r	TDF	TDF AUC ↑ 22%, C_{max} ↑ 24%, and C_{min} ↑ 37%	Clinical significance unknown. Monitor for TDF toxicity.
LPV/r	TDF	LPV/r AUC ↓ 15% TDF AUC ↑ 34%	Clinical significance unknown. Monitor for TDF toxicity.
TPV/r	ABC	ABC AUC ↓ 35%–44%	Appropriate doses for this combination have not been established.
	ddI	ddI-EC AUC ↔ and C_{min} ↓ 34% TPV/r ↔	Separate doses by at least 2 hours.
	TDF	TDF AUC ↔ TPV/r AUC ↓ 9%–18% and C_{min} ↓ 12%–21%	No dosage adjustment necessary.
	ZDV	ZDV AUC ↓ 35% TPV/r AUC ↓ 31%–43%	Appropriate doses for this combination have not been established.

Key to Abbreviations: 3TC = lamivudine, ABC = abacavir, ART = antiretroviral, ATV = atazanavir, ATV/r = atazanavir/ritonavir, AUC = area under the curve, C_{max} = maximum plasma concentration, C_{min} = minimum plasma concentration, d4T = stavudine, ddI = didanosine, DRV/r = darunavir/ritonavir, EC = enteric coated, LPV/r = lopinavir/ritonavir, NRTI = nucleoside reverse transcriptase inhibitor, PI = protease inhibitor, PK = pharmacokinetic, RAL = raltegravir, TDF = tenofovir, TPV/r = tipranavir/ritonavir, ZDV = zidovudine

Table 15d. Drug Interactions between Integrase Inhibitors and Other Drugs (Last updated February 12, 2013; last reviewed February 12, 2013) (page 1 of 6)

Raltegravir (RAL) is expected to have fewer drug interactions than elvitegravir/cobicistat (EVG/COBI) (see Drug Interactions text). In the following table, where RAL is not listed, no data currently exists and there is either no dosage recommendation or no dosage adjustment is necessary when RAL is used with the concomitant medication.

Concomitant Drug Class/Name	Integrase Inhibitor	Effect on Integrase Inhibitor or Concomitant Drug Concentrations	Dosing Recommendations and Clinical Comments
Acid Reducers			
Antacids	EVG/COBI/TDF/FTC	EVG AUC ↓ 15%–20% if given 2 hours before or after antacid; ↔ with 4-hour interval	Separate EVG/COBI/FTC/TDF and antacid administration by more than 2 hours
H2-Receptor Antagonists	EVG/COBI/TDF/FTC	No significant effect	No dosage adjustment necessary.
Proton Pump Inhibitors	EVG/COBI/TDF/FTC	No significant effect	No dosage adjustment necessary.
	RAL	RAL AUC ↑ 212%, C_{max} ↑ 315%, and C_{min} ↑ 46%	No dosage adjustment necessary.
Anticoagulants			
Warfarin	EVG/COBI/TDF/FTC	No data: but warfarin levels may be affected	Monitor INR and adjust warfarin dose accordingly.
Anticonvulsants			
Carbamazepine Oxcarbazepine Phenobarbital Phenytoin	EVG/COBI/TDF/FTC	↑ carbamazepine possible ↓ EVG possible ↓ COBI possible	Consider alternative anticonvulsant.
Ethosuximide	EVG/COBI/TDF/FTC	↑ ethosuximide possible	Clinically monitor for ethosuxamide toxicities.
Antidepressants			
Selective Serotonin Reuptake Inhibitors (SSRIs)	EVG/COBI/TDF/FTC	↑ SSRI possible	Initiate with lowest dose of SSRI and titrate dose carefully based on antidepressant response.
Tricyclic Antidepressants (TCAs) Amitriptyline Desipramine Imipramine Nortriptyline	EVG/COBI/TDF/FTC	Desipramine AUC ↑ 65%	Initiate with lowest dose and titrate dose of TCA carefully.
Trazodone	EVG/COBI/TDF/FTC	↑ trazodone possible	Initiate with lowest dose and titrate dose of trazodone carefully.

Concomitant Drug Class/Name	Integrase Inhibitor	Effect on Integrase Inhibitor or Concomitant Drug Concentrations	Dosing Recommendations and Clinical Comments
Antifungals			
Itraconazole	EVG/COBI/TDF/FTC	↑ itraconazole expected ↑ EVG and COBI possible	Consider monitoring itraconazole level to guide dosage adjustments. High doses (>200 mg/day) are not recommended unless dose is guided by itraconazole levels.
Posaconazole	EVG/COBI/TDF/FTC	↑EVG and COBI possible ↑ posaconazole possible	Monitor posaconazole concentrations with co-administration.
Voriconazole	EVG/COBI/TDF/FTC	↑ voriconazole expected ↑ EVG and COBI possible	Risk/benefit ratio should be assessed to justify use of voriconazole. If administered, consider monitoring voriconazole level. Adjust dose accordingly.
Antimycobacterials			
Clarithromycin	EVG/COBI/TDF/FTC	↑ clarithromycin possible ↑ COBI possible	<u>CrCl ≥60 mL/min</u>: No dose adjustment necessary <u>CrCl 50–60 mL/min</u>: Reduce clarithromycin dose by 50% <u>CrCl <50 mL/min</u>: EVG/COBI/TDF/FTC is not recommended.
Rifabutin	EVG/COBI/TDF/FTC	<u>Rifabutin (150 mg every other day)</u>: No significant change in rifabutin AUC; For 25-O-desacetyl-rifabutin, AUC ↑ 625% compared with rifabutin (300 mg daily) administered alone EVG AUC ↓ 21%, C_{min} ↓ 67%	Do not co-administer.
	RAL	RAL AUC ↑ 19%, C_{max} ↑ 39%, and C_{min} ↓ 20%	No dosage adjustment necessary.
Rifampin	EVG/COBI/TDF/FTC	Significant ↓ EVG and COBI expected	Do not co-administer.
	RAL	RAL 400 mg: RAL AUC ↓ 40% and C_{min} ↓ 61% Rifampin with RAL 800 mg BID compared with RAL 400 mg BID alone: RAL AUC ↑ 27% and C_{min} ↓ 53%	Dose: RAL 800 mg BID Monitor closely for virologic response or consider using rifabutin as an alternative rifamycin
Rifapentine	EVG/COBI/TDF/FTC	Significant ↓ EVG and COBI expected	Do not co-administer.
Benzodiazepines			
Clonazepam Clorazepate Diazepam Estazolam Flurazepam	EVG/COBI/TDF/FTC	↑ benzodiazepines possible	Dose reduction of benzodiazepine may be necessary. Initiate with low dose and clinically monitor. Consider alternative benzodiazepines to diazepam, such as lorazepam, oxazepam, or temazepam.
Midazolam Triazolam	EVG/COBI/TDF/FTC	↑ midazolam expected ↑ triazolam expected	Do not co-administer triazolam or oral midazolam and EVG/COBI. Parenteral midazolam can be used with caution in a closely monitored setting. Consider dose reduction, especially if >1 dose is administered.

Concomitant Drug Class/Name	Integrase Inhibitor	Effect on Integrase Inhibitor or Concomitant Drug Concentrations	Dosing Recommendations and Clinical Comments
Cardiac Medications			
Anti-Arrhythmics (amiodarone, bepridil, digoxin, disopyramide, dronedarone, flecainide, systemic lidocaine, mexilitine, propafenone, quinidine)	EVG/COBI/TDF/FTC	↑ anti-arrhythmics possible digoxin C_{max} ↑ 41%, AUC no significant change	Use anti-arrhythmics with caution. Therapeutic drug monitoring, if available, is recommended for anti-arrhythmics.
Bosentan	EVG/COBI/TDF/FTC	↑ bosentan possible	In patients on EVG/COBI/FTC/TDF ≥10 days: start bosentan at 62.5 mg once daily or every other day based on individual tolerability.
			In patients on bosentan who require EVG/COBI/FTC/TDF: stop bosentan ≥36 hours before EVG/COBI/FTC/TDF initiation. After at least 10 days following initiation of EVG/COBI/FTC/TDF, resume bosentan at 62.5 mg once daily or every other day based on individual tolerability.
Beta-blockers	EVG/COBI/TDF/FTC	↑ beta-blockers possible	Adjust beta-blockers according to clinical response. Beta-blocker dose may need to be decreased.
			Some beta-blockers are metabolized via CYP450 pathway (e.g., metoprolol, timolol). Consider using other beta-blockers (e.g., atenolol, labetalol, nadolol, sotalol) as these agents are not metabolized by CYP450 enzymes.
Dihydropyridine and Non-Dihydropyridine Calcium Channel Blockers	EVG/COBI/TDF/FTC	↑ CCBs possible	Co-administer with caution. Monitor for CCB efficacy and toxicities.
Corticosteroids			
Dexamethasone	EVG/COBI/TDF/FTC	↓ EVG and COBI possible	Co-administer with caution, monitor HIV virologic response
Fluticasone (inhaled/intranasal)	EVG/COBI/TDF/FTC	↑ fluticasone possible	Use alternative inhaled corticosteroid, particularly for long-term use
Hepatitis C NS3/4A—Protease Inhibitors			
Boceprevir	EVG/COBI/TDF/FTC	No data	**Do not co-administer.**
	RAL	No significant effect	No dosage adjustment necessary.
Telaprevir	EVG/COBI/TDF/FTC	No data	**Do not co-administer.**
	RAL	RAL AUC ↑ 31% Telaprevir ↔	No dosage adjustment necessary.

Concomitant Drug Class/Name	Integrase Inhibitor	Effect on Integrase Inhibitor or Concomitant Drug Concentrations	Dosing Recommendations and Clinical Comments
Hormonal Contraceptives			
Hormonal contraceptives	RAL	No clinically significant effect	Safe to use in combination
Norgestimate/ethinyl estradiol	EVG/COBI/TDF/FTC	Norgestimate AUC, C_{max}, C_{min} ↑ > 2-fold Ethinyl estradiol AUC ↓ 25%, C_{min} ↓ 44%	The effects of increases in progestin (norgestimate) are not fully known and can include insulin resistance, dyslipidemia, acne, and venous thrombosis. Weigh the risks and benefits of the drug, and consider alternative contraceptive method.
HMG-CoA Reductase Inhibitors			
Atorvastatin	EVG/COBI/TDF/FTC	↑ atorvastatin possible	Titrate statin dose slowly and use the lowest dose possible.
Lovastatin	EVG/COBI/TDF/FTC	Significant ↑ lovastatin expected	**Contraindicated. Do not co-administer.**
Pitavastatin Pravastatin	EVG/COBI/TDF/FTC	No data	No dosage recommendation
Rosuvastatin	EVG/COBI/TDF/FTC	Rosuvastatin AUC ↑ 38% and C_{max} ↑ 89%	Titrate statin dose slowly and use the lowest dose possible.
Simvastatin	EVG/COBI/TDF/FTC	Significant ↑ simvastatin expected	**Contraindicated. Do not co-administer.**
Immunosuppressants			
Cyclosporine Sirolimus Tacrolimus	EVG/COBI/TDF/FTC	↑ immunosuppressant possible	Initiate with an adjusted immunosuppressant dose to account for potential increased concentrations and monitor for toxicities. Therapeutic drug monitoring of immunosuppressant is recommended. Consult with specialist as necessary.
Narcotics/Treatment for Opioid Dependence			
Buprenorphine	EVG/COBI/TDF/FTC	Buprenorphine: AUC ↑ 35%, C_{max} ↑ 12%, C_{min} ↑ 66% Norbuprenorphine: AUC ↑ 42%, C_{max} ↑ 24%, C_{min} ↑ 57%	No dosage adjustment necessary. Clinical monitoring is recommended.
	RAL	No significant effect	No dosage adjustment necessary.
Methadone	EVG/COBI/TDF/FTC	No significant effect	No dosage adjustment necessary.
	RAL	No significant effect	No dosage adjustment necessary.
Neuroleptics			
Perphenazine Risperidone Thioridazine	EVG/COBI/TDF/FTC	↑ neuroleptic possible	Initiate neuroleptic at a low dose. Decrease in neuroleptic dose may be necessary.

Concomitant Drug Class/Name	Integrase Inhibitor	Effect on Integrase Inhibitor or Concomitant Drug Concentrations	Dosing Recommendations and Clinical Comments
Phosphodiesterase Type 5 (PDE5) Inhibitors			
Avanafil	EVG/COBI/TDF/FTC	No data	**Co-administration is not recommended.**
Sildenafil	EVG/COBI/TDF/FTC	↑ sildenafil expected	For treatment of erectile dysfunction: Start with sildenafil 25 mg every 48 hours and monitor for adverse effects of sildenafil. For treatment of PAH: **Contraindicated**
Tadalafil	EVG/COBI/TDF/FTC	↑ tadalafil expected	For treatment of erectile dysfunction: Start with tadalafil 5-mg dose and do not exceed a single dose of 10 mg every 72 hours. Monitor for adverse effects of tadalafil. For treatment of PAH: *In patients on a EVG/COBI >7 days:* Start with tadalafil 20 mg once daily and increase to 40 mg once daily based on tolerability. *In patients on tadalafil who require EVG/COBI:* Stop tadalafil ≥24 hours before EVG/COBI initiation. Seven days after EVG/COBI initiation restart tadalafil at 20 mg once daily, and increase to 40 mg once daily based on tolerability.
Vardenafil	EVG/COBI/TDF/FTC	↑ vardenafil expected	Start with vardenafil 2.5 mg every 72 hours and monitor for adverse effects of vardenafil.
Sedatives/Hypnotics			
Buspirone	EVG/COBI/TDF/FTC	↑ buspirone possible	Initiate buspirone at a low dose. Dose reduction may be necessary.
Zolpidem	EVG/COBI/TDF/FTC	↑ zolpidem possible	Initiate zolpidem at a low dose. Dose reduction may be necessary.

Table 15d. Drug Interactions between Integrase Inhibitors and Other Drugs (Last updated February 12, 2013; last reviewed February 12, 2013) (page 6 of 6)

Concomitant Drug Class/Name	Integrase Inhibitor	Effect on Integrase Inhibitor or Concomitant Drug Concentrations	Dosing Recommendations and Clinical Comments
Miscellaneous Interactions			
Colchicine	EVG/COBI/TDF/FTC	↑ colchicine expected	**Do not co-administer in patients with hepatic or renal impairment.** For treatment of gout flares: Colchicine 0.6 mg x 1 dose, followed by 0.3 mg 1 hour later. Do not repeat dose for at least 3 days. For prophylaxis of gout flares: If original regimen was colchicine 0.6 mg BID, the regimen should be decreased to 0.3 mg once daily. If regimen was 0.6 mg once daily, the regimen should be decreased to 0.3 mg every other day. For treatment of familial Mediterranean fever: Do not exceed colchicine 0.6 mg once daily or 0.3 mg BID.
Salmeterol	EVG/COBI/TDF/FTC	↑ salmeterol possible	**Do not co-administer** because of potential increased risk of salmeterol-associated cardiovascular events.

Key to Abbreviations: AUC = area under the curve, BID = twice daily, CCB = calcium channel blocker, COBI = cobicistat, C_{max} = maximum plasma concentration, C_{min} = minimum plasma concentration, EVG = elvitegravir, PAH = pulmonary arterial hypertension, RAL = raltegravir

Table 15e. Drug Interactions between CCR5 Antagonist and Other Drugs (Last updated March 27, 2012; last reviewed February 12, 2013)

This table provides information relating to pharmacokinetic (PK) interactions between maraviroc (MVC) and non-antiretroviral (ARV) drugs. For interactions between ARV agents and for dosing recommendations, please refer to Table 16b.

Concomitant Drug Class/Name	CCR5 Antagonist	Effect on CCR5 Antagonist or Concomitant Drug Concentrations	Dosing Recommendations and Clinical Comments
Anticonvulsants			
Carbamazepine Phenobarbital Phenytoin	MVC	↓ MVC possible	If used without a strong CYP3A inhibitor, use MVC 600 mg BID or an alternative antiepileptic agent.
Antifungals			
Itraconazole	MVC	↑ MVC possible	Dose: MVC 150 mg BID
Ketoconazole	MVC	MVC AUC ↑ 400%	Dose: MVC 150 mg BID
Voriconazole	MVC	↑ MVC possible	Consider dose reduction to MVC 150 mg BID
Antimycobacterials			
Clarithromycin	MVC	↑ MVC possible	Dose: MVC 150 mg BID
Rifabutin	MVC	↓ MVC possible	If used without a strong CYP3A inducer or inhibitor, use MVC 300 mg BID. If used with a strong CYP3A inhibitor, use MVC 150 mg BID.
Rifampin	MVC	MVC AUC ↓ 64%	**Co-administration is not recommended.** If co-administration is necessary, use MVC 600 mg BID. If co-administered with a strong CYP3A inhibitor, use MVC 300 mg BID.
Rifapentine	MVC	↓ MVC expected	**Do not co-administer.**
Herbal Products			
St. John's wort	MVC	↓ MVC possible	**Co-administration is not recommended.**
Hormonal Contraceptives			
Hormonal contraceptives	MVC	No significant effect on ethinyl estradiol or levonorgestrel	Safe to use in combination

Key to Abbreviations: ARV = antiretroviral, AUC = area under the curve, BID = twice daily, CYP = cytochrome P, MVC = maraviroc, PK = pharmacokinetic

Table 16a. Interactions Between Protease Inhibitors* (Last updated February 12, 2013; last reviewed February 12, 2013)

* Nelfinavir (NFV) and indinavir (IDV) are not included in this table. Refer to the NFV and IDV Food and Drug Administration package inserts for information regarding drug interactions.

Drug Affected	ATV	FPV	LPV/r	RTV	SQV	TPV
DRV	Dose: ATV 300 mg once daily + DRV 600 mg BID + RTV 100 mg BID	No data	Should not be co-administered because doses are not established	Dose: (DRV 600 mg + RTV 100 mg) BID or (DRV 800 mg + RTV 100 mg) once daily	Should not be co-administered because doses are not established	No data
FPV	Dose: Insufficient data	•	Should not be co-administered because doses are not established	Dose: (FPV 1400 mg + RTV [100 mg or 200 mg]) once daily or (FPV 700 mg + RTV 100 mg) BID	Dose: Insufficient data	Should not be co-administered because doses are not established
LPV/r	Dose: ATV 300 mg once daily + LPV/r 400/100 mg BID	Should not be co-administered because doses are not established	•	LPV is co-formulated with RTV and marketed as Kaletra.	Dose: SQV 1000 mg BID + LPV/r 400/100 mg BID	Should not be co-administered because doses are not established
RTV	Dose: (ATV 300 mg + RTV 100 mg) once daily	Dose: (FPV 1400 mg + RTV [100 mg or 200 mg]) once daily or (FPV 700 mg + RTV 100 mg) BID	LPV is co-formulated with RTV and marketed as Kaletra.	•	Dose: (SQV 1000 mg + RTV 100 mg) BID	Dose: (TPV 500 mg + RTV 200 mg) BID
SQV	Dose: Insufficient data	Dose: Insufficient data	Dose: SQV 1000 mg BID + LPV/r 400/100 mg BID	Dose: (SQV 1000 mg + RTV 100 mg) BID	•	Should not be co-administered because doses are not established

Key to Abbreviations: ATV = atazanavir, BID = twice daily, DRV = darunavir, FDA = Food and Drug Administration, FPV = fosamprenavir, IDV = indinavir, LPV/r = lopinavir/ritonavir, NFV = nelfinavir, PI = protease inhibitor, RTV = ritonavir, SQV = saquinavir, TPV = tipranavir

* Delavirdine (DLV), indinavir (IDV), and nelfinavir (NFV) are not included in this table. Refer to the DLV, IDV, and NFV Food and Drug Administration package inserts for information regarding drug interactions.

		EFV	ETR	NVP	RPV[a]
ATV +/– RTV	**PK data**	With unboosted ATV ATV: AUC ↓ 74% EFV: no significant change With (ATV 300 mg + RTV 100 mg) once daily with food ATV concentrations similar to those with unboosted ATV without EFV	With unboosted ATV ETR: AUC ↑ 50%, C_{max} ↑ 47%, and C_{min} ↑ 58% ATV: AUC ↓ 17% and C_{min} ↓ 47% With (ATV 300 mg + RTV 100 mg) once daily ETR: AUC, C_{max}, and C_{min} ↑ approximately 30% ATV: AUC ↓ 14% and C_{min} ↓ 38%	With (ATV 300 mg + RTV 100 mg) once daily ATV: AUC ↓ 42% and C_{min} ↓ 72% NVP: AUC ↑ 25%	With boosted and unboosted ATV ↑ RPV possible
	Dose	**Do not co-administer with unboosted ATV.** In ART-naive patients (ATV 400 mg + RTV 100 mg) once daily **Do not co-administer in ART-experienced patients.**	**Do not co-administer with ATV +/– RTV.**	**Do not co-administer with ATV +/– RTV.**	Standard
DRV (always use with RTV)	**PK data**	With (DRV 300 mg + RTV 100 mg) BID DRV: AUC ↓ 13%, C_{min} ↓ 31% EFV: AUC ↑ 21%	ETR 100 mg BID with (DRV 600 mg + RTV 100 mg) BID DRV: no significant change ETR: AUC ↓ 37%, C_{min} ↓ 49%	With (DRV 400 mg + RTV 100 mg) BID DRV: AUC ↑ 24%[b] NVP: AUC ↑ 27% and C_{min} ↑ 47%	RPV 150 mg once daily with (DRV 800 mg + RTV 100 mg) once daily DRV: no significant change RPV: AUC ↑ 130% and C_{min} ↑ 178%
	Dose	Clinical significance unknown. Use standard doses and monitor patient closely. Consider monitoring drug levels.	Standard (ETR 200 mg BID). Safety and efficacy of this combination, despite decreased ETR concentration, have been established in a clinical trial.	Standard	Standard
EFV	**PK data**	•	↓ ETR possible	NVP: no significant change EFV: AUC ↓ 22%	↓ RPV possible
	Dose		**Do not co-administer.**	**Do not co-administer.**	**Do not co-administer.**
ETR	**PK data**	↓ ETR possible	•	↓ ETR possible	↓ RPV possible
	Dose	**Do not co-administer.**		**Do not co-administer.**	**Do not co-administer.**

		EFV	ETR	NVP	RPVª
FPV	**PK data**	With (FPV 1400 mg + RTV 200 mg) once daily APV: C_{min} ↓ 36%	With (FPV 700 mg + RTV 100 mg) BID APV: AUC ↑ 69%, C_{min} ↑ 77%	With unboosted FPV 1400 mg BID APV: AUC ↓ 33% NVP: AUC ↑ 29% With (FPV 700 mg + RTV 100 mg) BID NVP: C_{min} ↑ 22%	With boosted and unboosted FPV ↑ RPV possible
	Dose	(FPV 1400 mg + RTV 300 mg) once daily or (FPV 700 mg + RTV 100 mg) BID EFV standard	**Do not co-administer with FPV +/– RTV.**	(FPV 700 mg + RTV 100 mg) BID NVP standard	Standard
LPV/r	**PK data**	With LPV/r tablets 500/125 mg BIDᶜ + EFV 600 mg LPV levels similar to LPV/r 400/100 mg BID without EFV	With LPV/r tablets ETR: AUC ↓ 35% (comparable to the decrease with DRV/r) LPV: AUC↓ 13%	With LPV/r capsules LPV: AUC ↓ 27% and C_{min} ↓51%	RPV 150 mg once daily with LPV/r capsules LPV: no significant change RPV: AUC ↑ 52% and C_{min} ↑ 74%
	Dose	LPV/r tablets 500/125 mgᶜ BID; LPV/r oral solution 533/133 mg BID EFV standard	Standard	LPV/r tablets 500/125 mgᶜ BID; LPV/r oral solution 533/133 mg BID NVP standard	Standard
NVP	**PK data**	NVP: no significant change EFV: AUC ↓ 22%	↓ ETR possible	•	↓ RPV possible
	Dose	**Do not co-administer.**	**Do not co-administer.**		**Do not co-administer.**
RPV	**PK data**	↓ RPV possible	↓ RPV possible	↓ RPV possible	•
	Dose	**Do not co-administer.**	**Do not co-administer.**	**Do not co-administer.**	
RTV	**PK data**	Refer to information for boosted PI.	Refer to information for boosted PI.	Refer to information for boosted PI.	Refer to information for boosted PI.
	Dose				
SQV (always use with RTV)	**PK data**	With SQV 1200 mg TID SQV: AUC ↓ 62% EFV: AUC ↓ 12%	With (SQV 1000 mg + RTV 100 mg) BID SQV: AUC unchanged ETR: AUC ↓ 33%, C_{min} ↓ 29% Reduced ETR levels similar to reduction with DRV/r	With 600 mg TID SQV: AUC ↓ 24% NVP: no significant change	↑ RPV possible
	Dose	(SQV 1000 mg + RTV 100 mg) BID	(SQV 1000 mg + RTV 100 mg) BID	Dose with SQV/r not established	Standard

Table 16b. Interactions between Non-Nucleoside Reverse Transcriptase Inhibitors, and Protease Inhibitors* (Last updated March 27, 2012; last reviewed February 2013) (page 3 of 3)

		EFV	ETR	NVP	RPV[a]
TPV (always use with RTV)	PK data	With (TPV 500 mg + RTV 100 mg) BID TPV: AUC ↓ 31%, C_{min} ↓ 42% EFV: no significant change With (TPV 750 mg + RTV 200 mg) BID TPV: no significant change EFV: no significant change	With (TPV 500 mg + RTV 200 mg) BID ETR: AUC ↓ 76%, C_{min} ↓ 82% TPV: AUC ↑ 18%, C_{min} ↑ 24%	With (TPV 250 mg + RTV 200 mg) BID and with (TPV 750 mg + RTV 100 mg) BID NVP: no significant change TPV: no data	↑ RPV possible
	Dose	Standard	**Do not co-administer.**	Standard	Standard

[a] Approved dose for RPV is 25 mg once daily. Most PK interaction studies were performed using 75 mg to 150 mg per dose.

[b] Based on between-study comparison.

[c] Use a combination of two LPV/r 200 mg/50 mg tablets + one LPV/r 100 mg/25 mg tablet to make a total dose of LPV/r 500 mg/125 mg.

Key to Abbreviations: APV = amprenavir, ART = antiretroviral therapy, ATV = atazanavir, AUC = area under the curve, BID = twice daily, C_{max} = maximum plasma concentration, C_{min} = minimum plasma concentration, CYP = cytochrome P, DLV = delavirdine, DRV = darunavir, DRV/r = darunavir/ritonavir, EFV = efavirenz, ETR = etravirine, FDA = Food and Drug Administration, FPV = fosamprenavir, IDV = indinavir, LPV = lopinavir, LPV/r = lopinavir/ritonavir, MVC = maraviroc, NFV = nelfinavir, NVP = nevirapine, PI = protease inhibitor, PK = pharmacokinetic, RAL = raltegravir, RPV = rilpivirine, RTV = ritonavir, SQV = saquinavir, SQV/r = saquinavir/ritonavir, TID = three times a day, TPV = tipranavir

Table 16c. Interactions between Integrase Inhibitors or Maraviroc and Non-Nucleoside Reverse Transcriptase Inhibitors or Protease Inhibitors* (Last updated February 12, 2013; last reviewed February 12, 2013) (page 1 of 2)

* Delavirdine (DLV), indinavir (IDV), and nelfinavir (NFV) are not included in this table. Refer to the DLV, IDV, and NFV Food and Drug Administration package inserts for information regarding drug interactions.

		EVG/COBI/TDF/FTC	RAL	MVC
ATV +/- RTV	PK Data	↑ or ↓ EVG, COBI, ATV possible	With unboosted ATV RAL: AUC ↑ 72% With (ATV 300 mg + RTV 100 mg) once daily RAL: AUC ↑ 41%	With unboosted ATV MVC: AUC ↑ 257% With (ATV 300 mg + RTV 100 mg) once daily MVC: AUC ↑ 388%
	Dose	Do not co-administer.	Standard	MVC 150 mg BID with ATV +/– RTV
DRV (always use with RTV)	PK Data	↑ or ↓ EVG, COBI, DRV possible	With (DRV 600 mg + RTV 100 mg) BID RAL: AUC ↓ 29% and C_{min} ↑ 38%	With (DRV 600 mg + RTV 100 mg) BID MVC: AUC ↑ 305% With (DRV 600 mg + RTV 100 mg) BID + ETR MVC: AUC ↑ 210%
	Dose	Do not co-administer.	Standard	MVC 150 mg BID
EFV	PK Data	↑ or ↓ EVG, COBI, EFV possible	EFV: AUC ↓ 36%	MVC: AUC ↓ 45%
	Dose	Do not co-administer.	Standard	MVC 600 mg BID
EVG/COBI/TDF/FTC	PK Data	•	No data	↑ MVC possible
	Dose		Do not co-administer.	Do not co-administer.
ETR	PK Data	↑ or ↓ EVG, COBI, ETR possible	ETR: C_{min} ↓ 17% RAL: C_{min} ↓ 34%	MVC: AUC ↓ 53%, C_{max} ↓ 60%
	Dose	Do not co-administer.	Standard	MVC 600 mg BID in the absence of a potent CYP3A inhibitor
FPV	PK Data	↑ or ↓ EVG, COBI, FPV possible	No significant effect	Unknown; ↑ MVC possible
	Dose	Do not co-administer.	Standard	MVC 150 mg BID
LPV/r	PK Data	↑ or ↓ EVG, COBI, LPV possible RTV and COBI have similar effects on CYP3A.	↓ RAL ↔ LPV/r	MVC: AUC ↑ 295% With LPV/r + EFV MVC: AUC ↑ 153%
	Dose	Do not co-administer.	Standard	MVC 150 mg BID
NVP	PK Data	↑ or ↓ EVG, COBI, NVP possible	No data	MVC: AUC ↔ and C_{max} ↑ 54%
	Dose	Do not co-administer.	Standard	Without PI MVC 300 mg BID With PI (except TPV/r) MVC 150 mg BID

		EVG/COBI/TDF/FTC	RAL	MVC
RAL	PK Data	No data	•	RAL: AUC ↓ 37% MVC: AUC ↓ 21%
	Dose	Do not co-administer.		Standard
RPV	PK Data	↑ or ↓ EVG, COBI, RPV possible	No data	No data
	Dose	Do not co-administer.	No data	No data
RTV	PK Data	↑ or ↓ EVG, COBI possible RTV and COBI have similar effects on CYP3A.	With RTV 100 mg BID RAL: AUC ↓ 16%	With RTV 100 mg BID MVC: AUC ↑ 161%
	Dose	Do not co-administer.	Standard	MVC 150 mg BID
SQV (always use with RTV)	PK Data	↑ or ↓ EVG, COBI, SQV possible RTV and COBI have similar effects on CYP3A.	No data	With (SQV 1000 mg + RTV 100 mg) BID MVC: AUC ↑ 877% With (SQV 1000 mg + RTV 100 mg) BID + EFV MVC: AUC ↑ 400%
	Dose	Do not co-administer.	Standard	MVC 150 mg BID
TPV (always use with RTV)	PK Data	↑ or ↓ EVG, COBI, TPV possible RTV and COBI have similar effects on CYP3A.	With (TPV 500 mg + RTV 200 mg) BID RAL: AUC ↓ 24%	With (TPV 500 mg + RTV 200 mg) BID MVC: No significant change in AUC TPV: No data
	Dose	Do not co-administer.	Standard	MVC 300 mg BID

Key to Abbreviations: APV = amprenavir, ART = antiretroviral therapy, ATV = atazanavir, AUC = area under the curve, BID = twice daily, COBI = cobicistat, C_{max} = maximum plasma concentration, C_{min} = minimum plasma concentration, CYP = cytochrome P, DLV = delavirdine, DRV = darunavir, DRV/r = darunavir/ritonavir, EFV = efavirenz, EVG = elvitegravir, ETR = etravirine, FDA = Food and Drug Administration, FPV = fosamprenavir, IDV = indinavir, LPV = lopinavir, LPV/r = lopinavir/ritonavir, MVC = maraviroc, NFV = nelfinavir, NVP = nevirapine, PI = protease inhibitor, PK = pharmacokinetic, RAL = raltegravir, RPV = rilpivirine, RTV = ritonavir, SQV = saquinavir, SQV/r = saquinavir/ritonavir, TID = three times a day, TPV = tipranavir

Preventing Secondary Transmission of HIV (Last updated March 27, 2012; last reviewed March 27, 2012)

Despite substantial advances in prevention and treatment of HIV infection in the United States, the rate of new infections has remained stable.[1-2] Although earlier prevention interventions mainly were behavioral, recent data demonstrate the strong impact of antiretroviral therapy (ART) on secondary HIV transmission. The most effective strategy to stem the spread of HIV will probably be a combination of behavioral, biological, and pharmacological interventions.[3]

Prevention Counseling

Counseling and related behavioral interventions for those living with HIV infection can reduce behaviors associated with secondary transmission of HIV. Each patient encounter offers the clinician an opportunity to reinforce HIV prevention messages, but multiple studies show that prevention counseling is frequently neglected in clinical practice.[4-5] Although delivering effective prevention interventions in a busy practice setting may be challenging, clinicians should be aware that patients often look to their providers for messages about HIV prevention. Multiple approaches to prevention counseling are available, including formal guidance from the Centers for Disease Control and Prevention (CDC) for incorporating HIV prevention into medical care settings. Such interventions have been demonstrated to be effective in changing sexual risk behavior[6-8] and can reinforce self-directed behavior change early after diagnosis.[9]

CDC has identified several prevention interventions for individuals infected with HIV that meet stringent criteria for efficacy and scientific rigor (http://www.cdc.gov/hiv/topics/research/prs/index.htm). The following three interventions have proven effective in treatment settings and can be delivered by providers as brief messages during clinic visits:

- Partnership for Health (http://effectiveinterventions.org/en/Interventions/PfH.aspx),
- Options (http://www.cdc.gov/hiv/topics/research/prs/resources/factsheets/options.htm),
- Positive Choice (http://www.cdc.gov/hiv/topics/research/prs/resources/factsheets/positive-choice.htm).

In addition, CDC's "Prevention Is Care" campaign (http://www.actagainstaids.org/provider/pic/index.html) helps providers (and members of a multidisciplinary care team) integrate simple methods to prevent transmission by HIV-infected individuals into routine care. These prevention interventions are designed to reduce the risk of secondary HIV transmission through sexual contact. The interventions are designed generally for implementation at the community or group level, but some can be adapted and administered in clinical settings by a multidisciplinary care team.

Need for Screening for High-Risk Behaviors

The primary care visit provides an opportunity to screen patients for ongoing high-risk drug and sexual behaviors for transmitting HIV infection. Routine screening and symptom-directed testing for and treatment of sexually transmitted diseases (STDs), as recommended by CDC,[10] remain essential adjuncts to prevention counseling. Genital ulcers may facilitate HIV transmission and STDs may increase HIV viral load in plasma and genital secretions.[7, 11-13] They also provide objective evidence of unprotected sexual activity, which should prompt prevention counseling.

The contribution of substance and alcohol use to HIV risk behaviors and transmission has been well established in multiple populations;[14-18] therefore, effective counseling for injection and noninjection drug users is essential to prevent HIV transmission. Identifying the substance(s) of use is important because HIV prevalence, transmission risk, risk behaviors, transmission rates, and potential for pharmacologic intervention all vary according to the type of substance used.[19-21] Risk-reduction strategies for injection drug users (IDUs), in addition to condom use, include needle exchange and instructions on cleaning drug paraphernalia. Evidence supporting the efficacy of interventions to reduce injection drug use risk behavior also exists. Interventions include both behavioral strategies[14-15, 22] and opiate substitution treatment with methadone or buprenorphine.[23-24] No successful pharmacologic interventions have been found for cocaine and methamphetamine users; cognitive and behavioral interventions demonstrate the greatest effect on reducing the risk behaviors of these users.[25-27] Given the significant impact of cocaine and methamphetamine on sexual risk behavior, reinforcement of sexual risk-reduction strategies is important.[14-18, 28]

Antiretroviral Therapy as Prevention

ART can play an important role in preventing HIV transmission. Lower levels of plasma HIV RNA have been associated with decreases in the concentration of virus in genital secretions.[29-32] Observational studies have demonstrated the association between low serum or genital HIV RNA and a decreased rate of HIV transmission among serodiscordant heterosexual couples.[29, 33-34] Ecological studies of communities with relatively high concentrations of men who have sex with men (MSM) and IDUs suggest increased use of ART is associated with decreased community viral load and reduced rates of new HIV diagnoses.[35-37] These data suggest that the risk of HIV transmission is low when an individual's viral load is below 400 copies/mL,[35, 38] but the threshold below which transmission of the virus becomes impossible is unknown. Furthermore, to be effective at preventing transmission it is assumed that: (1) ART is capable of durably and continuously suppressing viremia; (2) adherence to an effective ARV regimen is high; and (3) there is an absence of a concomitant STD. Importantly, detection of HIV RNA in genital secretions has been documented in individuals with controlled plasma HIV RNA and data describing a differential in concentration of most ARV drugs in the blood and genital compartments exist.[30, 39] At least one case of HIV transmission from a patient with suppressed plasma viral load to a monogamous uninfected sexual partner has been reported.[40]

In the HPTN 052 trial in HIV-discordant couples, the HIV-infected partners who were ART naive and had CD4 counts between 350 and 550 cells/mm³ were randomized to initiate or delay ART. In this study, those who initiated ART had a 96% reduction in HIV transmission to the uninfected partners.[3] Almost all of the participants were in heterosexual relationships, all participants received risk-reduction counseling, and the absolute number of transmission events was low: 1 among ART initiators and 27 among ART delayers. Over the course of the study virologic failure rates were less than 5%, a value much lower than generally seen in individuals taking ART for their own health. These low virologic failure rates suggest high levels of adherence to ART in the study, which may have been facilitated by the frequency of study follow-up (study visits were monthly) and by participants' sense of obligation to protect their uninfected partners. Therefore, caution is indicated when interpreting the extent to which ART for the HIV-infected partner protects seronegative partners in contexts where adherence and, thus, rates of continuous viral suppression, may be lower. Furthermore, for HIV-infected MSM and IDUs, biological and observational data suggest suppressive ART also should protect against transmission, but the actual extent of protection has not been established.

Rates of HIV risk behaviors can increase coincidently with the availability of potent combination ART, in some cases almost doubling compared with rates in the era prior to highly effective therapy.[9] A meta-analysis demonstrated that the prevalence of unprotected sex acts was increased in HIV-infected individuals who believed that receiving ART or having a suppressed viral load protected against transmitting HIV.[41] Attitudinal shifts away from safer sexual practices since the availability of potent ART underscore the role of provider-initiated HIV prevention counseling. With wider recognition that effective treatment decreases the risk of HIV transmission, it is particularly important for providers to help patients understand that a sustained viral load below the limits of detection will dramatically reduce but does not absolutely assure the absence of

HIV in the genital and blood compartments and, hence, the inability to transmit HIV to others.[41-42]

Maximal suppression of viremia not only depends on the potency of the ARV regimen used but also on the patient's adherence to prescribed therapy. Suboptimal adherence can lead to viremia that not only harms the patient but also increases his/her risk of transmitting HIV (including drug-resistant strains) via sex or needle sharing. Screening for and treating behavioral conditions that can impact adherence, such as depression and alcohol and substance use, improve overall health and reduce the risk of secondary transmission.

Summary

Consistent and effective use of ART resulting in a sustained reduction in viral load in conjunction with consistent condom usage, safer sex and drug use practices, and detection and treatment of STDs are essential tools for prevention of sexual and blood-borne transmission of HIV. Given these important considerations, medical visits provide a vital opportunity to reinforce HIV prevention messages, discuss sex- and drug-related risk behaviors, diagnose and treat intercurrent STDs, review the importance of medication adherence, and foster open communication between provider and patient.

References

1. Prejean J, Song R, Hernandez A, et al. Estimated HIV incidence in the United States, 2006-2009. *PLoS One.* 2011;6(8):e17502.

2. Centers for Disease Control and Prevention. HIV Surveillance Report http://www.cdc.gov/hiv/topics/surveillance/resources/reports/. 2009. Published February 2011. Accessed December 7, 2011.

3. Cohen MS, Chen YQ, McCauley M, et al. Prevention of HIV-1 infection with early antiretroviral therapy. *N Engl J Med.* Aug 11 2011;365(6):493-505.

4. Mayer KH, Safren SA, Gordon CM. HIV care providers and prevention: opportunities and challenges. *J Acquir Immune Defic Syndr.* Oct 1 2004;37(Suppl 2):S130-132.

5. Morin SF, Koester KA, Steward WT, et al. Missed opportunities: prevention with HIV-infected patients in clinical care settings. *J Acquir Immune Defic Syndr.* Aug 1 2004;36(4):960-966.

6. Metsch LR, McCoy CB, Miles CC, Wohler B. Prevention myths and HIV risk reduction by active drug users. *AIDS Educ Prev.* Apr 2004;16(2):150-159.

7. Johnson WD, Diaz RM, Flanders WD, et al. Behavioral interventions to reduce risk for sexual transmission of HIV among men who have sex with men. *Cochrane Database Syst Rev.* 2008(3):CD001230.

8. Centers for Disease Control and Prevention (CDC). Evolution of HIV/AIDS prevention programs—United States, 1981-2006. *MMWR Morb Mortal Wkly Rep.* Jun 2 2006;55(21):597-603.

9. Gorbach PM, Drumright LN, Daar ES, Little SJ. Transmission behaviors of recently HIV-infected men who have sex with men. *J Acquir Immune Defic Syndr.* May 2006;42(1):80-85.

10. Workowski KA, Berman S. Sexually transmitted diseases treatment guidelines, 2010. *MMWR Recomm Rep.* Dec 17 2010;59(RR-12):1-110.

11. Tanton C, Weiss HA, Le Goff J, et al. Correlates of HIV-1 genital shedding in Tanzanian women. *PLoS One.* 2011;6(3):e17480.

12. Wright TC, Jr., Subbarao S, Ellerbrock TV, et al. Human immunodeficiency virus 1 expression in the female genital tract in association with cervical inflammation and ulceration. *Am J Obstet Gynecol.* Feb 2001;184(3):279-285.

13. Schacker T, Ryncarz AJ, Goddard J, Diem K, Shaughnessy M, Corey L. Frequent recovery of HIV-1 from genital herpes simplex virus lesions in HIV-1-infected men. *JAMA.* Jul 1 1998;280(1):61-66.

14. Celentano DD, Latimore AD, Mehta SH. Variations in sexual risks in drug users: emerging themes in a behavioral context. *Curr HIV/AIDS Rep*. Nov 2008;5(4):212-218.

15. Mitchell MM, Latimer WW. Unprotected casual sex and perceived risk of contracting HIV among drug users in Baltimore, Maryland: evaluating the influence of non-injection versus injection drug user status. *AIDS Care*. Feb 2009;21(2):221-230.

16. Colfax G, Coates TJ, Husnik MJ, et al. Longitudinal patterns of methamphetamine, popper (amyl nitrite), and cocaine use and high-risk sexual behavior among a cohort of san francisco men who have sex with men. *J Urban Health*. Mar 2005;82(1 Suppl 1):i62-70.

17. Mimiaga MJ, Reisner SL, Fontaine YM, et al. Walking the line: stimulant use during sex and HIV risk behavior among Black urban MSM. *Drug Alcohol Depend*. Jul 1 2010;110(1-2):30-37.

18. Ostrow DG, Plankey MW, Cox C, et al. Specific sex drug combinations contribute to the majority of recent HIV seroconversions among MSM in the MACS. *J Acquir Immune Defic Syndr*. Jul 1 2009;51(3):349-355.

19. Sterk CE, Theall KP, Elifson KW. Who's getting the message? Intervention response rates among women who inject drugs and/or smoke crack cocaine. *Prev Med*. Aug 2003;37(2):119-128.

20. Sterk CE, Theall KP, Elifson KW, Kidder D. HIV risk reduction among African-American women who inject drugs: a randomized controlled trial. *AIDS Behav*. Mar 2003;7(1):73-86.

21. Strathdee SA, Sherman SG. The role of sexual transmission of HIV infection among injection and non-injection drug users. *J Urban Health*. Dec 2003;80(4 Suppl 3):iii7-14.

22. Copenhaver MM, Johnson BT, Lee IC, Harman JJ, Carey MP. Behavioral HIV risk reduction among people who inject drugs: meta-analytic evidence of efficacy. *J Subst Abuse Treat*. Sep 2006;31(2):163-171.

23. Hartel DM, Schoenbaum EE. Methadone treatment protects against HIV infection: two decades of experience in the Bronx, New York City. *Public Health Rep*. Jun 1998;113(Suppl 1):107-115.

24. Metzger DS, Navaline H, Woody GE. Drug abuse treatment as AIDS prevention. *Public Health Rep*. Jun 1998;113(Suppl 1):97-106.

25. Crawford ND, Vlahov D. Progress in HIV reduction and prevention among injection and noninjection drug users. *J Acquir Immune Defic Syndr*. Dec 2010;55(Suppl 2):S84-87.

26. Shoptaw S, Heinzerling KG, Rotheram-Fuller E, et al. Randomized, placebo-controlled trial of bupropion for the treatment of methamphetamine dependence. *Drug Alcohol Depend*. Aug 1 2008;96(3):222-232.

27. Heinzerling KG, Swanson AN, Kim S, et al. Randomized, double-blind, placebo-controlled trial of modafinil for the treatment of methamphetamine dependence. *Drug Alcohol Depend*. Jun 1 2010;109(1-3):20-29.

28. Centers for Disease Control and Prevention. Methamphetamine Use and Risk for HIV/AIDS. Atlanta, GA: Centers for Disease Control and Prevention, US Dept. of Health and Human Services. Last Modified: May 3, 2007.

29. Baeten JM, Kahle E, Lingappa JR, et al. Genital HIV-1 RNA predicts risk of heterosexual HIV-1 transmission. *Sci Transl Med*. Apr 6 2011;3(77):77ra29.

30. Sheth PM, Kovacs C, Kemal KS, et al. Persistent HIV RNA shedding in semen despite effective antiretroviral therapy. *AIDS*. Sep 24 2009;23(15):2050-2054.

31. Graham SM, Holte SE, Peshu NM, et al. Initiation of antiretroviral therapy leads to a rapid decline in cervical and vaginal HIV-1 shedding. *AIDS*. Feb 19 2007;21(4):501-507.

32. Vernazza PL, Troiani L, Flepp MJ, et al. Potent antiretroviral treatment of HIV-infection results in suppression of the seminal shedding of HIV. The Swiss HIV Cohort Study. *AIDS*. Jan 28 2000;14(2):117-121.

33. Hughes JP, Baeten JM, Lingappa JR, et al. Determinants of Per-Coital-Act HIV-1 Infectivity Among African HIV-1-Serodiscordant Couples. *J Infect Dis*. Feb 2012;205(3):358-365.

34. Quinn TC, Wawer MJ, Sewankambo N, et al. Viral load and heterosexual transmission of human immunodeficiency virus type 1. Rakai Project Study Group. *N Engl J Med*. Mar 30 2000;342(13):921-929.

35. Das M, Chu PL, Santos GM, et al. Decreases in community viral load are accompanied by reductions in new HIV infections in San Francisco. *PLoS One*. 2010;5(6):e11068.

36. Montaner JS, Lima VD, Barrios R, et al. Association of highly active antiretroviral therapy coverage, population viral load, and yearly new HIV diagnoses in British Columbia, Canada: a population-based study. *Lancet*. Aug 14 2010;376(9740):532-539.

37. Porco TC, Martin JN, Page-Shafer KA, et al. Decline in HIV infectivity following the introduction of highly active antiretroviral therapy. *AIDS*. Jan 2 2004;18(1):81-88.

38. Attia S, Egger M, Muller M, Zwahlen M, Low N. Sexual transmission of HIV according to viral load and antiretroviral therapy: systematic review and meta-analysis. *AIDS*. Jul 17 2009;23(11):1397-1404.

39. Cu-Uvin S, DeLong AK, Venkatesh KK, et al. Genital tract HIV-1 RNA shedding among women with below detectable plasma viral load. *AIDS*. Oct 23 2010;24(16):2489-2497.

40. Sturmer M, Doerr HW, Berger A, Gute P. Is transmission of HIV-1 in non-viraemic serodiscordant couples possible? *Antivir Ther*. 2008;13(5):729-732.

41. Crepaz N, Hart TA, Marks G. Highly active antiretroviral therapy and sexual risk behavior: a meta-analytic review. *JAMA*. Jul 14 2004;292(2):224-236.

42. Rice E, Batterham P, Rotheram-Borus MJ. Unprotected sex among youth living with HIV before and after the advent of highly active antiretroviral therapy. *Perspect Sex Reprod Health*. Sep 2006;38(3):162-167.

Conclusion (Last updated January 10, 2011; last reviewed January 10, 2011)

The Panel has carefully reviewed recent results from clinical trials in HIV therapy and considered how they inform appropriate care guidelines. The Panel appreciates that HIV care is highly complex and rapidly evolving. Guidelines are never fixed and must always be individualized. Where possible, the Panel has based recommendations on the best evidence from prospective trials with defined endpoints. When such evidence does not yet exist, the Panel attempted to reflect reasonable options in its conclusions.

HIV care requires, as always, partnerships and open communication. The provider can make recommendations most likely to lead to positive outcomes only if the patient's own point of view and social context are well known. Guidelines are only a starting point for medical decision making. They can identify some of the boundaries of high-quality care but cannot substitute for sound judgment.

As further research is conducted and reported, guidelines will be modified. The Panel anticipates continued progress in the simplicity of regimens, improved potency and barrier to resistance, and reduced toxicity. The Panel hopes the guidelines are useful and is committed to their continued adjustment and improvement.

Drug Name Abbreviations

Abbreviation	Full Name
3TC	lamivudine
ABC	abacavir
APV	amprenavir
ATV	atazanavir
ATV/r	ritonavir-boosted atazanavir
AZT	zidovudine
COBI	cobicistat
d4T	stavudine
ddI	didanosine
DLV	delavirdine
DRV	darunavir
DRV/r	ritonavir- boosted darunavir
EFV	efavirenz
ETR	etravirine
EVG	elvitegravir
FPV	fosamprenavir
FPV/r	ritonavir-boosted fosamprenavir
FTC	emtricitabine
GAZT	azidothymidine glucuronide
IDV	indinavir
LPV	lopinavir
LPV/r	ritonavir-boosted lopinavir
MVC	maraviroc
NFV	nelfinavir
NVP	nevirapine
RAL	raltegravir

RPV	rilpivirine
RTV	ritonavir
SQV	saquinavir
SQV/r	ritonavir-boosted saquinavir
T20	enfuvirtide
TDF	tenofovir disoproxil fumarate
TPV	tipranavir
TPV/r	ritonavir-boosted tipranavir
ZDV	zidovudine

General Terms

Abbreviation	Full Name
ACTG	AIDS Clinical Trials Group
AIDS	acquired immune deficiency syndrome
ALT	alanine aminotransferase
ART	antiretroviral therapy
ART-CC	ART Cohort Collaboration
ARV	antiretroviral
AST	aspartate aminotransferase
AUC	area under the curve
AV	atrioventricular
bDNA	branched DNA
BID	twice daily
BMD	bone mineral density
BMI	body mass index
BUN	blood urea nitrogen
cap	capsule
CAPD	chronic ambulatory peritoneal dialysis
CBC	complete blood count
CCB	calcium channel blocker
CDC	Centers for Disease Control and Prevention
CI	confidence interval
CKD	chronic kidney disease
C_{max}	maximum plasma concentration
CME	continuing medical education

C_{min}	minimum plasma concentration
CMV	cytomegalovirus
CNICS	Centers for AIDS Research Network of Integrated Clinical Systems
CNS	central nervous system
COC	combined oral contraceptives
CPK	creatine phosphokinase
CrCl	creatinine clearance
CSF	cerebrospinal fluid
CVD	cardiovascular disease
CYP	cytochrome P
D/M	dual or mixed (tropic)
D:A:D	Data Collection on Adverse Events of Anti-HIV Drugs Study
DILI	drug-induced liver injury
DM	diabetes mellitus
DMPA	depot medroxyprogesterone acetate
DOT	directly observed therapy
DR	delayed release
DXA	dual-energy x-ray absorptiometry
EBV	Epstein-Barr virus
EC	enteric coated
ECG	electrocardiogram
EI	entry inhibitor
EIA	enzyme immunoassay
FDA	Food and Drug Administration
FI	fusion inhibitor
GHB	gamma-hydroxybutyrate
GI	gastrointestinal
HAD	HIV-associated dementia
HAV	hepatitis A virus
HBeAg	hepatitis B e antigen
HBsAg	hepatitis B surface antigen
HBV	hepatitis B virus
HCV	hepatitis C virus
HD	hemodialysis
HDL	high-density lipoprotein

HELLP	hemolysis, elevated liver enzymes, low platelet count (syndrome)
HHS	Department of Health and Human Services
HHV	human herpes virus
HHV-8	human herpes virus-8
HIV	human immunodeficiency virus
HIV-1	human immunodeficiency virus type 1
HIV-2	human immunodeficiency virus type 2
HIVAN	HIV-associated nephropathy
HLA	human leukocyte antigen
HPV	human papilloma virus
HR	hazard ratio
HRSA	Health Resource Services Administration
hsCRP	high-sensitivity C-reactive protein
HSR	hypersensitivity reaction
HTLV	human T-cell leukemia virus
HTLV-1	human T-cell leukemia virus type 1
HTLV-2	human T-cell leukemia virus type 2
IAS-USA	International Antiviral Society-USA
IC	inhibitory concentration
IDU	injection drug user
IFN-γ	interferon-gamma
IGRA	interferon-gamma release assay
IL-2	interleukin-2
IL-6	interleukin-6
IL-7	interleukin-7
IND	investigational new drug
INH	isoniazid
inj	injection
INR	international normalized ratio
INSTI	integrase strand transfer inhibitor
IQ	inhibitory quotient
IRB	Institutional Review Board
IRIS	immune reconstitution inflammatory syndrome
IUD	intrauterine device
IV	Intravenous
LDL	low-density lipoprotein
LTBI	latent tuberculosis infection

Guidelines for the Use of Antiretroviral Agents in HIV-1-Infected Adults and Adolescents   O-4

MAC	*Mycobacterium avium* complex
MDMA	methylenedioxymethamphetamine
mDOT	modified directly observed therapy
MDR	multidrug-resistant
MDRD	modification of diet in renal disease (equation)
MHC	major histocompatability complex
MI	myocardial infarction
msec	milliseconds
MSM	men who have sex with men
MTB	*Mycobacterium tuberculosis*
MTCT	mother-to-child transmission
NA-ACCORD	The North American AIDS Cohort Collaboration on Research and Design
NIH	National Institutes of Health
NNRTI	non-nucleoside reverse transcriptase inhibitor
NRTI	nucleoside reverse transcriptase inhibitor
OAR	Office of AIDS Research
OARAC	Office of AIDS Research Advisory Council
OI	opportunistic infection
PAH	pulmonary arterial hypertension
PCP	*Pneumocystis jiroveci* pneumonia
PDE5	phosphodiesterase type 5
PegIFN	peginterferon
p-gp	p-glycoprotein
PI	protease inhibitor
PK	pharmacokinetic
PMTCT	prevention of mother-to-child transmission
PNS	peripheral nervous system
PO	orally
PPI	proton pump inhibitor
PR	protease (gene)
PrEP	pre-exposure HIV prophylaxis
PT	prothrombin time
QTc	QT corrected for heart rate
RT	reverse transcriptase (gene)

RT-PCR	reverse transcriptase-polymerase chain reaction
SJS	Stevens-Johnson syndrome
soln	solution
SPT	skin patch test
STD	sexually transmitted disease
SVR	sustained virologic response
SWP	suggested wholesale price
$t_{1/2}$	half-life
tab	tablet
TAM	thymidine analogue mutation
TB	tuberculosis
TCA	tricyclic antidepressant
TDM	therapeutic drug monitoring
TEN	toxic epidermal necrosis
TG	triglyceride
the Panel	Panel on Antiretroviral Guidelines for Adults and Adolescents
TID	three times daily
TST	tuberculin skin test
UDP	uridine diphosphate
UGT	uridine diphosphate gluconyltransferase
UGT1A1	uridine diphosphate glucuronosyltransferase 1A1
ULN	upper limit of normal
VPA	valproic acid
WBC	white blood cell
WHO	World Health Organization
WITS	Women and Infants Transmission Study
XDR	extensively drug-resistant
XR	extended release

Generic Name (Abbreviation)/ Trade Name	Formulations	Dosing Recommendations (For dosage adjustment in renal or hepatic insufficiency, see Appendix B, Table 7.)	Elimination	Serum/ Intracellular Half-Lives	Adverse Events (Also see Table 13.)
Abacavir (ABC)/ Ziagen Generic available in tablet formulation **Also available as a component of fixed-dose combinations:**	Ziagen • 300 mg tablets • 20 mg/mL oral solution	Ziagen 300 mg BID or 600 mg once daily Take without regard to meals	Metabolized by alcohol dehydrogenase and glucuronyl transferase Renal excretion of metabolites 82% Dosage adjustment for ABC is recommended in patients with hepatic insufficiency (see Appendix B, Table 7)	1.5 hours/ 12–26 hours	• HSRs: Patients who test positive for HLA-B*5701 are at highest risk. HLA screening should be done before initiation of ABC. Re-challenge is not recommended. • Symptoms of HSR may include fever, rash, nausea, vomiting, diarrhea, abdominal pain, malaise, or fatigue or respiratory symptoms such as sore throat, cough, or shortness of breath. • Some cohort studies suggest increased risk of MI with recent or current use of ABC, but this risk is not substantiated in other studies.
Trizivir ABC with ZDV + 3TC	Trizivir (ABC 300 mg + ZDV 300 mg + 3TC 150 mg) tablet	Trizivir 1 tablet BID			
Epzicom ABC with 3TC	Epzicom (ABC 600 mg + 3TC 300 mg) tablet	Epzicom 1 tablet once daily			
Didanosine (ddI)/ Videx EC Generic available; dose same as Videx EC	Videx EC 125, 200, 250, and 400 mg capsules Videx 10 mg/mL oral solution	**Body weight ≥60kg:** 400 mg once daily *With TDF:* 250 mg once daily **Body weight <60kg:** 250 mg once daily *With TDF:* 200 mg once daily Take 1/2 hour before or 2 hours after a meal Note: Preferred dosing with oral solution is BID (total daily dose divided into 2 doses)	Renal excretion 50% Dosage adjustment in patients with renal insufficiency is recommended (see Appendix B, Table 7).	1.5 hours/ >20 hours	• Pancreatitis • Peripheral neuropathy • Retinal changes, optic neuritis • Lactic acidosis with hepatic steatosis +/- pancreatitis (rare but potentially life-threatening toxicity) • Nausea, vomiting • Potential association with non-cirrhotic portal hypertension, in some cases, patients presented with esophageal varices • One cohort study suggested increased risk of MI with recent or current use of ddI, but this risk is not substantiated in other studies. • Insulin resistance/diabetes mellitus

Generic Name (Abbreviation)/ Trade Name	Formulations	Dosing Recommendations (For dosage adjustment in renal or hepatic insufficiency, see Appendix B, Table 7.)	Elimination	Serum/ Intracellular Half-Lives	Adverse Events (Also see Table 13.)
Emtricitabine (FTC)/ Emtriva **Also available as a component of fixed-dose combinations:**	Emtriva • 200 mg hard gelatin capsule • 10 mg/mL oral solution	Emtriva *Capsule:* 200 mg once daily *Oral solution:* 240 mg (24 mL) once daily Take without regard to meals	Renal excretion 86% Dosage adjustment in patients with renal insufficiency is recommended (see Appendix B, Table 7).	10 hours/ >20 hours	• Minimal toxicity • Hyperpigmentation/skin discoloration • Severe acute exacerbation of hepatitis may occur in HBV-co-infected patients who discontinue FTC.
Atripla FTC with EFV + TDF	Atripla (FTC 200 mg + EFV 600 mg + TDF 300 mg) tablet	Atripla 1 tablet at or before bedtime Take on an empty stomach to reduce side effects.			
Complera FTC with RPV+TDF	Complera (FTC 200 mg + RPV 25 mg + TDF 300 mg) tablet	Complera 1 tablet once daily with a meal			
Stribild FTC with EVG + COBI + TDF	Stribild (FTC 200 mg + EVG 150 mg + COBI 150 mg + TDF 300 mg) tablet	Stribild 1 tablet once daily with food			
Truvada FTC with TDF	Truvada (FTC 200 mg + TDF 300 mg) tablet	Truvada 1 tablet once daily			

Generic Name (Abbreviation)/ Trade Name	Formulations	Dosing Recommendations (For dosage adjustment in renal or hepatic insufficiency, see Appendix B, Table 7.)	Elimination	Serum/ Intracellular Half-Lives	Adverse Events (Also see Table 13.)
Lamivudine (3TC)/ Epivir Generic available in tablet formulation **Also available as a component of fixed-dose combinations:**	Epivir • 150 and 300 mg tablets • 10 mg/mL oral solution	Epivir 150 mg BID or 300 mg once daily Take without regard to meals	Renal excretion 70% Dosage adjustment in patients with renal insufficiency is recommended (see Appendix B, Table 7).	5–7 hours/ 18–22 hours	• Minimal toxicity • Severe acute exacerbation of hepatitis may occur in HBV-co-infected patients who discontinue 3TC.
Combivir 3TC with ZDV Generic available	Combivir (3TC 150 mg + ZDV 300 mg) tablet	Combivir 1 tablet BID			
Epzicom 3TC with ABC	Epzicom (3TC 300 mg + ABC 600 mg) tablet	Epzicom 1 tablet once daily			
Trizivir 3TC with ZDV+ABC	Trizivir (3TC 150 mg + ZDV 300 mg + ABC 300 mg) tablet	Trizivir 1 tablet BID			
Stavudine (d4T)/ Zerit Generic available	Zerit • 15, 20, 30, and 40 mg capsules • 1 mg/mL oral solution	**Body weight ≥60 kg:** 40 mg BID **Body weight <60 kg:** 30 mg BID Take without regard to meals Note: WHO recommends 30 mg BID dosing regardless of body weight.	Renal excretion 50% Dosage adjustment in patients with renal insufficiency is recommended (see Appendix B, Table 7).	1 hours/ 7.5 hours	• Peripheral neuropathy • Lipoatrophy • Pancreatitis • Lactic acidosis/severe hepatomegaly with hepatic steatosis (rare but potentially life-threatening toxicity) • Hyperlipidemia • Insulin resistance/diabetes mellitus • Rapidly progressive ascending neuromuscular weakness (rare)

Generic Name (Abbreviation)/ Trade Name	Formulations	Dosing Recommendations (For dosage adjustment in renal or hepatic insufficiency, see Appendix B, Table 7.)	Elimination	Serum/ Intracellular Half-Lives	Adverse Events (Also see Table 13.)
Tenofovir Disoproxil Fumarate (TDF)/ Viread **Also available as a component of fixed-dose combinations:**	Viread • 150, 200, 250, 300 mg tablets • 40 mg/g oral powder	Viread 300 mg once daily or 7.5 scoops once daily Take without regard to meals Mix oral powder with 2–4 ounces of soft food that does not require chewing (e.g., applesauce, yogurt). **DO NOT MIX ORAL POWDER WITH LIQUID.**	Renal excretion Dosage adjustment in patients with renal insufficiency is recommended (see Appendix B, Table 7).	17 hours/ >60 hours	• Renal insufficiency, Fanconi syndrome, proximal tubulopathy • Osteomalacia, decrease in bone mineral density • Potential decrease in bone mineral density • Severe acute exacerbation of hepatitis may occur in HBV-co-infected patients who discontinue TDF. • Asthenia, headache, diarrhea, nausea, vomiting, and flatulence
Atripla TDF with EFV+FTC	Atripla (TDF 300 mg + EFV 600 mg + FTC 200 mg) tablet	Atripla 1 tablet at or before bedtime Take on an empty stomach to reduce side effects			
Complera TDF with RPV+FTC	Complera (TDF 300 mg + RPV 25 mg + FTC 200 mg) tablet	Complera 1 tablet once daily Take with a meal			
Stribild TDF with EVG+COBI+ FTC	Stribild (TDF 300 mg + EVG 150 mg + COBI 150 mg + FTC 200 mg) tablet	Stribild 1 tablet once daily with food			
Truvada TDF with FTC	Truvada (TDF 300 mg + FTC 200 mg) tablet	Truvada 1 tablet once daily Take without regard to meals			

Generic Name (Abbreviation)/ Trade Name	Formulations	Dosing Recommendations (For dosage adjustment in renal or hepatic insufficiency, see Appendix B, Table 7.)	Elimination	Serum/ Intracellular Half-Lives	Adverse Events (Also see Table 13.)
Zidovudine (ZDV)/ Retrovir Generic available **Also available as a component of fixed-dose combinations**	Retrovir • 100 mg capsule • 300 mg tablet (generic only) • 10 mg/mL intravenous solution • 10 mg/mL oral solution	Retrovir 300 mg BID or 200 mg TID Take without regard to meals	Metabolized to GAZT Renal excretion of GAZT Dosage adjustment in patients with renal insufficiency is recommended (see Appendix B, Table 7).	1.1 hours/ 7 hours	• Bone marrow suppression: macrocytic anemia or neutropenia • Nausea, vomiting, headache, insomnia, asthenia • Nail pigmentation • Lactic acidosis/severe hepatomegaly with hepatic steatosis (rare but potentially life-threatening toxicity) • Hyperlipidemia • Insulin resistance/diabetes mellitus • Lipoatrophy • Myopathy
Combivir ZDV with 3TC Generic available	Combivir (ZDV 300 mg + 3TC 150 mg) tablet	Combivir 1 tablet BID			
Trizivir ZDV with 3TC+ ABC	Trizivir (ZDV 300 mg + 3TC 150 mg + ABC 300 mg) tablet	Trizivir 1 tablet BID			

Key to Abbreviations: 3TC = lamivudine, ABC = abacavir, BID = twice daily, COBI = cobicistat, d4T = stavudine, ddI = didanosine, EC = enteric coated, EFV = efavirenz, EVG = elvitegravir, FTC = emtricitabine, GAZT = azidothymidine glucuronide, HBV = hepatitis B virus, HLA = human leukocyte antigen, HSR = hypersensitivity reaction, MI = myocardial infarction, RPV = rilpivirine, TDF = tenofovir disoproxil fumarate, TID = three times a day, WHO = World Health Organization, ZDV = zidovudine

Appendix B, Table 2. Characteristics of Non-Nucleoside Reverse Transcriptase Inhibitors* (Last updated February 12, 2013; last reviewed February 12, 2013) (page 1 of 2)

* Delavirdine (DLV) is not included in this table. Please refer to the DLV FDA package insert for related information.

Generic Name (Abbreviation)/ Trade Name	Formulations	Dosing Recommendations (For dosage adjustment in renal or hepatic insufficiency, see Appendix B, Table 7.)	Elimination	Serum Half-Life	Adverse Events (Also see Table 13.)
Efavirenz (EFV)/ Sustiva **Also available as a component of fixed-dose combination:**	• 50 and 200 mg capsules • 600 mg tablet	600 mg once daily, at or before bedtime Take on an empty stomach to reduce side effects.	Metabolized by CYPs 2B6 and 3A4 CYP3A4 mixed inducer/inhibitor (more an inducer than an inhibitor)	40–55 hours	• Rash[a] • Neuropsychiatric symptoms[b] • Increased transaminase levels • Hyperlipidemia • False-positive results with some cannabinoid and benzodiazepine screening assays reported. • Teratogenic in non-human primates and potentially teratogenic in humans
Atripla EFV with TDF + FTC	(EFV 600 mg + FTC 200 mg + TDF 300 mg) tablet	1 tablet once daily, at or before bedtime			
Etravirine (ETR)/ Intelence	• 25, 100, and 200 mg tablets	200 mg BID Take following a meal.	CYP3A4, 2C9, and 2C19 substrate 3A4 inducer; 2C9 and 2C19 inhibitor	41 hours	• Rash, including Stevens-Johnson syndrome[a] • HSRs, characterized by rash, constitutional findings, and sometimes organ dysfunction, including hepatic failure, have been reported. • Nausea

Nevirapine (NVP)/ Viramune or Viramine XR Generic available for 200 mg tablets	• 200 mg tablet
	 • 400 mg XR tablet
	 • 50 mg/5 mL oral suspension
		200 mg once daily for 14 days (lead-in period); thereafter, 200 mg BID, or 400 mg (Viramune XR tablet) once daily
		
		 Take without regard to meals
		
		 Repeat lead-in period if therapy is discontinued for more than 7 days
		
		 In patients who develop mild-to-moderate rash without constitutional symptoms, continue lead-in period until rash resolves but not longer than 28 days total.
			CYP450 substrate, inducer of 3A4 and 2B6; 80% excreted in urine (glucuronidated metabolites, <5% unchanged); 10% in feces	25–30 hours	• Rash, including Stevens-Johnson syndrome[a]
					 • Symptomatic hepatitis, including fatal hepatic necrosis, has been reported:
					   • Rash reported in approximately 50% of cases
					   • Occurs at significantly higher frequency in ARV-naive female patients with pre-NVP CD4 counts >250 cells/mm³ and in ARV-naive male patients with pre-NVP CD4 counts >400 cells/mm³. NVP should not be initiated in these patients unless the benefit clearly outweighs the risk.

Appendix B, Table 2. Characteristics of Non-Nucleoside Reverse Transcriptase Inhibitors* (Last updated February 12, 2013; last reviewed February 12, 2013) (page 2 of 2)

* Delavirdine (DLV) is not included in this table. Please refer to the DLV FDA package insert for related information.

Generic Name (Abbreviation)/ Trade Name	Formulations	Dosing Recommendations (For dosage adjustment in renal or hepatic insufficiency, see Appendix B, Table 7.)	Elimination	Serum Half-Life	Adverse Events (Also see Table 13.)
Rilpivirine (RPV)/ Edurant **Also available as a component of fixed-dose combination:**	• 25 mg tablet	25 mg once daily Take with a meal	CYP3A4 substrate	50 hours	• Rash[a] • Depression, insomnia, headache • Hepatotoxicity
Complera RPV with TDF + FTC	Complera (RPV 25 mg + TDF 300 mg + FTC 200 mg) tablet	1 tablet once daily with a meal			

Key to Abbreviations: ARV = antiretroviral, BID = twice daily, CYP = cytochrome P, DLV = delavirdine, EFV = efavirenz, ETR = etravirine, FDA = Food and Drug Administration, FTC = emtricitabine, HSR = hypersensitivity reaction, NNRTI = non-nucleoside reverse transcriptase inhibitor, NVP = nevirapine, RPV = rilpivirine, TDF = tenofovir disoproxil fumarate, XR = extended release

[a] Rare cases of Stevens-Johnson syndrome have been reported with most NNRTIs; the highest incidence of rash was seen with NVP.

[b] Adverse events can include dizziness, somnolence, insomnia, abnormal dreams, confusion, abnormal thinking, impaired concentration, amnesia, agitation, depersonalization, hallucinations, and euphoria. Approximately 50% of patients receiving EFV may experience any of these symptoms. Symptoms usually subside spontaneously after 2 to 4 weeks but may necessitate discontinuation of EFV in a small percentage of patients.

Generic Name (Abbreviation)/ Trade Name	Formulations	Dosing Recommendations (For dosage adjustment in hepatic insufficiency, see Appendix B, Table 7.)	Elimination	Serum Half-Life	Storage	Adverse Events (Also see Table 13.)
Atazanavir (ATV)/ Reyataz	100, 150, 200, and 300 mg capsules	ARV-naive patients: 400 mg once daily, or (ATV 300 mg + RTV 100 mg) once daily With TDF or in ARV-experienced patients: (ATV 300 mg + RTV 100 mg) once daily With EFV in ARV-naive patients: (ATV 400 mg + RTV 100 mg) once daily **For recommendations on dosing with H2 antagonists and PPIs, refer to Table 16a.** Take with food	CYP3A4 inhibitor and substrate Dosage adjustment in patients with hepatic insufficiency is recommended. (see Appendix B, Table 7).	7 hours	Room temperature (up to 25ºC or 77ºF)	• Indirect hyperbilirubinemia • PR interval prolongation: First degree symptomatic AV block reported. Use with caution in patients with underlying conduction defects or on concomitant medications that can cause PR prolongation. • Hyperglycemia • Fat maldistribution • Possible increased bleeding episodes in patients with hemophilia • Cholelithiasis • Nephrolithiasis • Skin rash (20%) • Serum transaminase elevations • Hyperlipidemia (especially with RTV boosting)
Darunavir (DRV)/ Prezista	75, 150, 300, 400, 600, and 800 mg tablets 100 mg/mL oral suspension	ARV-naive patients or ARV-experienced patients with no DRV mutations: (DRV 800 mg + RTV 100 mg) once daily ARV-experienced patients with at least one DRV mutation: (DRV 600 mg + RTV 100 mg) BID Unboosted DRV is **not** recommended. Take with food	CYP3A4 inhibitor and substrate	15 hours (when combined with RTV)	Room temperature (up to 25ºC or 77ºF)	• Skin rash (10%): DRV has a sulfonamide moiety; Stevens-Johnson syndrome, toxic epidermal necrolysis, acute generalized exanthematous pustulosis, and erythrema multiforme have been reported. • Hepatotoxicity • Diarrhea, nausea • Headache • Hyperlipidemia • Serum transaminase elevation • Hyperglycemia • Fat maldistribution • Possible increased bleeding episodes in patients with hemophilia

Generic Name (Abbreviation)/ Trade Name	Formulations	Dosing Recommendations (For dosage adjustment in hepatic insufficiency, see Appendix B, Table 7.)	Elimination	Serum Half-Life	Storage	Adverse Events (Also see Table 13.)
Fosamprenavir (FPV)/ Lexiva (a prodrug of amprenavir [APV])	• 700 mg tablet • 50 mg/mL oral suspension	<u>ARV-naive patients:</u> FPV 1400 mg BID, or (FPV 1400 mg + RTV 100–200 mg) once daily, or (FPV 700 mg + RTV 100 mg) BID <u>PI-experienced patients (once-daily dosing **not** recommended):</u> (FPV 700 mg + RTV 100 mg) BID <u>With EFV:</u> (FPV 700 mg + RTV 100 mg) BID, or (FPV 1400 mg + RTV 300 mg) once daily *Tablet:* Take without regard to meals (if not boosted with RTV tablet) *Suspension:* Take without food *FPV with RTV tablet:* Take with meals	APV is a CYP3A4 substrate, inhibitor, and inducer. Dosage adjustment in patients with hepatic insufficiency is recommended (see Appendix B, Table 7).	7.7 hours (APV)	Room temperature (up to 25°C or 77°F)	• Skin rash (12%–19%): FPV has a sulfonamide moiety. • Diarrhea, nausea, vomiting • Headache • Hyperlipidemia • Serum transaminase elevation • Hyperglycemia • Fat maldistribution • Possible increased bleeding episodes in patients with hemophilia • Nephrolithiasis
Indinavir (IDV)/ Crixivan	100, 200, and 400 mg capsules	800 mg every 8 hrs Take 1 hour before or 2 hours after meals; may take with skim milk or low-fat meal <u>With RTV:</u> (IDV 800 mg + RTV 100–200 mg) BID Take without regard to meals	CYP3A4 inhibitor and substrate Dosage adjustment in patients with hepatic insufficiency is recommended (see Appendix B, Table 7).	1.5–2 hours	Room temperature (15°–30°C/ 59°–86°F) Protect from moisture	• Nephrolithiasis • GI intolerance, nausea • Hepatitis • Indirect hyperbilirubinemia • Hyperlipidemia • Headache, asthenia, blurred vision, dizziness, rash, metallic taste, thrombocytopenia, alopecia, and hemolytic anemia • Hyperglycemia • Fat maldistribution • Possible increased bleeding episodes in patients with hemophilia

Generic Name (Abbreviation)/ Trade Name	Formulations	Dosing Recommendations (For dosage adjustment in hepatic insufficiency, see Appendix B, Table 7.)	Elimination	Serum Half-Life	Storage	Adverse Events (Also see Table 13.)
Lopinavir + Ritonavir LPV/r)/ Kaletra	Tablets: (LPV 200 mg + RTV 50 mg), or (LPV 100 mg + RTV 25 mg) Oral solution: Each 5 mL contains (LPV 400 mg + RTV 100 mg) Oral solution contains 42% alcohol	LPV/r 400 mg/100 mg BID or LPV/r 800 mg/200 mg once daily Once-daily dosing is not recommended for patients with ≥3 LPV-associated mutations, pregnant women, or patients receiving EFV, NVP, FPV, NFV, carbamazepine, phenytoin, or phenobarbital. With EFV or NVP (PI-naive or PI-experienced patients): LPV/r 500 mg/125 mg tablets BID (Use a combination of two LPV/r 200 mg/50 mg tablets + one LPV/r 100 mg/25 mg tablet to make a total dose of LPV/r 500 mg/125 mg.) or LPV/r 533 mg/133 mg oral solution BID _Tablet_: Take without regard to meals _Oral solution_: Take with food	CYP3A4 inhibitor and substrate	5–6 hours	Oral tablet is stable at room temperature. Oral solution is stable at 2°–8°C (36°–46°F) until date on label and is stable for up to 2 months when stored at room temperature (up to 25°C or 77°F).	• GI intolerance, nausea, vomiting, diarrhea • Pancreatitis • Asthenia • Hyperlipidemia (especially hypertriglyceridemia) • Serum transaminase elevation • Hyperglycemia • Insulin resistance/diabetes mellitus • Fat maldistribution • Possible increased bleeding episodes in patients with hemophilia • PR interval prolongation • QT interval prolongation and torsades de pointes have been reported; however, causality could not be established.
Nelfinavir (NFV)/ Viracept	• 250 and 625 mg tablets • 50 mg/g oral powder	1250 mg BID or 750 mg TID Dissolve tablets in a small amount of water, mix admixture well, and consume immediately. Take with food	CYP2C19 and 3A4 substrate— metabolized to active M8 metabolite; CYP 3A4 inhibitor	3.5–5 hours	Room temperature (15°–30°C/ 59°–86°F)	• Diarrhea • Hyperlipidemia • Hyperglycemia • Fat maldistribution • Possible increased bleeding episodes in patients with hemophilia • Serum transaminase elevation

Generic Name (Abbreviation)/ Trade Name	Formulations	Dosing Recommendations (For dosage adjustment in hepatic insufficiency, see Appendix B, Table 7.)	Elimination	Serum Half-Life	Storage	Adverse Events (Also see Table 13.)
Ritonavir (RTV)/ Norvir	• 100 mg tablet • 100 mg soft gel capsule • 80 mg/mL oral solution Oral solution contains 43% alcohol	As pharmacokinetic booster for other PIs: 100–400 mg per day in 1–2 divided doses (refer to other PIs for specific dosing recommendations) *Tablet*: Take with food *Capsule and oral solution:* To improve tolerability, take with food if possible.	CYP3A4 >2D6 substrate; potent 3A4, 2D6 inhibitor	3–5 hours	Tablets do not require refrigeration. Refrigerate capsules. Capsules can be left at room temperature (up to 25°C or 77°F) for up to 30 days. Oral solution should **not** be refrigerated; store at room temperature (20°–25°C/ 68°–77°F).	• GI intolerance, nausea, vomiting, diarrhea • Paresthesias (circumoral and extremities) • Hyperlipidemia (especially hypertriglyceridemia) • Hepatitis • Asthenia • Taste perversion • Hyperglycemia • Fat maldistribution • Possible increased bleeding episodes in patients with hemophilia
Saquinavir (SQV)/ Invirase	• 500 mg tablet • 200 mg hard gel capsule	(SQV 1000 mg + RTV 100 mg) BID Unboosted SQV is **not** recommended. Take with meals or within 2 hours after a meal	CYP3A4 inhibitor and substrate	1–2 hours	Room temperature (15°–30°C/ 59°–86°F)	• GI intolerance, nausea, and diarrhea • Headache • Serum transaminase elevation • Hyperlipidemia • Hyperglycemia • Fat maldistribution • Possible increased bleeding episodes in patients with hemophilia • PR interval prolongation • QT interval prolongation, torsades de pointes have been reported. Patients with pre-SQV QT interval >450 msec should not receive SQV (see Table 5b).

Generic Name (Abbreviation)/ Trade Name	Formulations	Dosing Recommendations (For dosage adjustment in hepatic insufficiency, see Appendix B, Table 7.)	Elimination	Serum Half-Life	Storage	Adverse Events (Also see Table 13.)
Tipranavir (TPV)/ Aptivus	• 250 mg capsule • 100 mg/mL oral solution	(TPV 500 mg + RTV 200 mg) BID Unboosted TPV is **not** recommended. *TPV taken with RTV **tablets**:* Take with meals *TPV taken with RTV **capsules** or **solution**:* Take without regard to meals	CYP P450 3A4 inducer and substrate Net effect when combined with RTV (CYP 3A4, 2D6 inhibitor)	6 hours after single dose of TPV/r	Refrigerate capsules. Capsules can be stored at room temperature (25°C or 77°F) for up to 60 days. Oral solution should **not** be refrigerated or frozen and should be used within 60 days after bottle is opened.	• Hepatotoxicity: Clinical hepatitis (including hepatic decompensation and hepatitis-associated fatalities) has been reported; monitor patients closely, especially those with underlying liver diseases. • Skin rash (3%–21%): TPV has a sulfonamide moiety; use with caution in patients with known sulfonamide allergy. • Rare cases of fatal and nonfatal intracranial hemorrhages have been reported. Risks include brain lesion, head trauma, recent neurosurgery, coagulopathy, hypertension, alcoholism, use of anti-coagulant or anti-platelet agents (including vitamin E). • Hyperlipidemia • Hyperglycemia • Fat maldistribution • Possible increased bleeding episodes in patients with hemophilia

Key to Abbreviations: APV = amprenavir, ARV = antiretroviral, ATV = atazanavir, AV = atrioventricular, BID = twice daily, CYP = cytochrome P, DRV = darunavir, EFV = efavirenz, FPV = fosamprenavir, GI = gastrointestinal, IDV = indinavir, LPV = lopinavir, LPV/r = lopinavir + ritonavir, msec = millisecond, NFV = nelfinavir, NVP = nevirapine, PI = protease inhibitor, PPI = proton pump inhibitor, RTV = ritonavir, SQV = saquinavir, TDF = tenofovir disoproxil fumarate, TID = three times a day, TPV = tipranavir

Appendix B, Table 4. Characteristics of Integrase Inhibitors (Last updated February 12, 2013; last reviewed February 12, 2013)

Generic Name (Abbreviation)/ Trade Name	Formulations	Dosing Recommendations (For dosage adjustment in hepatic insufficiency, see Appendix B, Table 7.)	Serum Half-Life	Route of Metabolism	Adverse Events (Also see Table 13.)
Raltegravir (RAL)/ Isentress	400 mg tablet 25 and 100 mg chewable tablets	400 mg BID With rifampin: 800 mg BID Take without regard to meals	~9 hours	UGT1A1-mediated glucuronidation	• Rash, including Stevens-Johnson syndrome, HSR, and toxic epidermal necrolysis • Nausea • Headache • Diarrhea • Pyrexia • CPK elevation, muscle weakness, and rhabdomyolysis
Elvitegravir (EVG) Currently only available as a co-formulated product with: **Cobicistat** (COBI)/ TDF/FTC Stribild	(EVG 150 mg + COBI 150 mg + TDF 300 mg + FTC 200 mg) tablet	1 tablet once daily with food **Not recommended** for patients with baseline CrCl< 70 mL/min. See Appendix B, Table 7 for the equation for calculating CrCl. **Not recommended for use with other antiretroviral drugs**	~13 hours	EVG: CYP3A, UGT1A1/3 COBI: CYP3A, CYP2D6 (minor)	• Nausea • Diarrhea • New onset or worsening renal impairment • Potential decrease in bone mineral density • Severe acute exacerbation of hepatitis may occur in HBV-coinfected patients who discontinue FTC and TDF.

Key to Abbreviations: BID = twice daily, COBI = cobicistat, CPK = creatine phosphokinase, CrCl = creatinine clearance, EVG = elvitegravir, FTC = emtricitabine, HSR = hypersensitivity reaction, RAL = raltegravir, TDF = tenofovir, UGT = uridine diphosphate gluconyltransferase

Appendix B, Table 5. Characteristics of Fusion Inhibitor (Last updated January 29, 2008; last reviewed February 12, 2013)

Generic Name (Abbreviation)/ Trade Name	Formulations	Dosing Recommendations	Serum Half-Life	Elimination	Storage	Adverse Events (Also see Table 13.)
Enfuvirtide (T20)/ Fuzeon	• Injectable; supplied as lyophilized powder • Each vial contains 108 mg of T20; reconstitute with 1.1mL of sterile water for injection for delivery of approximately 90 mg/1 mL.	90 mg (1 mL) subcutaneously BID	3.8 hours	Expected to undergo catabolism to its constituent amino acids, with subsequent recycling of the amino acids in the body pool	Store at room temperature (up to 25°C or 77°F). Re-constituted solution should be refrigerated at 2°C–8°C (36°F–46°F) and used within 24 hours.	• Local injection site reactions (e.g., pain, erythema, induration, nodules and cysts, pruritus, ecchymosis) in almost 100% of patients • Increased incidence of bacterial pneumonia • HSR (<1% of patients): Symptoms may include rash, fever, nausea, vomiting, chills, rigors, hypotension, or elevated serum transaminases. Re-challenge is not recommended.

Key to Abbreviations: BID = twice daily, HSR = hypersensitivity reaction, T20 = enfuvirtide

Appendix B, Table 6. Characteristics of CCR5 Antagonist (Last updated March 27, 2012; last reviewed February 12, 2013)

Generic Name (Abbreviation)/ Trade Name	Formulation	Dosing Recommendations (For dosage adjustment in hepatic insufficiency, see Appendix B, Table 7.)	Serum Half-Life	Elimination	Adverse Events (Also see Table 13.)
Maraviroc (MVC)/ Selzentry	150 and 300 mg tablets	**150 mg BID** when given with drugs that are strong CYP3A inhibitors (with or without CYP3A inducers) including PIs (except TPV/r) **300 mg BID** when given with NRTIs, T20, TPV/r, NVP, RAL, and other drugs that are not strong CYP3A inhibitors or inducers **600 mg BID** when given with drugs that are CYP3A inducers, including EFV, ETR, etc. (without a CYP3A inhibitor) Take without regard to meals	14–18 hours	CYP3A4 substrate	• Abdominal pain • Cough • Dizziness • Musculoskeletal symptoms • Pyrexia • Rash • Upper respiratory tract infections • Hepatotoxicity, which may be preceded by severe rash or other signs of systemic allergic reactions • Orthostatic hypotension, especially in patients with severe renal insufficiency

Key to Abbreviations: BID = twice daily, CYP = cytochrome P, EFV = efavirenz, ETR = etravirine, MVC = maraviroc, NRTI = nucleoside reverse transcriptase inhibitor, NVP = nevirapine, PI = protease inhibitor, RAL = raltegravir, T20 = enfuvirtide, TPV/r = tipranavir + ritonavir

Guidelines for the Use of Antiretroviral Agents in HIV-1-Infected Adults and Adolescents

Appendix B, Table 7. Antiretroviral Dosing Recommendations in Patients with Renal or Hepatic Insufficiency (Last updated February 12, 2013; last reviewed February 12, 2013) (page 1 of 5)

See the reference section following Table 7 for creatinine clearance (CrCl) calculation formulas and criteria for Child-Pugh classification.

Antiretrovirals Generic Name (Abbreviation)/ Trade Name	Usual Daily Dose (Refer to Appendix B, Tables 1–6 for additional dosing information.)	Dosing in Renal Insufficiency (Including with chronic ambulatory peritoneal dialysis and hemodialysis)	Dosing in Hepatic Impairment
Nucleoside Reverse Transcriptase Inhibitors			
Stribild should not be initiated in patients with CrCl <70 mL/min. Use of the following fixed-dose combinations is not recommended in patients with CrCl <50 mL/min: Atripla, Combivir, Stribild, Trizivir, or Epzicom. Use of Truvada is not recommended in patients with CrCl <30 mL/min.			
Abacavir (ABC)/ Ziagen	300 mg PO BID	No dosage adjustment necessary	Child-Pugh Score Dose 5–6 200 mg PO BID (use oral solution) >6 Contraindicated
Didanosine EC (ddI)/ Videx EC	Body weight ≥60 kg: 400 mg PO once daily Body weight <60 kg: 250 mg PO once daily	**Dose (once daily)** CrCl (mL/min) ≥60 kg <60 kg 30–59 200 mg 125 mg 10–29 125 mg 125 mg <10, HD, CAPD 125 mg use ddI oral solution	No dosage adjustment necessary
Didanosine oral solution (ddI)/ Videx	Body weight ≥60 kg: 200 mg PO BID or 400 mg PO once daily Body weight <60 kg: 250 mg PO once daily or 125 mg PO BID	**Dose (once daily)** CrCl (mL/min) ≥60 kg <60 kg 30–59 200 mg 150 mg 10–29 150 mg 100 mg <10, HD, CAPD 100 mg 75 mg	No dosage adjustment necessary
Emtricitabine (FTC)/ Emtriva	200 mg oral capsule once daily or 240 mg (24 mL) oral solution once daily	**Dose** CrCl (mL/min) Capsule Solution 30–49 200 mg q48h 120 mg q24h 15–29 200 mg q72h 80 mg q24h <15 or on HD* 200 mg q96h 60 mg q24h *On dialysis days, take dose after HD session.	No dosage recommendation
Lamivudine (3TC)/ Epivir	300 mg PO once daily or 150 mg PO BID	CrCl (mL/min) Dose 30–49 150 mg q24h 15–29 1 x 150 mg, then 100 mg q24h 5–14 1 x 150 mg, then 50 mg q24h <5 or on HD* 1 x 50 mg, then 25 mg q24h *On dialysis days, take dose after HD session.	No dosage adjustment necessary

See the reference section following Table 7 for creatinine clearance (CrCl) calculation formulas and criteria for Child-Pugh classification.

Antiretrovirals Generic Name (Abbreviation)/ Trade Name	Usual Daily Dose (Refer to Appendix B, Tables 1–6 for additional dosing information.)	Dosing in Renal Insufficiency (Including with chronic ambulatory peritoneal dialysis and hemodialysis)	Dosing in Hepatic Impairment
Stavudine (d4T)/ Zerit	Body weight ≥60 kg: 40 mg PO BID Body weight <60 kg: 30 mg PO BID	Dose CrCl (mL/min) ≥60 kg <60 kg 26–50 20 mg q12h 15 mg q12h 10–25 or on HD* 20 mg q24h 15 mg q24h *On dialysis days, take dose after HD session.	No dosage recommendation
Tenofovir (TDF)/ Viread	300 mg PO once daily	CrCl (mL/min) Dose 30–49 300 mg q48h 10–29 300 mg twice weekly (every 72–96 hours) <10 and not on HD Not recommended On HD* 300 mg q7d *On dialysis days, take dose after HD session.	No dosage adjustment necessary
Emtricitabine (FTC) + Tenofovir (TDF)/ Truvada	1 tablet PO once daily	CrCl (mL/min) Dose 30–49 1 tablet q48h <30 or on HD Not recommended	No dosage recommendation
Zidovudine (AZT, ZDV)/ Retrovir	300 mg PO BID	CrCl (mL/min) Dose <15 or HD* 100 mg TID or 300 mg once daily *On dialysis days, take dose after HD session.	No dosage recommendation
Non-Nucleoside Reverse Transcriptase Inhibitors			
Delavirdine (DLV)/ Rescriptor	400 mg PO TID	No dosage adjustment necessary	No dosage recommendation; use with caution in patients with hepatic impairment.
Efavirenz (EFV)/ Sustiva	600 mg PO once daily, at or before bedtime	No dosage adjustment necessary	No dosage recommendation; use with caution in patients with hepatic impairment.
Efavirenz (EFV) + Tenofovir (TDF) + Emtricitabine (FTC)/ Atripla	1 tablet PO once daily	Not recommended for use in patients with CrCl <50 mL/min. Instead use the individual drugs of the fixed-dose combination and adjust TDF and FTC doses according to CrCl level.	
Etravirine (ETR)/ Intelence	200 mg PO BID	No dosage adjustment necessary	Child-Pugh Class A or B: No dosage adjustment Child-Pugh Class C: No dosage recommendation

See the reference section following Table 7 for creatinine clearance (CrCl) calculation formulas and criteria for Child-Pugh classification.

Antiretrovirals Generic Name (Abbreviation)/ Trade Name	Daily Dose (Refer to Appendix B, Tables 1–6 for additional dosing information.)	Dosing in Renal Insufficiency (Including with chronic ambulatory peritoneal dialysis and hemodialysis)	Dosing in Hepatic Impairment
Non-Nucleoside Reverse Transcriptase Inhibitors, continued			
Nevirapine (NVP)/ Viramune or Viramune XR	200 mg PO BID or 400 mg PO once daily (using Viramune XR formulation)	<u>Patients on HD</u>: limited data; no dosage recommendation	<u>Child-Pugh Class A</u>: No dosage adjustment <u>Child-Pugh Class B or C</u>: Contraindicated
Rilpivirine (RPV)/ Edurant	25 mg PO once daily	No dosage adjustment necessary	<u>Child-Pugh Class A or B</u>: No dosage adjustment <u>Child-Pugh Class C</u>: No dosage recommendation
Rilpivirine (RPV) + **Tenofovir** (TDF) + **Emtricitabine** (FTC)/ Complera	1 tablet PO once daily	Not recommended for use in patients with CrCl <50 mL/min. Instead use the individual drugs of the fixed-dose combination and adjust TDF and FTC doses levels according to CrCl level.	<u>Child-Pugh Class A or B</u>: No dosage adjustment <u>Child-Pugh Class C</u>: No dosage recommendation
Protease Inhibitors			

Atazanavir (ATV)/ Reyataz	400 mg PO once daily or (ATV 300 mg + RTV 100 mg) PO once daily	No dosage adjustment for patients with renal dysfunction not requiring HD
		
		<u>ARV-naive patients on HD</u>: (ATV 300 mg + RTV 100 mg) once daily
		
		<u>ARV-experienced patients on HD</u>: ATV or RTV-boosted ATV not recommended
			Child-Pugh Class **Dose**
			   B 300 mg once daily
			   C Not recommended
			
			RTV boosting is **not** recommended in patients with hepatic impairment (Child-Pugh Class B or C).

Darunavir (DRV)/ Prezista	(DRV 800 mg + RTV 100 mg) PO once daily (ARV-naive patients only) or (DRV 600 mg + RTV 100 mg) PO BID	No dosage adjustment necessary	<u>Mild-to-moderate hepatic impairment</u>: No dosage adjustment <u>Severe hepatic impairment</u>: Not recommended

Fosamprenavir (FPV)/ Lexiva	1400 mg PO BID or (FPV 1400 mg + RTV 100–200 mg) PO once daily or (FPV 700 mg + RTV 100 mg) PO BID	No dosage adjustment necessary	<u>PI-naive patients only</u>:
			Child-Pugh Score **Dose**
			   5–9 700 mg BID
			  10–15 350 mg BID
			
			<u>PI-naive or PI-experienced patients</u>:
			Child-Pugh Score **Dose**
			   5–6 700 mg BID + RTV 100 mg once daily
			   7–9 450 mg BID + RTV 100 mg once daily
			  10–15 300 mg BID + RTV 100 mg once daily

Guidelines for the Use of Antiretroviral Agents in HIV-1-Infected Adults and Adolescents

See the reference section following Table 7 for creatinine clearance (CrCl) calculation formulas and criteria for Child-Pugh classification.

Antiretrovirals Generic Name (Abbreviation)/ Trade Name	Daily Dose (Refer to Appendix B, Tables 1–6 for additional dosing information.)	Dosing in Renal Insufficiency (Including with chronic ambulatory peritoneal dialysis and hemodialysis)	Dosing in Hepatic Impairment
Protease Inhibitors, continued			
Indinavir (IDV)/ Crixivan	800 mg PO q8h	No dosage adjustment necessary	Mild-to-moderate hepatic insufficiency because of cirrhosis: 600 mg q8h
Lopinavir/ritonavir (LPV/r) Kaletra	400/100 mg PO BID or 800/200 mg PO once daily	Avoid once-daily dosing in patients on HD	No dosage recommendation; use with caution in patients with hepatic impairment.
Nelfinavir (NFV)/ Viracept	1250 mg PO BID	No dosage adjustment necessary	Mild hepatic impairment: No dosage adjustment Moderate-to-severe hepatic impairment: Do not use
Ritonavir (RTV)/ Norvir	As a PI-boosting agent: 100–400 mg per day	No dosage adjustment necessary	Refer to recommendations for the primary PI.
Saquinavir (SQV)/ Invirase	(SQV 1000 mg + RTV 100 mg) PO BID	No dosage adjustment necessary	Mild-to-moderate hepatic impairment: Use with caution Severe hepatic impairment: Contraindicated
Tipranavir (TPV)/ Aptivus	(TPV 500 mg + RTV 200 mg) PO BID	No dosage adjustment necessary	Child-Pugh Class A: Use with caution Child-Pugh Class B or C: Contraindicated
Integrase Inhibitors			
Raltegravir (RAL)/ Isentress	400 mg BID	No dosage adjustment necessary	Mild-to-moderate hepatic insufficiency: No dosage adjustment necessary Severe hepatic insufficiency: No recommendation
Elvitegravir (EVG)/ **Cobicistat** (COBI)/ **Tenofovir** (TDF)/ **Emtricitabine** (FTC)/ Stribild (only available as a co-formulated product)	1 tablet once daily	EVG/COBI/TDF/FTC **should not be initiated** in patients with CrCl <70 mL/min. Discontinue EVG/COBI/TDF/FTC if CrCl declines to <50 mL/min while patient is on therapy.	Mild-to-moderate hepatic insufficiency: No dosage adjustment necessary Severe hepatic insufficiency: Not recommended

See the reference section following Table 7 for creatinine clearance (CrCl) calculation formulas and criteria for Child-Pugh classification.

Antiretrovirals Generic Name (Abbreviation)/ Trade Name	Daily Dose (Refer to Appendix B, Tables 1–6 for additional dosing information.)	Dosing in Renal Insufficiency (Including with chronic ambulatory peritoneal dialysis and hemodialysis)	Dosing in Hepatic Impairment
Fusion Inhibitor			
Enfuvirtide (T20)/ Fuzeon	90 mg subcutaneous BID	No dosage adjustment necessary	No dosage adjustment necessary
CCR5 Antagonist			
Maraviroc (MVC)/ Selzentry	The recommended dose differs based on concomitant medications and potential for drug-drug interactions. See Appendix B, Table 6 for detailed dosing information.	**CrCl <30 mL/min or on HD** Without potent CYP3A inhibitors or inducers: 300 mg BID; reduce to 150 mg BID if postural hypotension occurs With potent CYP3A inducers or inhibitors: Not recommended	No dosage recommendations. Concentrations will likely be increased in patients with hepatic impairment.

Key to Abbreviations: 3TC = lamivudine, ABC = abacavir, ARV = antiretroviral, ATV = atazanavir, AZT = zidovudine, BID = twice daily, CAPD = chronic ambulatory peritoneal dialysis, COBI = cobicistat, CrCl = creatinine clearance, CYP = cytochrome P, d4T = stavudine, ddI = didanosine, DLV = delavirdine, DRV = darunavir, EC = enteric coated, EFV = efavirenz, ETR = etravirine, EVG= elvitegravir, FPV = fosamprenavir, FTC = emtricitabine, HD = hemodialysis, IDV = indinavir, LPV/r = lopinavir/ritonavir, MVC = maraviroc, NFV = nelfinavir, NNRTI = non-nucleoside reverse transcriptase inhibitor, NRTI = nucleoside reverse transcriptase inhibitor, NVP = nevirapine, PI = protease inhibitor, PO = orally, RAL = raltegravir, RPV = rilpivirine, RTV = ritonavir, SQV = saquinavir, T20 = enfuvirtide, TDF = tenofovir, TID = three times daily, TPV = tipranavir, XR = extended release, ZVD = zidovudine

Creatinine Clearance Calculation

Male:	$\dfrac{(140 - \text{age in years}) \times (\text{weight in kg})}{72 \times (\text{serum creatinine})}$	Female:	$\dfrac{(140 - \text{age in years}) \times (\text{weight in kg}) \times (0.85)}{72 \times (\text{serum creatinine})}$

Child-Pugh Score

Component	Points Scored		
	1	2	3
Encephalopathy[a]	None	Grade 1–2	Grade 3–4
Ascites	None	Mild or controlled by diuretics	Moderate or refractory despite diuretics
Albumin	>3.5 g/dL	2.8–3.5 g/dL	<2.8 g/dL
Total bilirubin or	<2 mg/dL (<34 µmol/L)	2–3 mg/dL (34 µmol/L to 50 µmol/L)	>3 mg/dL (>50 µmol/L)
Modified total bilirubin[b]	<4 mg/dL	4–7 mg/dL	>7 mg/dL
Prothrombin time (seconds prolonged) or	<4	4–6	>6
International normalized ratio (INR)	<1.7	1.7–2.3	>2.3

[a] Encephalopathy Grades

    Grade 1: Mild confusion, anxiety, restlessness, fine tremor, slowed coordination

    Grade 2: Drowsiness, disorientation, asterixis

    Grade 3: Somnolent but rousable, marked confusion, incomprehensible speech, incontinence, hyperventilation

    Grade 4: Coma, decerebrate posturing, flaccidity

[b] Modified total bilirubin used for patients who have Gilbert's syndrome or who are taking indinavir or atazanavir

Child-Pugh Classification	Total Child-Pugh Score[c]
Class A	5–6 points
Class B	7–9 points
Class C	>9 points

[c] Sum of points for each component

Appendix B Table 8: Monthly Suggested Wholesale Price (SWP)ᵃ of Antiretroviral Drugs (Last updated February 12, 2013; last reviewed February 12, 2013) (page 1 of 3)

Antiretroviral Drug (Generic and Brand Names)	Strength	Dosing	Tabs/Capsules/mLs per Month	SWPᵃ (Monthly)
Nucleoside Reverse Transcriptase Inhibitors (NRTIs)				
abacavir				
• generic	300 mg tab	2 tabs daily	60 tabs	$602.66
• Ziagen	300 mg tab	2 tabs daily	60 tabs	$670.37
• Ziagen	20 mg/mL soln	30 mL daily	900 mL	$674.60
didanosine delayed-release				
• generic	400 mg cap	1 cap daily	30 caps	$368.72
• Videx EC	400 mg cap	1 cap daily	30 caps	$478.08
emtricitabine				
• Emtriva	200 mg cap	1 cap daily	30 tabs	$574.14
• Emtriva	10 mg/mL soln	24 mL daily	680 mL (28-day supply)	$542.32
lamivudine				
• generic	300 mg tab	1 tab daily	30 tabs	$429.66
• Epivir	300 mg tab	1 tab daily	30 tabs	$498.89
• Epivir	10 mg/mL soln	30 mL daily	900 mL	$498.90
stavudine				
• generic	40 mg cap	1 cap twice daily	60 caps	$403.70
• Zerit	40 mg cap	1 cap twice daily	60 caps	$512.62
tenofovir				
• Viread	300 mg tab	1 tab daily	30 tabs	$998.80
zidovudine				
• generic	300 mg tab	1 tab twice daily	60 tabs	$360.97
• Retrovir	300 mg tab	1 tab twice daily	60 tabs	$557.83
Combination NRTI Products				
abacavir/lamivudine				
• Epzicom	600/300 mg tab	1 tab daily	30 tabs	$1,118.90
tenofovir/emtricitabine				
• Truvada	300/150 mg tab	1 tab daily	30 tabs	$1,467.97
zidovudine/lamivudine				
• generic	300/150 mg tab	1 tab twice daily	60 tabs	$931.61
• Combivir	300/150 mg tab	1 tab twice daily	60 tabs	$1,081.70
abacavir/zidovudine/ lamivudine				
• Trizivir	300/300/150 mg tab	1 tab twice daily	60 tabs	$1,839.66

Appendix B Table 8: Monthly Suggested Wholesale Price (SWP)[a] of Antiretroviral Drugs (Last updated February 12, 2013; last reviewed February 12, 2013) (page 2 of 3)

Antiretroviral Drug (Generic and Brand Names)	Strength	Dosing	Tabs/Capsules/mLs per Month	SWP[a] (Monthly)
Non-Nucleoside Reverse Transcriptase Inhibitors (NNRTIs)				
efavirenz • Sustiva	600 mg tab	1 tab daily	30 tabs	$785.90
etravirine • Intelence	200 mg tab	1 tab twice daily	60 tabs	$978.64
nevirapine • generic	200 mg tab	1 tab twice daily	60 tabs	$650.48
• Viramune	200 mg tab	1 tab twice daily	60 tabs	$723.08
• Viramune XR (nevirapine extended release)	400 mg tab	1 tab daily	30 tabs	$670.63
rilpivirine • Endurant	25 mg tab	1 tab daily	30 tabs	$804.38
Protease Inhibitors (PIs)				
atazanavir • Reyataz	150 mg cap[b]	2 caps daily	60 caps	$1,222.10
• Reyataz	200 mg cap	2 caps daily	60 caps	$1,222.10
• Reyataz	300 mg cap[b]	1 cap daily	30 caps	$1,210.56
darunavir • Prezista	400 mg tab[b]	2 tabs daily	60 tabs	$1,230.20
• Prezista	600 mg tab[b]	1 tab twice daily	60 tabs	$1,230.20
fosamprenavir • Lexiva	700 mg tab	2 tabs twice daily	120 tabs	$1,988.96
• Lexiva	700 mg tab	1 tab twice daily[b]	60 tabs	$994.48
• Lexiva	700 mg tab	2 tabs once daily[b]	60 tabs	$994.48
lopinavir/ritonavir • Kaletra	200 mg/50 mg tab	2 tabs twice daily or 4 tabs once daily	120 tabs	$871.36
• Kaletra	400 mg/100 mg per 5 mL soln	5 mL twice daily	300 mL	$871.34
ritonavir (total daily dose depends on concomitant PI) • Norvir	100 mg tab	1 tab once daily	30 tabs	$308.60
• Norvir	100 mg tab	1 tab twice daily	60 tabs	$617.20
• Norvir	100 mg tab	2 tabs twice daily	120 tabs	$1,234.40
saquinavir • Invirase	500 mg tab[b]	2 tabs twice daily	120 tabs	$1,088.84
tipranavir • Aptivus	250 mg cap[b]	2 caps twice daily	120 caps	$1,335.14

Appendix B Table 8: Monthly Suggested Wholesale Price (SWP)[a] of Antiretroviral Drugs (Last updated February 12, 2013; last reviewed February 12, 2013) (page 3 of 3)

Antiretroviral Drug (Generic and Brand Names)	Strength	Dosing	Tabs/Capsules/mLs per Month	SWP[a] (Monthly)
Integrase Strand Transfer Inhibitor (INSTI) (Please refer to Co-formulated Combination Antiretroviral Drugs for cost of elvitegravir/cobicistat/tenofovir/emtricitabine [Stribild])				
raltegravir • Isentress	400 mg tab	1 tab twice daily	60 tabs	$1,228.69
Fusion Inhibitor				
enfuviritide • Fuzeon	90 mg injection kit	1 injection twice daily	60 doses (1 kit)	$3,248.72
CR5 Antagonist				
maraviroc • Selzentry	150 mg tab	1 tab twice daily	60 tabs	$1,259.82
• Selzentry	300 mg tab	1 tab twice daily	60 tabs	$1,259.82
Co-formulated Combination Products as Complete Antiretroviral Regimens				
efavirenz/tenofovir/ emtricitabine • Atripla	600/300/200 mg tab	1 tab daily	30 tabs	$2,253.88
rilpivirine/tenofovir/ emtricitabine • Complera	25/300/200 mg tab	1 tab daily	30 tabs	$2,195.83
elvitegravir/cobicistat/ tenofovir/emtricitabine • Stribild	150/150/300/200 mg tab	1 tab daily	30 tabs	$2,810.96

[a] SWP = Suggested Wholesale Price (source: AmerisourceBergen, accessed December 2012/January 2013) Note that this price may not represent the pharmacy acquisition price or the price paid by consumers.

[b] Should be used in combination with ritonavir. Please refer to Appendix B, Table 3 for ritonavir doses.

Key to Abbreviations: cap = capsule, DR = delayed release, EC = enteric coated, soln = solution, SWP = suggested wholesale price, tab = tablet, XR = extended release

www.ingramcontent.com/pod-product-compliance
Lightning Source LLC
Chambersburg PA
CBHW080238180526
45167CB00006B/2321